Techniques in Spinal Fusion and Stabilization

PATRICK W. HITCHON, M.D.
Professor of Neurosurgery
Division of Neurosurgery
The University of Iowa Hospitals and Clinics
Iowa City, Iowa

VINCENT C. TRAYNELIS, M.D.
Department of Surgery
Division of Neurosurgery
The University of Iowa Hospitals and Clinics
Iowa City, Iowa

SETTI S. RENGACHARY, M.D.
Professor
Department of Neurosurgery
University of Minnesota Medical School
Minneapolis, Minnesota

1995
Thieme Medical Publishers, Inc., New York
Georg Thieme Verlag, Stuttgart · New York

Thieme Medical Publishers, Inc.
381 Park Avenue South
New York, New York 10016

TECHNIQUES IN SPINAL FUSION AND STABILIZATION
Patrick W. Hitchon

Techniques in spinal fusion and stabilization/edited by Patrick W. Hitchon, Setti S. Rengachary, Vincent C. Traynelis.
         p   cm.
    Includes bibliographical references and index.
    ISBN 0-86577-523-0 (Thieme Medical Publishers).—ISBN3-13-100131-3 (G. Thieme Verlag)
    1. Spinal fushion.   2. Spinal implants.   I. Hitchon, Patrick W.
 II. Rengachary, Setti S.   III. Traynelis, Vincent C. (Vincent Charles)
    [DNLM: 1. Spinal Fusion--instrumentation.   2. Spinal Fusion-methods.   WE 725 T255 1995)
 RD533.T42 1995
 617.3'75059—dc20
 DNLM/DLC
 for Library of Congress
                                                                                      94-
                                                                                      95-36947
                                                                                      CIP

Important note: Medicine is an ever-changing science. Research and clinical experience are continually broadening our knowledge, in particular our knowledge of proper treatment and drug therapy. Insofar as this book mentions any dosage or applications, readers may rest assured that the authors, editors, and publishers have made every effort to ensure that such references are strictly in accordance with the state of knowledge at the time of production of the book. Nevertheless, every user is requested to carefully examine the manufacturers' leaflets accompanying each drug to check on his own responsibility whether the dosage schedules recommended therein or the contraindications stated by the manufacturers differ from the statements made in the present book. Such examination is particularly important with drugs that are either rarely used or have been newly released on the market.

Some of the product names, patents, and registered designs referred to in this book are in fact registered trademarks or proprietary names even though specific reference to this fact is not always made in the text. Therefore, the appearance of a name without designation as proprietary is not to be construed as a representation by the publisher that it is in the public domain.

Printed in the United States of America.

5 4 3 2 1

TMP ISBN 0-86577-523-0
GTV ISBN 3-13-100131-3

This book is dedicated to our families
Patrick W. Hitchon, Setti S. Rengachary, and Vincent C. Traynelis

Contents

Contributors

Ronald C. Allen, Ph.D.
Department of Research and Development
Advanced Medicine and Surgery
Hayward, California

Nevan G. Baldwin, M.D.
Division of Neurosurgery
University of New Mexico School of Medicine
Albuquerque, New Mexico

Perry A. Ball, M.D.
Division of Neurosurgery
Dartmouth-Hitchcock Medical Center
Lebanon, New Hampshire

Ronald A. Bergman, Ph.D.
Professor of Anatomy
Department of Anatomy
College of Medicine
University of Iowa
Iowa City, Iowa

Gregory J. Bennett, M.D.
Assistant Professor of Neurosurgery
School of Medicine and Biomedical Sciences
State University of New York at Buffalo
Buffalo, New York

Edward C. Benzel, M.D., F.A.C.S.
Professor and Chief
Division of Neurosurgery
University of New Mexico School of Medicine
Albuquerque, New Mexico

Jen-Yuh Chen, M.D.
Department of Orthopaedic Surgery
Taipei Medical College Hospital
Taipei, Taiwan
Republic of China

John D. Clausen, B.S.
Graduate Research Assistant
Department of Biomedical Engineering
University of Iowa
Iowa City, Iowa

Mitchell G. Cohen, M.D.
Private Practice
Comprehensive Orthopaedic Practice
Fountain Valley, California

Curtis A. Dickman, M.D.
Associate Chief, Spine Section
Director of Spinal Research
Division of Neurological Surgery
Barrow Neurological Institute
St. Joseph's Hospital and Medical Center
Phoenix, Arizona

Thomas A. Duff, M.D.
Department of Neurological Surgery
University of Wisconsin
Madison, Wisconsin

Derek A. Duke, M.D.
Resident in Neurological Surgery
Mayo Clinic
Rochester, Minnesota

Kenneth J. Easton, M.D.
Department of Orthopedics
State University of New York
Health Science Center
Syracuse, New York

Georges Y. El-Khoury, M.D.
Professor of Radiology
University of Iowa Hospitals and Clinics
Iowa City, Iowa

Emad A. El-Mehy, M.D.
Department of Orthopedics
State University of New York
Health Science Center
Syracuse, New York

Eric Flores, M.D.
Resident Physician
Department of Neurosurgery
University of Minnesota Medical School
Minneapolis, Minnesota

Kenneth A. Follett, M.D., Ph.D.
Department of Surgery
Division of Neurosurgery
The University of Iowa Hospitals and Clinics
Iowa City, Iowa

Fred H. Geisler, M.D., Ph.D.
Director, Spinal Services
Chicago Neurosurgical Center
Chicago, Illinois

Vijay K. Goel, Ph.D.
Professor and Chairman
Department of Biomedical Engineering
College of Engineering
University of Iowa
Iowa City, Iowa

Souheil S. Haddad, M.D.
Department of Surgery
Division of Neurosurgery
The University of Iowa Hospitals and Clinics
Iowa City, Iowa

Regis W. Haid, M.D.
Assistant Professor of Neurosurgery
Department of Neurosurgery
Emory University School of Medicine
Atlanta, Georgia

Kurt G. Harris, M.D.
Assistant Professor
Neuroradiology
Department of Radiology
University of Iowa College of Medicine
Iowa City, Iowa

Steven J. Harrison, M.S., F.A.M.I.
Department of Medical Illustration
Medical College of Georgia
Augusta, Georgia

Patrick W. Hitchon, M.D.
Professor of Neurosurgery
Division of Neurosurgery
The University of Iowa Hospitals and Clinics
Iowa City, Iowa

Robert Jacobson, M.D.
Neurological Spine Surgery
South Miami, Florida

Paul M. Lin, M.D.
Emeritus Clinical Professor of Neurosurgery
Department of Neurosurgery
Temple University Health Sciences Center
Philadelphia, Pennsylvania

Gary L. Lowery, M.D., Ph.D.
Research Institute International, Inc.
Gainesville, Florida

Paul C. McAfee, M.D.
Chief of Spinal Reconstructive Surgery
St. Joseph's Hospital
Baltimore, Maryland

Dennis E. McDonnell, M.D., F.A.C.S.
Department of Surgery
Section of Neurosurgery
Medical College of Georgia
Augusta, Georgia

Arnold H. Menezes, M.D.
Professor and Vice Chairman
Division of Neurosurgery
The University of Iowa College of Medicine
   and the University of Iowa Hospitals and Clinics
Iowa City, Iowa

Loren J. Mouw, M.D.
Division of Neurosurgery
University of Iowa Hospitals and Clinics
Iowa City, Iowa

Sally A. Oklund, Ph.D.
Executive Director
Western Transportation Services
San Jose, CA

Richard K. Osenbach, M.D.
Attending Neurosurgeon
Walter Reed Army Medical Center
Washington, DC

Noel I. Perin, M.D., F.R.C.S. (E.D.I.N.)
Assistant Professor
Department of Neurosurgery
University of Cincinnati Medical Center
Cincinnati, Ohio

Donald J. Prolo, M.D.
Clinical Associate Professor of Neurosurgery
Stanford University School of Medicine
San Jose, CA

Setti S. Rengachary, M.D.
Professor
Department of Neurosurgery
University of Minnesota Medical School
Minneapolis, Minnesota

Abraham Rogozinski, M.D.
Rogozinski Orthopaedic Clinic
Jacksonville, Florida

Chaim Rogozinski, M.D.
Rogozinski Orthopaedic Clinic
Jacksonville, Florida

Timothy C. Ryken, M.D.
Department of Surgery
Division of Neurosurgery
College of Medicine
University of Iowa
Iowa City, Iowa

James W. Simmons, M.D., F.A.C.S.
Orthopaedic Surgeon
Alamo Bone and Joint Clinic
San Antonio, Texas

Volker K.H. Sonntag, M.D.
Clinical Professor of Surgery
University of Arizona
Tucson, Arizona

Chester E. Sutterlin III, M.D.
Spinal Associates of North Central Florida
Gainesville, Florida

James C. Torner, Ph.D.
Department of Preventive Medicine and
    Environmental Health
Division of Epidemiology
The University of Iowa Hospitals and Clinics
Iowa City, Iowa

Vincent C. Traynelis, M.D.
Department of Surgery
Division of Neurosurgery
College of Medicine
University of Iowa
Iowa City, Iowa

John C. VanGilder, M.D.
Professor and Chairman
Division of Neurological Surgery
The University of Iowa Hospitals and Clinics
Iowa City, Iowa

Thoru Yamada, M.D.
Professor
University of Iowa College of Medicine
Iowa City, Iowa
and
Chief
Division of Clinical Electrophysiology
University of Iowa Hospitals and Clinics
Iowa City, Iowa

Hansen A. Yuan, M.D.
Professor of Orthopedic and Neurological Surgery
Departments of Orthopedics and Neurosurgery
State University of New York
Health Science Center
Syracuse, New York

Thomas A. Zdeblick, M.D.
Assistant Professor
Division of Orthopedic Surgery
University of Wisconsin
Madison, Wisconsin

Introduction

When I was invited to write an introduction for this book, I was flattered and I promptly accepted. Then came the problem of what to say about a book on spinal surgery, considering that there have been numerous publications on the subject. This phenomenon is not new: "Of making many books there is no end" (Ecclesiastes {12:12}). One definition of introduction is "a preface, as in a book," and a definition of preface is "a statement, introducing a book, and explaining its scope, intention, or background." The chapter titles of this book attest to the burgeoning techniques for spinal fusion; 21 present methods and devices generally not available more than a decade ago. Although spinal fusions can be classified as posterior, intertransverse, and interbody, and fixation as intraosseous or extraosseous, the means by which these functions are accomplished have become progressively more diverse. To those who decry the development of multitudinous devices for vertebral fixation, it should be pointed out that a substantially greater variety of automobiles is available for movement from one place to another without walking, a process that is less complicated than stabilization of the unstable spinal column. This proliferation of devices and techniques is laudable and reflects the intense interest and significant advances in spinal surgery. Development has been rapid; consequently, a surgeon finds it difficult to decide which technique to employ on the basis of personal experience. To a significant extent, we must rely on the observations of those who have developed and used a particular method for a sufficient time to become familiar with its advantages and disadvantages. Therefore, a collection of descriptions and analyses of currently employed methods for spinal fusion represents a valuable service. With this book, the editors and authors have admirably met a real need that even King Solomon would have approved.

Foreword

To the spine surgeon, fractures and diseases of the spine constitute challenging problems, owing to issues of biomechanical instability and neural injury. These two problems are often inseparable: Spinal cord decompression often entails manipulation of the spine to a degree that affects stability; and, the treating physician must be adept at managing both instability and optimizing neurological recovery.

Spinal fusion and instrumentation are often necessary for the restoration of alignment and stability. Recently, a surge of interest in spinal instrumentation and a plethora of devices have occurred. Undoubtedly, some devices achieve the desired ends better than others, either through different approaches or mechanisms of fixation. The importance of careful analysis of the spine fracture or pathologic process for the selection of the optimal approach or instrumentation cannot be overemphasized.

This text provides the reader with a description of the instrumentation currently as presented by experienced surgeons. Each chapter identifies the patient population most suited for such a device, followed by description of the actual operative procedure. A section in each chapter is dedicated to expected results and complications.

The reader is forewarned that the presence of instability does not always necessitate the implantation of spinal instrumentation. Stability can—and sometimes should—be achieved by nonoperative means, allowing for bony fusion to take place. The choice of surgery or recumbency creates a challenge to the spinal surgeon as can be appreciated from many sources as well as Chapter 34. The literature is replete with evidence in favor of surgical or nonsurgical treatment of spinal fractures, with neurological improvement in both. This text gives the reader some guidelines regarding the optimal modality of treatment.

Spine reconstruction and neural decompression do not exclude pharmacological intervention. Surgery or recumbency in the treatment of spinal fractures is to be undertaken in conjunction with the recommendations of the *National Acute Spinal Cord Injury Study—Part II*. In patients with acute neurological deficit arising from spinal cord injury, methylprednisolone should be administered. Randomized clinical studies published by Bracken et al. (N Engl J Med, pp 1405–1411, May 17, 1990) have shown a significant improvement in neurological deficit associated with methylprednisolone treatment over those treated with placebo or naloxone. A too mechanistic approach in the management of spinal cord injuries may be inadequate if not provided in conjunction with current accepted pharmacological treatment.

Lastly, I wish to acknowledge the support of my colleagues from the Division of Neurosurgery in referring patients with spinal fractures to my care. I wish also to acknowledge the generosity of Doctors Sanford Larson and Dennis Maiman in sharing their experience and advice in the management of complicated cases.

Needless to say, this book would not have been possible were it not for the joint efforts of Vince and Setti, to whom I am grateful.

Patrick W. Hitchon, M.D.

1 Anatomy of the Spine

Loren J. Mouw, M.D., Ronald A. Bergman, Ph.D.

INTRODUCTION

The vertebral column provides a stable platform for anchoring the limb girdles, bony support for the trunk, multiple attachment sites for axial muscles, and a hard protective case for the spinal cord as well as its nerve roots. The vertebrae are attached firmly to each other by fibrous and elastic ligaments. This allows only limited movement between adjacent vertebrae but nevertheless provides the column, as a whole, with a high degree of flexibility. Even so, stability is maintained by the unique structural form, intervertebral articular joints, paraspinal muscles, and the controlling check ligaments, which are of great strength.

Classically, the vertebral column is divided into the cervical (Latin for "neck"), thoracic or dorsal (Greek for "breast plate"), lumbar (Latin for "loin"), sacral (Latin for "sacred"), and coccygeal (Greek for "cuckoo") regions with 7, 12, 5, 5, and 4 vertebrae at each level, respectively. In children, there are 33 vertebrae of which the first 24 normally retain their individuality throughout life and are called movable vertebrae. The succeeding five vertebrae fuse to form the sacrum, and the remaining four most distal vertebrae form the coccyx. The sacrum and coccyx, because their components are fused, are known as fixed vertebrae. There is a great deal of variation in numbers, especially in the lower spine (Fig. 1–1). The normal curvatures of the adult spine include the cervical and lumbar lordosis as well as the thoracic and sacral kyphosis (Fig. 1–2).[1,2,3,4]

DEVELOPMENT

At birth, most vertebrae are composed of three bony regions: the body and two lateral masses, which will constitute the neural arch. These regions correspond to three initial centers of ossification that are joined by hyaline cartilage. The point of union between the body and the arch (pedicles) is known as the neurocentral synchondrosis. This synchondrosis may persist for several years (Fig. 1–3).

In cervical vertebrae, the lateral ossification centers form a greater amount of the body than they do in the vertebrae of other regions. The fifth, sixth, and seventh cervical vertebrae have additional ossification centers for the costal processes. In the remaining cervical vertebrae, the costal processes ossify by growth of the lateral ossification centers. If the costal processes of the seventh cervical vertebra remain separate, they will develop into cervical ribs.[5]

In regard to the atlas, the lateral masses and the posterior arch form from three ossification centers (Fig. 1–4), these appear about the third fetal month. The anterior arch becomes ossified from one center, which appears several months into the postnatal period. Posteriorly, union of the lateral masses occurs in the third year of life. Complete fusion of the lateral masses with the anterior arch occurs in about the sixth postnatal year.[5]

The arch of the axis and its associated processes are formed by two lateral centers of ossication. These appear roughly in the third fetal month (Fig. 1–5). The cartilage that constitutes the body and the dens of the axis is ossified by four or five centers. One or two of these centers give rise to the body of C2 in the fourth fetal month. Two centers are found laterally and will form the lower portion of the dens at four and one half months. The final ossification center is found in the apex of the dens. With regard to fusion, the dens joins to the body of C2 between the fourth to sixth years of life. This line of union of dens and body may be marked occasionally even into middle age by a small disk of cartilage. The arch fuses dorsally and ventrally at approximately the same time. The apical cartilage of the dens unites with the main portion of the dens in early adolescence.

The thoracic vertebrae have articulations for the heads of the ribs situated dorsal to the neurocentral joint. The arch is united with the vertebra body by the fifth year. The laminae fuse in the dorsal midline during the first and second postnatal years. Ossification of various vertebral processes is often not complete until young adulthood. Secondary sites of ossification include the spinous and transverse processes as well as the cartilaginous endplates. Vertebral epiphyses appear between puberty and the 25th year and are generally completely ossified by the 25th year.

COMMON CHARACTERISTICS

In Figure 1–6, the basic structure of the vertebra can be reviewed. It is composed of a ventrally placed body and a dorsal arch. The body is responsible for carrying the weight of the trunk and head. The dimensions of the body increase in a gradual progression from cervical to lumbar regions. One of the specimens increased in width from 1.5 cm at C2 to 5.0 cm at L5 and in height from 1.5 cm at C2 to 3.0 cm at L5. The rostral and caudal surfaces of the body are irregular and covered by the intervertebral disk. The ventral and lateral sides of the body have a variable concavity that is more

1

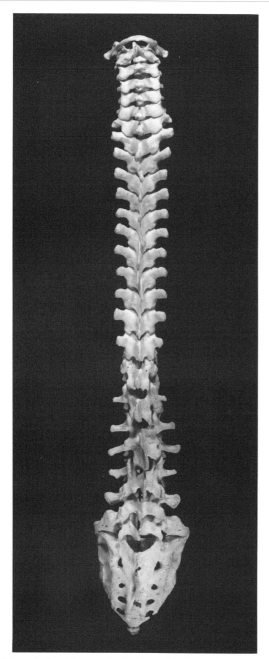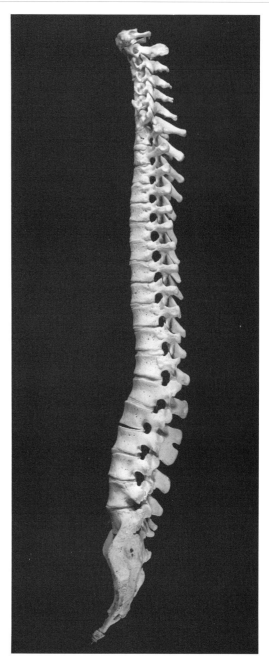

Figure 1–1. The vertebral column is viewed from the posterior and left lateral aspect. These columns do not show the typical lordotic and kyphotic curvatures. The vertebral column is the most variable part of the body. This column has defects in the lumbar spine, including fusion of the posterior elements of L2 to L3, incomplete fusion of S1 to the sacrum and lack of fusion of the embryonic laminae of S1, and lack of fusion of the S3 pedicle and lamina.

pronounced in the lower thoracic and lumbar spine. The body has greater height dorsally than ventrally. The rostral and caudal endplates are slightly concave. The body is perforated by numerous vascular foramina (Fig. 1–7).

The vertebral arch covers the spinal cord dorsally and is formed by two pedicles laterally and two laminae posteriorly. It has seven processes: one spinous, two transverse, and four articular. The pedicles are short pillars of bone projecting dorsally from the dorsal aspect of the body. Each pedicle has notches on its rostral and caudal surfaces. In anatomic position, these adjacent notches form the intervertebral foramen, which is the exit or entrance for spinal nerve

roots and radicular vessels. The laminae are usually symmetrical broad plates of bone that complete the arch dorsally. The spinous process arises from the junction of the two laminae. Each laminae has a roughened rostral and a roughened ventral caudal surface. The ligamenta flava or yellow ligaments attach to these irregular surfaces of adjacent vertebrae. The laminae are typically sloped and may even overlap somewhat, much like shingles on a roof. Posteriorly, spinous processes provide attachment sites for paraspinal muscles, interspinous, and supraspinous ligaments. The transverse processes extend laterally and dorsally from the junction of the laminae and pedicles.

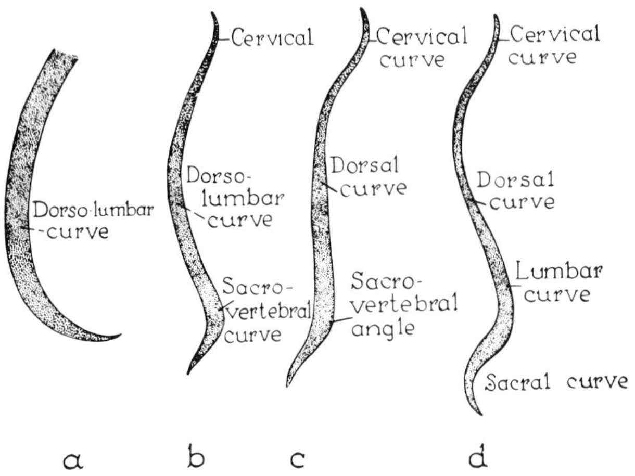

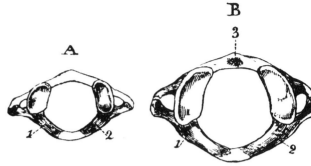

Figure 1–2. The development of the curves of the vertebrae column. (**a**). A single dorso-lumbar curve is present until the third fetal month. (**b**). Cervical, dorsolumbar (thoracolumbar), and sacrovertebral curves appear about the fourth month. (**c**). At birth the three curves include the cervical and dorsal (thoracic) and the sacrovertebral angle. (**d**). The adult curves are the cervical, dorsal (thoracic), lumbar, and sacral.[4]

There are four posterior articulating processes (facets), two superior and two inferior. They arise and project from the arch at the level of the transverse processes. The orientation of the facets changes in position within each region of the spine. Initially they are nearly horizontal in the upper cervical spine (Fig. 1–9); however, they rotate gradually to become almost vertical in an anteroposterior plane in the lower lumbar region (Fig. 1–15). More details of facet orientation will be given in subsequent sections.

The vertebral foramen or spinal canal is formed by the body ventrally and the arch of each vertebra posteriorly. The shape of the canal is triangular in the cervical and lumbar spines and is oval in the thoracic region. The inside diameter of the thoracic spine is smaller than either of the other two regions. The results of an examination of the dimensions of the spinal canal of 30 dried vertebral columns (source unknown) are shown in Figure 1–8. In every instance (except C1) the width (coronal diameter) exceeds

Figure 1–4. Ossification centers of the atlas. (**A**). Before birth, two ossification centers develop. (**B**). During the first postnatal year, a third ossification center develops. Two are lateral centers (1, 2) and the third center arises in the anterior arch (3).[5]

the height (sagittal diameter) of the canal. The cervical enlargement of the spinal cord begins at the level of the third cervical vertebra and continues to the level of the second thoracic vertebra. The cord has its greatest width (12 to 14 mm), thickness (9 mm), and circumference (38 mm) adjacent to the body of the fifth cervical vertebra. The cord is smallest in the midthoracic level, measuring 10 mm in width and 8 mm in thickness. The lumbar enlargement (width of 11 to 13 mm and thickness of 8.5 mm) occurs at the 10th thoracic vertebra but tapers quickly to form the conus medullaris at the 12th thoracic vertebra.

CERVICAL VERTEBRAE

The axial skeleton of the neck, composed of seven cervical vertebrae, permits great flexibility and movement (Figs. 1–9 and 1–10). This ability arises from the specific conformation of vertebrae and the characteristics of the facets.

The body is smaller than those in the thoracic and lumbar regions and is oval in shape. The rostral surface is concave from side to side and slopes anteriorly slightly. The lateral margins of the rostral surface of the body form prominent lips with small articular surfaces. The caudal surface is also concave in shape. The inferior and lateral margins are

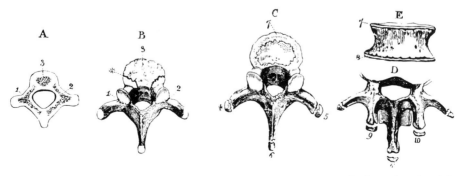

Figure 1–3. Ossification of vertebrae. (**A**). The three primary centers of ossification in a fetal vertebra: 1 and 2 are the neural arch ossification centers, 3 is the central (body) ossification center. (**B**). Thoracic vertebra in a 2-year-old child: The neural arch ossification centers have encroached on the central (body) center (at asterisk). The neurocentral synchondroses have extended into the articular and transverse processes and have united in the spinous processes, leaving the ends cartilaginous. (**C**). Thoracic vertebra in a 17-year-old person. The epiphyses are seen on the transverse processes (4, 5), spinous process (6), and the upper epiphyseal plate of the body (7). (**D**) and (**E**). Lumnbar vertebra of a 17-year-old person. This shows similar development to C, in addition, the lower epiphyseal plate of the body (8).[5]

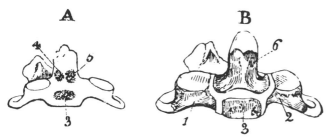

Figure 1–5. The ossification centers of the axis. (**A**). The axis from a fetus of 7 months: the vertebra has three centers, one for the body (3) and two centers in the base of the dens (4, 5). (**B**). The axis shortly after birth: the centers for the vertebral arch (1, 2), body (3), and dens (6).[5]

known as uncinate processes and articulate with the superior and lateral margins of the vertebral body immediately caudal. This interlocking mechanism provides some degree of stability to adjacent vertebra.

The pedicles are short (±3 mm) and are directed laterally and dorsally. They arise from the body just behind the prominent uncinate processes. Two vertebral notches are found in the pedicles. They form, with the adjacent vertebra, the intervertebral foramen. The superior notch is usually smaller than the inferior notch.

The superior and inferior articular processes (facets) are located at the junction of the pedicles and the lamina. The articular surfaces are ovoid and essentially horizontal in orientation in the upper cervical spine. The superior articular process faces rostrally and dorsally whereas the inferior faces caudally and ventrally.

The transverse process is poorly defined but possesses, near its base, a circular transverse foramen. This foramen provides for the passage of the vertebral artery, veins, and the plexus of sympathetic nerve fibers associated with the vertebral artery. In addition, each transverse process has a groove for a cervical spinal nerve. The transverse process is bifid at its distal end; hence, each possesses an anterior and posterior tubercle. The vertebral artery typically enters the transverse foramen at C6 and exits at C1 (Table 1–1). The transverse foramen is bounded medially by the pedicles, dorsally by the lateral process, ventrally by the costal process, and laterally by the costotransverse lamella.

The vertebral foramen is roughly semicircular or triangular with rounded corners. As seen in Figure 1–12, the vertebral foramina are largest in the cervical region to accommodate the cervical enlargement of the spinal cord as well as to allow for the greater flexibility and movement of the cervical region of the vertebral column.

The structural differences of the third through sixth cervical vertebrae are limited primarily to the direction of the costotransverse lamellae, size and level of the tubercles of the transverse process, and orientation of the superior and inferior facets.

ATLAS

The first cervical vertebra, or atlas, is unique in that it has no body. The atlas takes the shape of an irregular circle and consists of two symmetrical lateral masses (transverse processes and facets). The lateral masses are interposed between the anterior and posterior arches (Fig. 1–11). The anterior arch is smaller than the posterior arch and constitutes only about one fifth of the circumference of the ring of bone. On the ventral surface of the anterior arch a small median anterior tubercle is formed, which is the attachment site of the longus colli muscle and the anterior longitudinal ligament. The circular fovea dentis is found on its dorsal surface and articulates with the dens of the axis. The rostral and caudal borders of the anterior arch provide attachment sites for the ligaments anchoring the atlas to the occipital bone and the axis.

The two lateral masses are thick and possess superior as well as inferior facets that articulate with the occipital condyles of the skull and axis, respectively. The superior facets are oval to somewhat triangular and slightly concave. The pits are sloped medially with the lateral rim higher than the medial rim. The inferior articular pits are circular and concave in the sagittal plane and slightly concave in the transverse direction. The inferior pits are directed caudally and medially to articulate with the superior facets of the axis. The facet joint between the atlas and axis is ventral to the exit path of the second cervical nerve.

Within the bony ring on the medial aspect of the lateral mass, a rounded tubercle can be found signifying the attachment site of the transverse ligament of the atlas. The transverse ligament divides the spinal canal into a smaller ventral part containing the dens and a larger dorsal part containing the spinal cord, its membranes, and the blood vessels and nerves.

The transverse processes of the atlas extend for a greater distance (±1 cm) than that of the axis and the remaining cervical vertebrae. They are flattened rostrocaudally and perforated by the transverse foramen. They serve as an attachment site for muscles. The posterior arch unites the lateral masses and constitutes about two fifths of the circumference of the atlas. The rostral surface of the posterior arch, at its junction with the lateral masses, contains a groove for the

Table 1–1. Point of the Entrance of Vertebral Artery into the Transverse Foramina of Cervical Vertebrae.[9]

| VERTEBRAL ARTERY | PERCENTAGE ENTERING TRANSVERSE FORAMEN AT | | | |
	C4	C5	C6	C7
Left side	0.5	9.3	87.9	3.1
Right side	0.5	4.9	91.5	3.1

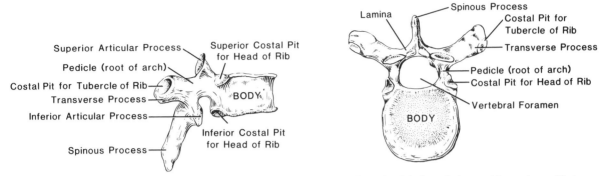

Figure 1–6. Parts of a typical thoracic vertebra (T6), which is shown from the right lateral view and from above. Photo taken from Bergman anatomy collection.

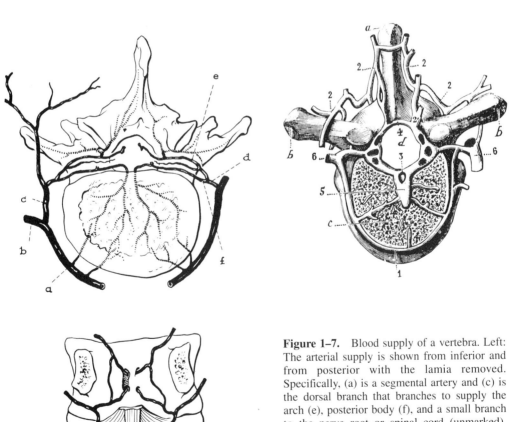

Figure 1–7. Blood supply of a vertebra. Left: The arterial supply is shown from inferior and from posterior with the lamia removed. Specifically, (a) is a segmental artery and (c) is the dorsal branch that branches to supply the arch (e), posterior body (f), and a small branch to the nerve root or spinal cord (unmarked). Lower: Dorsal branches supplying the posterior aspect of the body. Note that the vessels perforate the posterior longitudinal ligament. Right: The venous drainage of the vertebra. Venous communications exist between the body, epidural space, and articular processes. Batson's plexus is noted by 3 and 4. After Anson,[1] Augier,[6] and Testut.[7]

VERTEBRAL CANAL

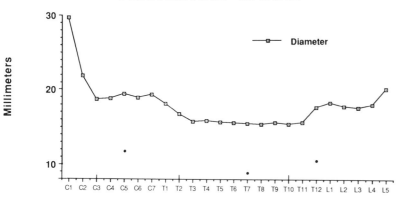

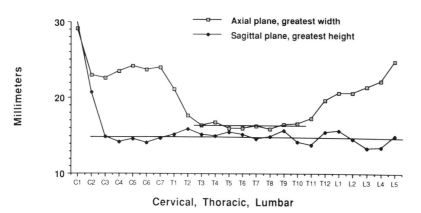

Cervical, Thoracic, Lumbar

Figure 1–8. The vertebral foramen and canal. The illustration (above) is an average diameter (AP and Lat) of the canal throughout the spinal column. Two block dots at the upper and lower end of the group indicate the area at which the so-called cervical and lumbar enlargements begin. The middle of the three dots represents the thinnest area of the spinal cord. The lower graph compares the height and width of the vertebral foramen. Note that the width (transverse plane) of a vertebral foramen exceeds its height (sagittal plane) and that the height (anterior/posterior plane) of the foramen is almost constant in size throughout the vertebral column.

vertebral artery and first spinal nerve (suboccipital nerve). There is another shallow notch on the inferior surface to allow the passage of the second spinal nerve. Finally, the rostral and caudal surfaces of the posterior arch provide attachment sites for ligaments, securing the atlas to the occiput and axis.

AXIS

The axis is the thickest and strongest of the cervical vertebrae (Fig. 1–12). The occipitoatlantoaxial junctions account for a relatively large percentage of rotational movement of the cervical spine. The ventral surface has a median ridge

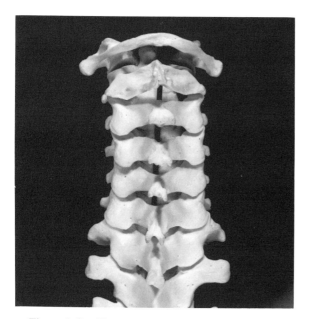

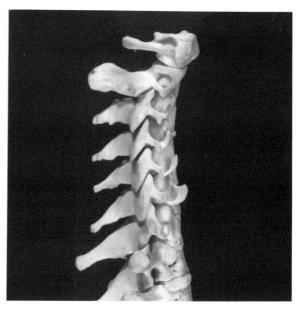

Figure 1–9. The seven cervical vertebrae are shown from a posterior and right lateral view. Note the change in facet orientation as well as the bifid nature of most of the posterior spinous processes.

separating two lateral grooves that are the insertion sites for the longus colli muscles. The superior articular surfaces are uniquely located partly on the pedicles and partly on the vertebral body. The surfaces are oval and convex in the sagittal plane. Positioned rostrally and laterally, they articulate with the inferior articular facets of the atlas. The inferior facets resemble in form and position those of the succeeding vertebrae. The dens is large and blunt and is considered by some investigators as the displaced body of the atlas. On its ventral surface, the dens has an oval, saddle-shaped facet that articulates with the fovea dentis on the dorsal surface of the anterior arch of the atlas. Dorsally, it may have a smooth groove that receives the transverse ligament of the atlas, which provides stability between the atlas and the axis. The apical ligament attaches to the apex of the dens. The alar ligaments attach to the irregular lateral surface of the dens. Together the apical and alar ligaments provide stabilization to the cranial base. The pedicles are thick and broadly grooved on their cranial margins for the passage of the second spinal nerve. The laminae are also relatively thick. The spinous process is large, broad, and deeply concave on its caudal aspect. It is almost uniformly bifid.

SEVENTH CERVICAL VERTEBRA

The seventh cervical vertebra is a transitional vertebra in that it possesses some features of both the cervical and the thoracic regions.

The spinous process is usually the longest of the cervical series. It usually is not bifid but ends bluntly, producing a characteristic palpable subcutaneous bulge, and is commonly referred to as the vertebra prominens. The transverse processes are massive and end bluntly. The transverse foramina are variable in size and transmit the vertebral artery in only about 3% of cases (Table 1–2) but commonly permit the passage of a vertebral vein.

Variations

The spinous processes show considerable variation in regard to their distal end.[3,5,10] Generally in northern Europeans, the second through fifth vertebrae have bifid spinous processes. An accessory transverse foramen is commonly found posterior to and is smaller than the primary foramen in the sixth vertebra. The structural characteristics of the atlas suggest that the vertebra is a degenerate bone in humans. The ossification of the anterior and posterior arches may be incomplete, and the arch may be incomplete anteriorly.

Assimilation of the atlas with the occiput or axis may occur. The dens may exist separately (os odontoideum) or may articulate with a third occipital condyle. An ossicle is present occasionally in the apical ligament.

The spinous processes of C6 or T1 produce the most prominent palpable bulge on the dorsum rather than C7. Occasionally the costal process may be replaced by a cervical rib. However, only rarely is there a complete pair of cervical ribs that articulate with the sternum.

THORACIC VERTEBRAE

The typical features of members of this series of 12 vertebrae have already been considered. In summary, the most important distinguishing features of the bones of this group are the costal pits of the transverse processes and sides of the bodies, which articulate with the tubercles and heads of the ribs, respectively (Fig. 1–13).

Specialized Vertebrae

As with the seventh cervical, the first thoracic is a transitional vertebra and its body is similar to that of the seventh cervical.

The ninth thoracic vertebra has only superior costal pits but no inferior pits. The 10th vertebra usually has a com-

Table 1–2.   Summary of Primary Points of Difference between Typical Vertebrae of the Three Presacral Groups.

VERTEBRAL PART	REGION		
	Cervical	*Thoracic*	*Lumbar*
Body	Broad	Diameters are most equal; concave behind	Broad
	Cranial surface with raised sides and rounded anterior border	Flat	Flat
	No facets	Costal semifacets	No facets
Vertebral foramen	Triangular, greatest diameter transverse	Circular	Triangular, Diameters almost equal
Pedicles	Notches above or below almost equal	Arising from top of body; large notch below	Small notch above, large notch below
Laminae	Narrow, with spaces between	Broad, no space between	Extending downward; large spaces between
Transverse processes	Double foramen at root; two tubercles	Strong, with articular facet	Slender
Superior articular processes	Nearly flat, face upward and backward	Flat, vertical; face almost backward	Concave, vertical, face chiefly inward

Redrawn and modified from Huber.[3]

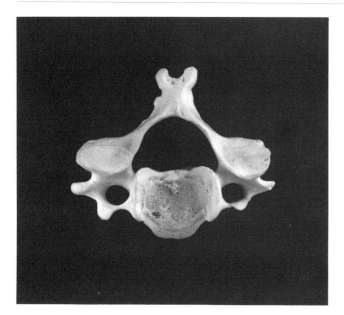

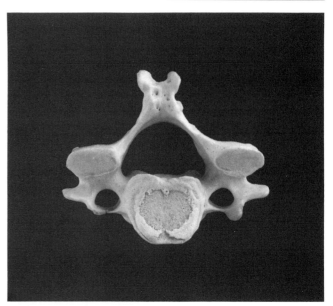

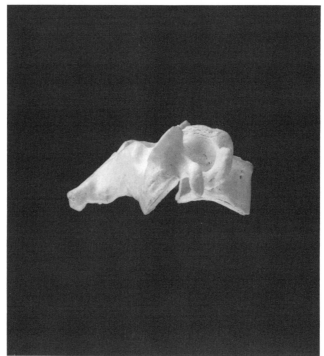

Figure 1–10. The fourth cervical vertebra. The third through sixth cervical vertebra can be considered typical. The 1st, 2nd, and 7th, 8th, 9th, 10th, 11th, and 12th all have unusual characteristics.[1,3,8]

plete costal pit near the cranial margin of the body on each side.

The 11th vertebra has a large body similar to those in the lumbar series of vertebrae. The costal pits are located on the pedicles of the vertebra. The transverse processes are short and do not have costal pits.

The 12th thoracic vertebra is similar to the 11th with the exception of the superior facets, which are oriented in the anteroposterior axis (Fig. 1–14). The inferior facet surfaces face laterally and are convex. The transverse processes are rudimentary.

Notable Variations

The head of the first rib may articulate with the body of C7. An aortic impression consists of a variable but notable flattening of the left side of the thoracic vertebrae. T9 to 11 may also take on transitional lumbar characteristics. Vertebral hemibodies may exist and are often ankylosed.[3,5,10]

LUMBAR VERTEBRAE

The lumbar region is sufficiently flexible to allow a wide range of motion in spite of the necessity of carrying the

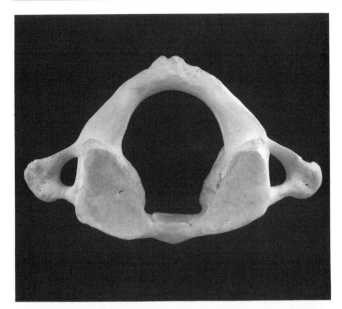

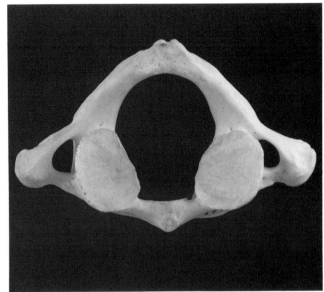

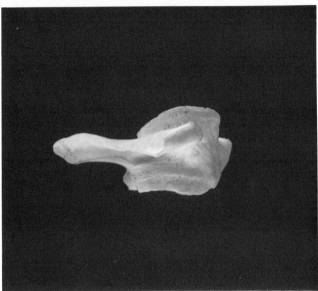

Figure 1–11. The atlas or first cervical vertebra. The atlas is shown from a superior, inferior, and right lateral view.

weight of the head, trunk, and upper limb. In addition to their size, the lumbar vertebrae are recognized from the cervical and thoracic vertebrae by the absence of transverse foramina (cervical) and costal pits (thoracic) (Fig. 1–15).

With the exception of the fifth, the bodies of the lumbar vertebrae are kidney shaped (Fig. 1–16). The fifth is oval. Because of its shape, the lumbar body is longer in the transverse plane than in the sagittal plane. The body is flat both cranially and caudally. In contrast to the cervical and thoracic bodies, the ventral height is greater than the dorsal in L1 to L4. The pedicles, transverse processes, and lamina are more heavily constructed as compared to the cervical and thoracic regions. The facets are oriented in a sagittal plane. The superior facet is concave and faces dorsally and medially, whereas the inferior facets face laterally.

Specialized Lumbar Vertebrae

The fifth lumbar vertebra represents a transitional vertebra (Fig. 1–16). The vertebra articulates with the sacrum, forming the sacrovertebral angle. Its transverse processes are short and thick, and they arise from both the pedicles and the body. The spinous process of the fifth lumbar vertebra is the shortest in the lumbar series.

Variations

A lumbar rib may be present at the first lumbar vertebra. If present, it is joined to the ventral surface or to the distal end of the transverse process. The fifth lumbar vertebra may be sacralized (ie, fused with the sacral vertebrae).[4,7,8]

Defects can occur in the pedicles between the facets (pars interarticularis). This results in the body, pedicles,

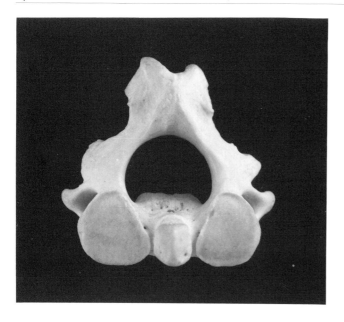

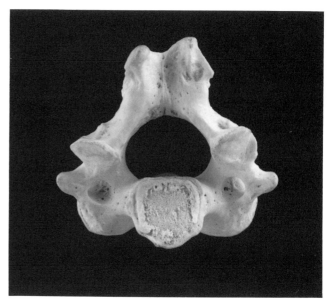

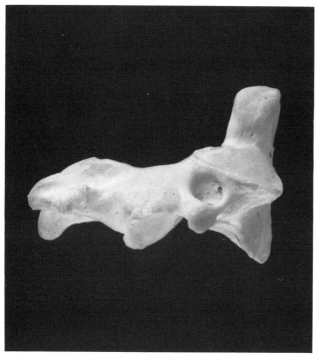

Figure 1–12. The axis or second cervical vertebra. The axis is shown from a superior, inferior, and right lateral view.

transverse processes, and superior facets in one unit and the laminae, spinous process, and inferior facets in another. This can occur unilaterally or bilaterally, and its incidence is approximately 4.2% based on a study of 4200 skeletons.[11]

ARTHROLOGY

The joints of the vertebral column are of three varieties: Those between vertebral bodies are cartilaginous; those between the laminae, spinous processes, and transverse processes are fibrous joints; and those between the facets are synovial joints.

The components that unite the vertebral bodies are the intervertebral disks as well as the anterior and posterior longitudinal ligaments (Figs. 1–17 and 1–18). The intervertebral disks are strong, extensible, and compressible. They are composed of fibrocartilage and are adherent to the cancellous bony endplates. The disk is divided into a fibrous ring of type I collagen and fibrocartilage, which is arranged in concentric layers. These fibers pass obliquely between the bodies of adjacent vertebrae and are attached securely to them. The fibrous ring is thinner posteriorly; hence, some of the circumferential layers are incomplete posteriorly. The more central layers are incomplete as well, and the dense fibrous collagen gives way to a firm, gel-like fibrocartilage.

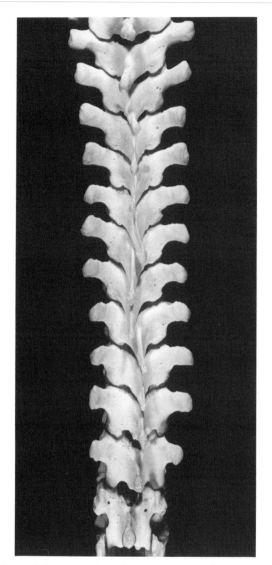 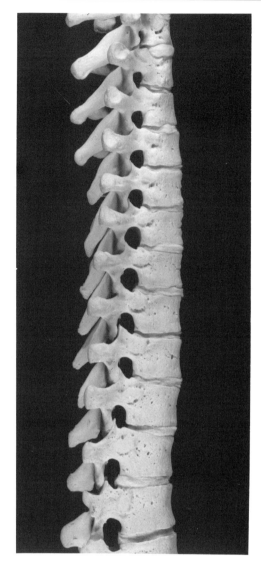

Figure 1–13.   The thoracic vertebrae. Note that the spinous processes tend to flatten between T4 and T10. Also note that the transverse processes move progressively in a dorsal direction from the transverse plane and that they diminish in size in T10 and T11.

The nucleus pulposus is located eccentrically and is nearer the dorsal aspect of the disk. The nucleus forms an elastic ball of highly compressed material with a high concentration of keratin sulfate (glycosamine). The nucleus pulposus and the more central fibrous layers of annulus are separated from any contact with the bony vertebral surfaces by a thin layer of hyaline or articular cartilage.

The intervertebral disks vary with the shape and size of opposing vertebral bodies. They are thickest and widest in the lumbar region. In both the cervical and lumbar regions, they are thicker ventrally than dorsally and contribute to the anterior convexity of the cervical and lumbar regions. The posterior convexity of the thoracic region is due, almost entirely, to the shape of the vertebral bodies. The disks play a much smaller role in the thoracic region.

Disks are responsible for about one fourth of the length of the vertebral column. The relative proportion of disk to body varies according to the region. The disks constitute about 40% in the cervical region, 20% in the thorax, and 33% in the lumbar region of the overall length of the spine.[1,3] Topographically, the disks are adjacent to the anterior longitudinal ligament ventrally, the posterior longitudinal ligament dorsally, and the interarticular, and radiate ligaments of the ribs laterally.

In the cervical region, small synovial joints (uncinate processes) are located on each side of the disk. They are small and are contained within the intervals between the prominent lateral lips of the cranial surface of the body and the beveled, lateral edges of the caudal surface of the body cranially.

ANTERIOR LONGITUDINAL LIGAMENT

The anterior longitudinal ligament begins as a band attached to the inferior surface of the occipital bone in the midline (Fig. 1–17). The ligament is fixed securely to the anterior

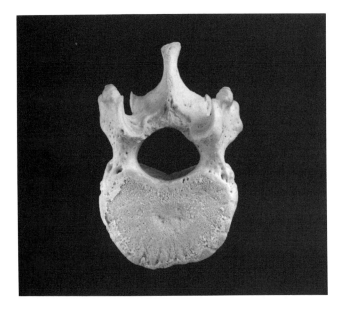
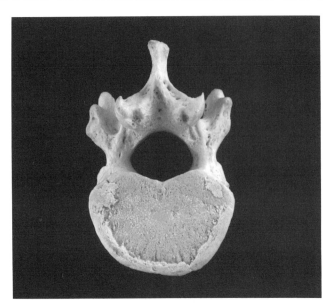
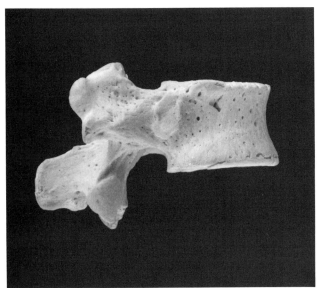
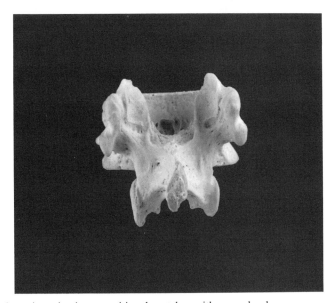

Figure 1–14. The 12th thoracic vertebra. The last of the thoracic series is a transitional vertebra with some lumbar characteristics. Notice the articular processes and the tripartite transverse process.

tubercle of the atlas and to the anterior surface of the succeeding vertebral bodies. Its lateral edges are blended with the periosteum except where blood vessels pass. The ligament widens until it reaches about 4 cm in the lumbar region (Fig. 1–18). The anterior longitudinal ligament is attached firmly to the first segment of the sacrum.

POSTERIOR LONGITUDINAL LIGAMENT

Also known as the PLL, the posterior longitudinal ligament extends from the occipital bone to the coccyx (Fig. 1–17). It is widest cranially and narrows as it travels caudally. It is attached firmly to the posterior aspect of the body in the cervical spine and fans out laterally to cover a portion of the intervertebral disk. The tectorial membrane is a cranial extension of the superficial layer (Fig. 1–18). The dura

mater is attached firmly to the PLL at the margin of the foramen magnum. In the thoracic and lumbar regions, the PLL is separated from the posterior aspect of the body by loose areolar connective tissue. Finally, it joins the filum of the dura at the caudal part of the sacrum.

LIGAMENTUM FLAVUM

The ligamenta flava or yellow ligaments are thick, dense bands of elastic connective tissue fibers attached to the laminae of adjacent vertebrae (Fig. 1–19). They form a series of elastic syndesmoses. Typically they are thicker and have greater strength in the midline. Because they extend to the medial portion of the facets, they participate in the formation of the facet capsule. They also extend between the bases of the spinous processes, where they thin into the interspinal

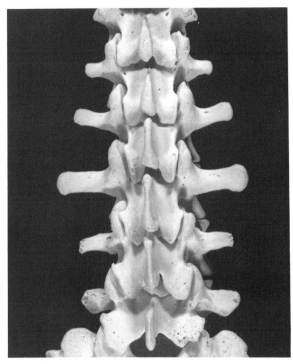
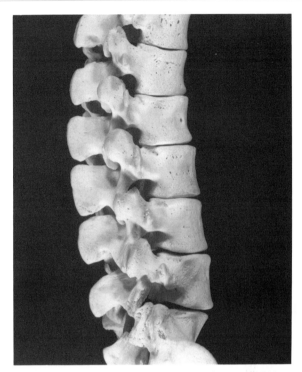

Figure 1–15. The lumbar vertebrae. Note the change in facet orientation from the thoracolumbar junction to the fifth lumbar vertebra.

ligament. They are thickest in the lumbar region and almost membranous in the cervical spine.

SUPRA- AND INTERSPINAL LIGAMENTS

The spinous processes are joined by the supraspinal and interspinal ligaments and the ligamentum nuchae. The supraspinal ligament is a strong, well-marked band of con-

nective tissue fibers along the tips of the spinous processes of C7 to the sacrum.

The ligamentum nuchae has the same position in the neck as the supraspinal ligament, although it is structurally different. The ligamentum nuchae is a thin septum that extends from the occipital protuberance and crest of the occipital bone to the spinous process of C7. The anterior margin of the ligament is joined to the occipital bone, the posterior tubercle of the atlas, and all of the tips of the cervical verte-

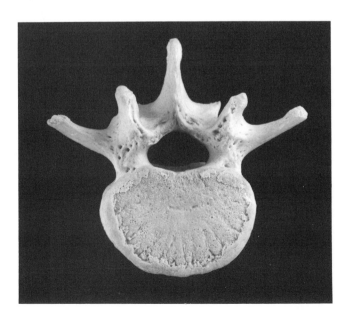
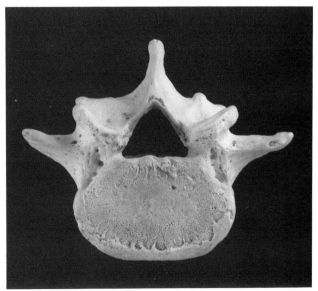

Figure 1–16. Lumbar vertebrae. This shows that the shape of the bodies changes between L1 and L5. The L1 vertebral body is kidney shaped (left side) whereas the L5 vertebra body is oval in shape (right side) and more massive overall.

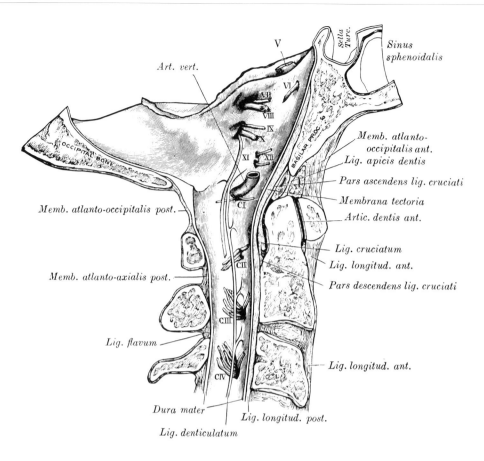

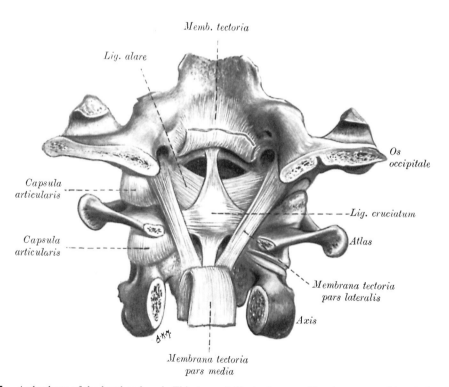

Figure 1–17.   Arthrology of the head and neck. This (upper) illustration provides the topographic relationships of various articular ligaments. Note in particular the anterior and posterior longitudinal ligaments and ligamentum flavum. The lower illustration also demonstrates two articular capsules and other ligaments of the upper cervical region.[5]

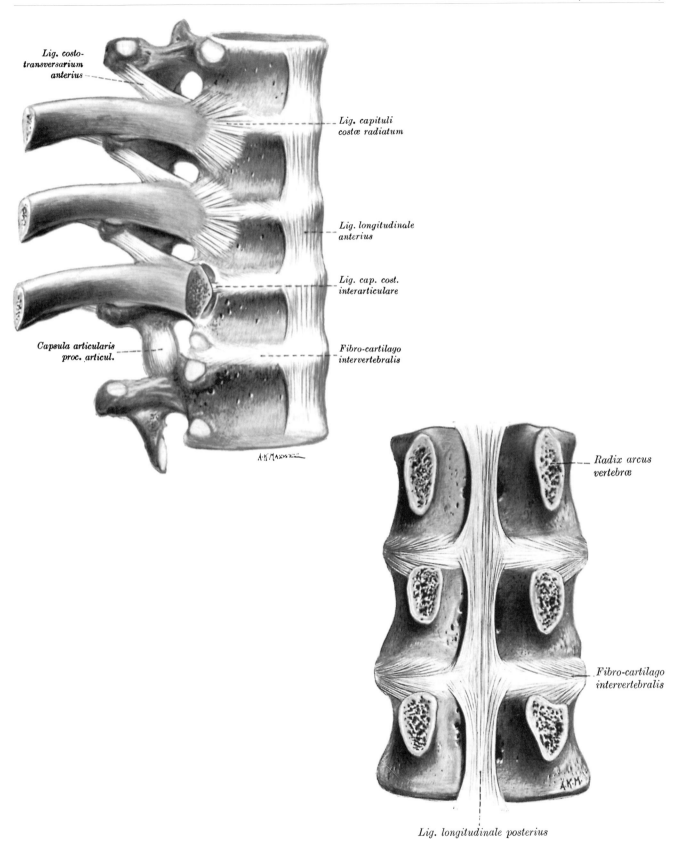

Lig. costo-
transversarium
anterius

Lig. capituli
costæ radiatum

Lig. longitudinale
anterius

Lig. cap. cost.
interarticulare

Capsula articularis
proc. articul.

Fibro-cartilago
intervertebralis

Radix arcus
vertebræ

Fibro-cartilago
intervertebralis

Lig. longitudinale posterius

Figure 1–18.   Anterior and posterior longitudinal ligaments, intervertebral disks, and articular capsules. On the left side the lowest rib has been removed to show the articular capsule of two thoracic vertebrae. Note also the costotransverse ligament and the anterior longitudinal ligament with its relationship to the fibrocartilage of the intervertebral disks. Posteriorly, the posterior longitudinal ligament blends laterally with the annulus fibrosus at each intervertebral space.[5]

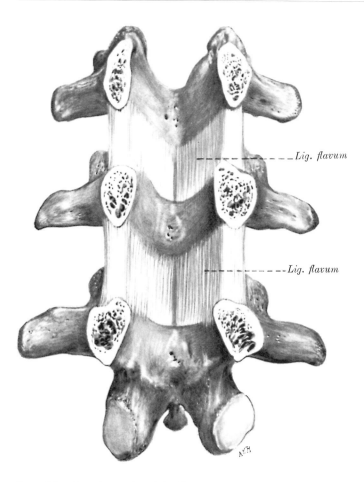

Lig. flavum

Lig. flavum

Figure 1–19. Ligamentum flavum. The body has been removed and the anterior surfaces of the laminae are shown.[5]

brae. The dorsal margin of the ligament provides the site of origin of the trapezius muscles. The lateral surfaces also provide sites of attachment for the dorsal muscles of the head and neck.

The interspinal ligaments are membranous connections between the spinous processes of adjacent vertebrae. They are poorly developed in the cervical spine.

ARTICULAR CAPSULES

Articular capsules surrounding the articular facets are composed of both yellow elastic fibers and white collagenous connective tissue fibers. They provide both extensibility and stability. In the cervical region, only the medial portion is composed of the ligamentum flavum. In the thoracic and lumbar regions, the ligamentum flavum extends further anteriorly to the margins of the intervertebral foramina.

TRANSVERSE LIGAMENT OF THE ATLAS

This ligament is approximately 6 mm in its vertical dimension and slightly thickened in the midline. It is attached, at each end, to a tubercle on the medial side of the lateral mass of the atlas. It is the major restraining ligament binding the dens of the atlas and, as such, keeps the dens positioned against the anterior arch of the atlas and thus protects the spinal cord from injury (Fig. 1–17).

Acknowledgment.   The authors acknowledge the help of Dina Abu-Yousef, research assistant in Dr. Bergman's laboratory, who painstakingly performed the spinal measurements given in Figure 1–8.

REFERENCES

1. Anson BJ, ed. *Morris' Human Anatomy.* 12th ed. New York, NY: McGraw-Hill; 1966.
2. Clemente CD. *Gray's Anatomy of the Human Body.* 30th ed. Philadelphia, Pa: Lea & Febiger; 1985.
3. Huber CG, ed. *Piersol's Human Anatomy.* 9th ed. Philadelphia, Pa: JB Lippincott; 1930.
4. Coventry MB. The American Academy of Orthopedic Surgeons, Instructional Course Lectures. Vol 6, 1949:218–227. Ann Arbor, Mich.: J. W. Edwards.
5. Schafer EA, Symington J, Bryce TH, eds. *Quain's Elements of Anatomy.* 11th ed. London: Longmans, Green, and Co.; 1915.
6. Augier M. Constitution generale du squelette. In: Poirier M, Charpy, eds. *Traite d'Anatomie Humaine.* 4th ed. Vol 1. Paris: Masson et Cie; 1931:79–88.
7. Testut L. *Traite d'Anatomie Humaine.* Vol 2. Paris: Doin; 1891.
8. Williams PL, Warwick R, Dyson M, et al. *Gray's Anatomy.* 27th ed. Edinburgh: Churchill Livingstone; 1989.
9. Çavdar S, Arisan L. Variations in the extra cranial origin of the human vertebral artery. *Acta Anat.* 1989;135:236–238.
10. Bergman RA, Thompson SA, Afifi AK, et al. *Compendium of Human Anatomic Variation.* Baltimore, Md: Urban and Schwarzenberg; 1988.
11. Roche MB, Rowe GG. The incidence of separate neural arch and coincident bond variation. *Anat Rec.* 1951;109:233–252.

2 Spine Imaging

Kurt G. Harris, M.D., Georges Y. El-Khoury, M.D.

INTRODUCTION

Only a few years ago this chapter might have been titled "Spine Radiography." In the last decade or so, there has been a change in the hierarchy of our imaging tools, with radiography occupying the same clinical territory but myelography being largely displaced by magnetic resonance imaging (MRI). Spine imaging is an impossibly broad subject for one chapter, so this discussion will necessarily be a limited one. The various imaging techniques available will be described, and in keeping with the purpose of this book, their roles will be defined with special emphasis on their application to trauma and spinal instability.

IMAGING TECHNIQUES

Radiography

Radiography is a technique that has been in use for almost 100 years. The basic principle is differential attenuation of photons in the x-ray portion of the electromagnetic spectrum by the object one is imaging.[1] This differential attenuation depends primarily on the electron density of the object.

Radiography is limited in its ability to display differences in density between different soft tissues, but it is outstanding at differentiating bone from soft tissue. In addition, the spatial resolution of radiography remains unexceeded by digital imaging techniques such as computed tomography (CT) or MRI. Low cost, high spatial resolution, and excellent definition of bone, as well as the advantage of a projected image of a large area of the spine, have maintained radiography as the core technique in spine imaging (Figs. 2–1 and 2–2).

Computed Tomography

Computed tomography or CT is a digital imaging technique whose clinical use was pioneered in the early 1970s by Sir Geoffrey Hounsfield.[2] It is based on the same physical principle as radiography: the differential attenuation of photons in the x-ray spectrum by tissues of different density. CT overcomes the limitations of radiography by employing unique scanner geometry and computerized image formation and display. With CT, a thin, fan-shaped beam of x-rays is rotated about the patient. An array of detectors oriented opposite the x-ray source registers the amount of radiation, which is recorded digitally for each projection (degree of rotation) of the rotating source. The data from multiple pro-

jections are then manipulated mathematically to form an image matrix. The resulting matrix of picture elements (pixels), each with a different gray scale value, constitutes the image from a single scan, representing an axial slice of tissue whose thickness can be varied (Figs. 2–2 to 2–4).

The combination of an array of sensitive detectors and digital recording of attenuation coefficients gives CT extraordinary dynamic range. Because a 256-level gray scale can be assigned to represent an arbitrary range of the attenuation coefficients resolved by the detectors (referred to as a window), high contrast resolution may be obtained, making discrimination of small differences in density possible.

The spatial resolution of CT depends on various parameters but is generally lower than that of radiography yet higher than that of MRI, with a lower limit of about 0.3 mm within the scan plane.[1] A principal limitation of CT is that images can only be obtained in a plane perpendicular to the axis of the scanner, so image orientation is limited by the physical configuration of the patient within the machine. This can be partially overcome by computer reformatting of axial images to create reformatted parasagittal or coronal images, but the spatial resolution of these is limited to the slice thickness of the axial images, usually no more than 2 mm (Fig. 2–5). In addition, there are often significant artifacts introduced by interscan motion.

MRI

Radiography and CT rely on the single parameter of electron density as the physical basis for image contrast. MRI depends on a whole host of parameters for image contrast, some of which are user definable. This makes MRI complex to master but gives it extraordinary flexibility and power. The physics of MRI allows tomographic images to be acquired in any arbitrary plane, a significant advantage over CT. In practice, the in-plane spatial resolution is usually less than that of CT, but contrast resolution is superior, especially for soft tissues.

Clinical MRI is actually hydrogen nucleus or proton MRI. It is based on the nuclear magnetic resonance properties of protons in the body. The nuclear magnetic dipole moments of hydrogen nuclei are oriented at random when there is no external magnetic field present. When a strong static magnetic field is applied, the magnetic dipole moments precess with a frequency proportional to the magnetic field strength about an axis parallel to the field, with slightly more of the

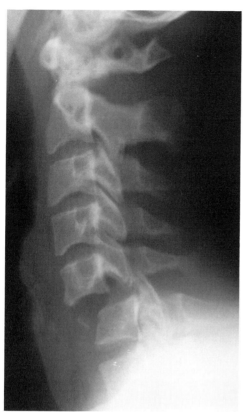

Figure 2–1. Bilateral interfacetal dislocation with "locked facets." This 25-year-old male was quadriplegic after a diving accident. Lateral radiograph shows C5 to C6 interfacetal dislocation—a three-column injury. Note fracture of anterosuperior corner of C6.

nuclei oriented parallel than anti-parallel to the field. This results in a net vector of longitudinal magnetization along the bore of the magnet (z-axis). This magnetization does not by itself provide any signal from which to construct an image. Imaging requires application of radiofrequency (RF) pulses to this net vector in order to perturb it. In the generic MRI sequence, the vector is perturbed or tipped toward the transverse plane by an RF pulse. The net transverse vector component then begins to precess about the z-axis, giving rise to a radiofrequency signal whose magnitude can be measured with an RF antenna or coil. The coil is critical in determining the signal-to-noise ratio of the final image. High-quality spine imaging requires the use of surface coils close to the area of interest to optimize the signal-to-noise ratio. Changes in magnitude of the RF signal received by the coil are the basis for computerized image reconstruction. The principal intrinsic tissue parameters determining the strength of the RF signal, and hence image contrast, are the spin-lattice relaxation time (T1) and spin-spin relaxation time (T2).[3] T1 reflects the time it takes for longitudinal or z-axis magnetization to return after perturbation by the applied RF pulse. T2 reflects the rapidity of decay in the transverse magnetization due to loss of phase coherence between the precessing nuclear magnetic dipole moments. T2* is also a parameter that reflects loss of phase coherence but that in addition reflects phase losses due to factors in addition to spin-spin interactions. All these parameters depend on the local chemical and nuclear magnetic environment. Proton density has a smaller but significant effect on signal and image contrast as well. The power of MRI lies in the ability to emphasize selectively the effect of each of these parameters on image contrast. Signal is acquired following specific pulse sequences that consist of RF pulses and the application of magnetic field gradients (in addition to the main field) to specify slice thickness and slice orientation and to localize the signal in space. The repetition time (TR) and echo time (TE) influence the relative weighting of the image toward the intrinsic parameters. For spin-echo imaging, long TR, long TE images are relatively T2-weighted. Short TR, short TE images are relatively T1 weighted. Long TR, short TE images are often referred to as proton-density–weighted images. All images contain some influence from all the intrinsic parameters, however, and thus *weighting* is always a relative term. Motion has complex effects on signal intensity that modify the effects of intrinsic tissue parameters. These effects are important and may even be clinically useful when imaging flowing blood or cerebrospinal fluid.[4] Although spin-echo imaging remains the workhorse of MRI, there is a plethora of available pulse sequences. Gradient recalled echo (GRE) sequences allow fast imaging with the advantage of very bright cerebrospinal fluid for a "myelographic effect". This is useful for defining the effect of extradural pathology on the intraspinal contents. GRE techniques are especially useful in the cervical spine, which lacks the natural extradural contrast provided by fat in the lumbar region (Fig. 2–6). GRE sequences are influenced more by T2* relaxation than by T2 and thus tend to be more artifact-prone than spin-echo sequences. Another recent innovation is the introduction of fast spin-echo sequences. These are particularly useful in the spine because shorter examination times reduce motion artifact (Fig. 2–7). Fast spin-echo sequences allow long TR sequences to be performed in a fraction of the time required previously but with identical signal-to-noise ratio. There are minor differences in image contrast, such as accentuation of fat. In addition, there are fewer magnetic susceptibility artifacts, which may be advantageous at times.

Paramagnetic contrast agents such as gadopentetate dimeglumine are used to increase the sensitivity of MRI to pathology that has abnormal vasculature or breakdown in the blood/central nervous system barrier. These agents work by altering the local environment to shorten spin-lattice relaxation times (T1 values). Thus, T1-weighted images (T1WI) following intravenous paramagnetic contrast administration show abnormal areas as increased signal intensity (Fig. 2–8). The physiology of paramagnetic contrast enhancement is not fundamentally different from enhancement with iodinated contrast for CT imaging. However, because such small concentrations of paramagnetic contrast agent are required to influence the local magnetic environment, contrast-enhanced MRI is very sensitive.

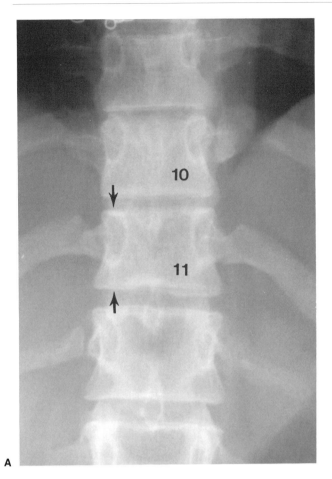

A

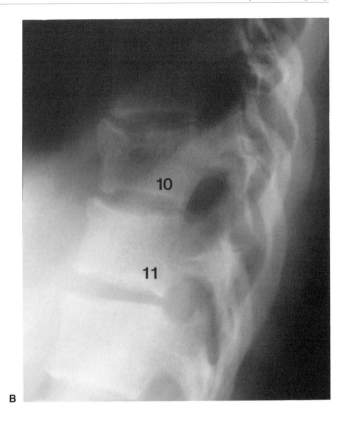

B

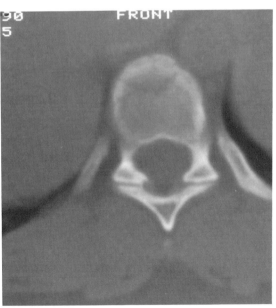

C

Figure 2–2. Compression fractures of T10 and T11. Sixteen-year-old girl in a motor vehicle accident, neurologically intact. (**A**). AP radiograph shows loss of height of right aspect of T11 and normal interpediculate distances. (**B**). Lateral view shows compression fractures of T10 and T11. Note characteristic buckling of anterior cortex of T11 and anterior displacement of fracture fragment from T10. (**C**). Axial CT shows anterior column disruption affecting T10.

Contraindications to MRI include cardiac pacemakers, intracranial aneurysm clips, cochlear implants, and intraorbital ferromagnetic metal. In patients with ferromagnetic metal near the anatomy of interest, MRI is not necessarily dangerous but may be uninterpretable due to artifact. Examination of the postoperative spine is greatly aided by using non-ferromagnetic (titanium) hardware or wire when-

ever practical.[5,6] Obese, large, or claustrophobic persons may be difficult, if not impossible, to image.

Myelography and CT Myelography
The primary role for myelography today is in imaging the intraspinal contents of patients with contraindications to MRI or with technically inadequate MRI studies. The bore

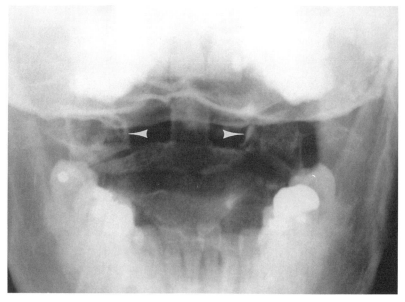

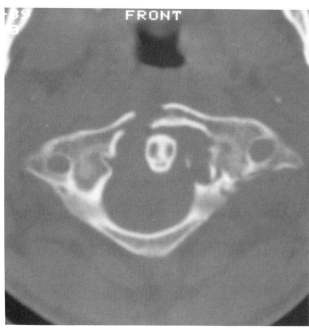

Figure 2–3. Jefferson fracture. This 30-year-old man dove into shallow water. (**A**). Open-mouth view demonstrates displacement (arrows) of lateral masses of C1. (**B**). Axial CT at C1 shows fractures of both anterior and posterior arches of C1.

of high-field magnets may exclude some patients due to excessive size or weight. Such large patients may not be well imaged with conventional or CT myelography for the same reasons. Another area in which myelography is still useful is in evaluating the integrity of the dural envelope and where direct visualization of the subarachnoid nerve roots is desired.[7] This is the case in patients with lower motor neuron lesions who have had cervical and–or upper extremity trauma. Although both CT myelography and MRI are capable of demonstrating posttraumatic pseudomeningoceles (Fig. 2–9), the presence of these is neither completely sensitive nor specific for subarachnoid nerve root avulsion.[7] Therefore, conventional myelography remains the procedure of choice for demonstrating subarachnoid (preganglionic) nerve root avulsion. The distinction between this

and more peripheral injuries is important because more peripheral injuries may be amenable to surgical repair.

Conventional Tomography

Conventional tomography, or planigraphy, has been a mainstay of spine imaging for many years. By performing radiography with reciprocal motion of both the x-ray source and the film, a tomographic image can be created by blurring structures above and below the desired focal plane. A typical examination consists of a series of stepwise acquisitions to produce a stack of images in coronal or parasagittal planes. This technique has lower contrast resolution than an axial CT image but is useful for imaging the spine in the parasagittal and coronal planes because the interscan motion artifact and low resolution of reformatted CT images are

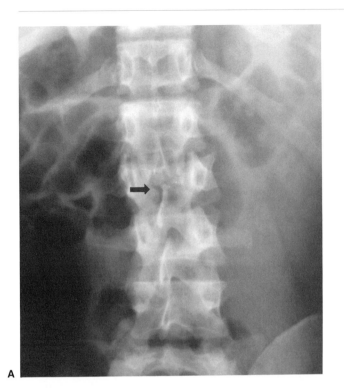

A

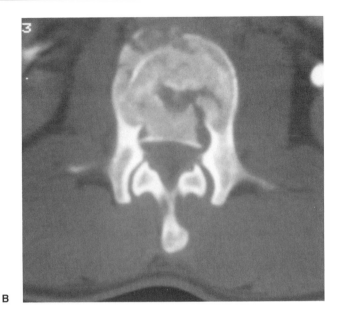

B

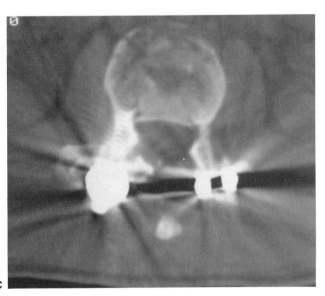

C

Figure 2–4. L2 burst fracture. Twenty-five-year-old man with incomplete cauda equina injury. (**A**). AP radiograph with increased interpediculate distance, loss of vertebral body height, and laminar fracture (arrow). (**B**). Axial CT image shows bursting of the centrum, the laminar fracture, and about 50% canal compromise by the retropulsed fragment. (**C**). Postoperative CT shows reduction of retropulsed fragment.

avoided. Applications include congenital vertebral anomalies, trauma (especially of the dens and cervical spine), and demonstration of pseudarthroses or failed fusion (Fig. 2–10).

Sonography

Sonography, or ultrasound, employs sound waves with frequencies in the megahertz range to image structures composed primarily of fluid and soft tissue. Bone reflects essentially all incident sound waves at the usable frequencies, so the applicability of sonography to the adult spine is confined mainly to the intraoperative state, where a window can be created in the normal anatomy to allow visualization of the

intraspinal contents and the inner contours of the spinal canal. Real-time imaging with a small, movable transducer is ideal for intraoperative monitoring of the physical configuration of the spinal cord and spinal canal and for assessing the adequacy of fracture reduction before the wound is closed.[8,9]

TRAUMA AND INSTABILITY

Instability, in the engineering sense, refers to a loss in the mechanical stiffness of a structure such that small applied loads may result in unusually large or catastrophic displacements.[10] The spine has obvious support functions that may

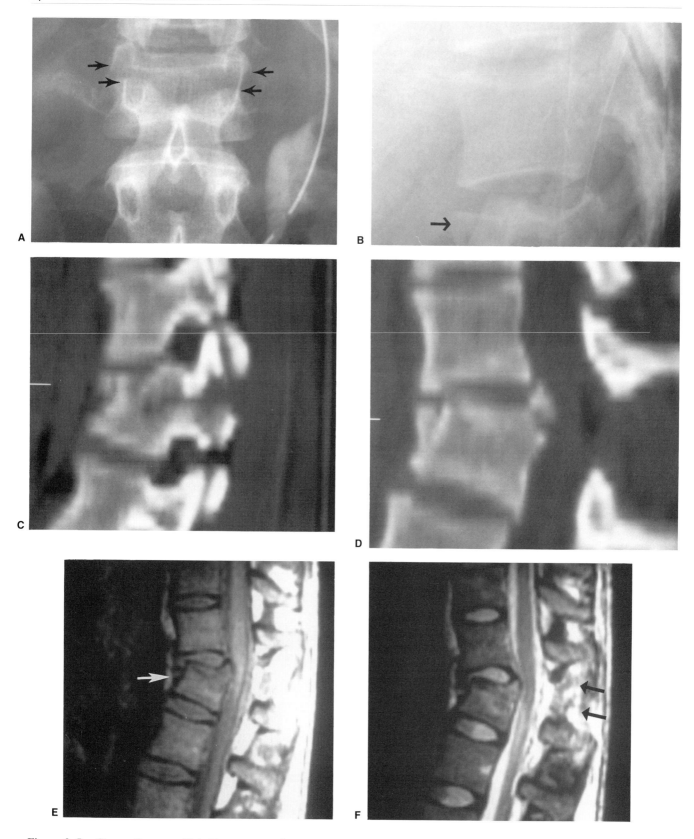

Figure 2–5.   Chance fracture of L1. Young woman in a motor vehicle accident. (**A**). Classic horizontal splitting of the pedicles at L1 (arrows). (**B**). Lateral view shows widening of L1 pedicles. Partial disruption of anterior column is indicated by subluxation of T12 and fracture fragment arising from anterosuperior body of L1. (**C**) and (**D**). Left parasagittal and midsagittal images reformatted from axial CT images provide an excellent demonstration of the horizontal fracture plane through the pedicles and upper body of L1. (**E**). Sagittal T1-weighted MRI shows stripping of anterior longitudinal ligament from body of L1 (arrow). (**F**). Parasagittal T2-weighted images show interspinous ligament disruption with bright signal due to hemorrhage and edema (double arrows) and disruption of posterior longitudinal ligament with avulsion of posterosuperior corner of L1 body.

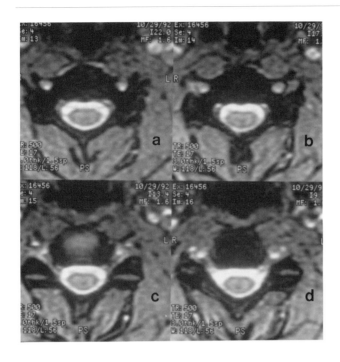

Figure 2–6. Normal cervical spine MRI. (**A–D**). Sequential axial gradient echo (GRE) images of midcervical spine. Three-millimeter slice thickness with 1.5-mm interscan spacing. Note excellent contrast between spinal cord and cerebrospinal fluid, faintly visualized ventral and dorsal roots arising from cord, bright signal from normal water content of disk (**C**), and excellent definition of neural foramina (**C** and **D**).

become compromised by pathologic processes. Trauma, neoplasm, and some iatrogenic states may all impart instability to the spine in the true mechanical sense. However, we are more concerned with the role of the spine in protecting the vulnerable neural tissue it contains than with catastrophic loss of support. Thus, for this chapter we will adhere to the definition of clinical instability by White and Panjabi as "the loss of the ability of the spine under physiologic loads to maintain its pattern of displacement so that there is no initial or additional neurologic deficit, no major deformity, and no incapacitating pain."[11] This definition emphasizes the function of the spine as a neural conduit and therefore encompasses most entities requiring spine fusion and instrumentation. In addition to true mechanical instability, then, degenerative and congenital deformity with neural compromise are included. Although precise quantitation of spine motion behavior in the clinical setting remains difficult,[12] imaging the spine is critical to evaluating instability in the clinical sense.

Trauma

Trauma is the most common and most obvious cause of spinal instability. The imaging evaluation of spine trauma has evolved in the past few years, although radiography remains the core technique. A general approach to detection and definition of injury in the cervical and thoracolumbar spine follows, with emphasis on the roles of the imaging techniques rather than complete classification of injury.

Cervical Spine Trauma: Diagnostic Approach

When evaluating the cervical spine of the trauma patient, it is useful to divide patients into groups based on a priori likelihood of injury. A patient with head injury who is sober, neurologically intact, and lacking neck pain does not even

need radiography because the chance of missing a significant neck injury is vanishingly small.[13] The other extreme is the patient with obvious neurologic deficit consistent with significant spine injury. Such a patient should be evaluated with imaging, including CT and MRI, until pathology accounting for the deficit is revealed. The intermediate levels of a priori probability of injury include those who have pain or subjective changes without physical evidence of neurologic deficit and those in whom complete neurologic assessment is impossible due to unconsciousness. Evaluation of all these patient groups should begin with a screening trauma series of radiographs.

At the University of Iowa, the trauma series comprises anteroposterior (AP), lateral, oblique, and open-mouth views. A high-quality lateral view is particularly important because at least two thirds of injuries will be evident on this view.[14] The lateral view should include the craniovertebral junction and clivus at its rostral extent and the C7 to T1 articulation caudally. Attempts to visualize the lower cervical levels are aided by gentle traction on the arms to lower the shoulders if the patient is supine. If this is not successful, a "swimmer's view," with one arm abducted to uncover the cervicothoracic junction, often demonstrates the lower cervical vertebrae to good advantage, as well as the upper thoracic levels. Oblique views demonstrate the articular pillars and facet joints and may be obtained upright with a Philadelphia collar if the patient was ambulatory to begin with. In the patient who is unconscious or who has suffered multiple trauma, supine oblique views are obtained. Supine images lack the aesthetics of the upright views but provide useful information. The open-mouth view is an AP view taken to demonstrate the atlantoaxial relationship and the dens (Fig. 2–3A).

In those with intermediate probability of significant injury, the exhaustiveness of evaluation will depend on

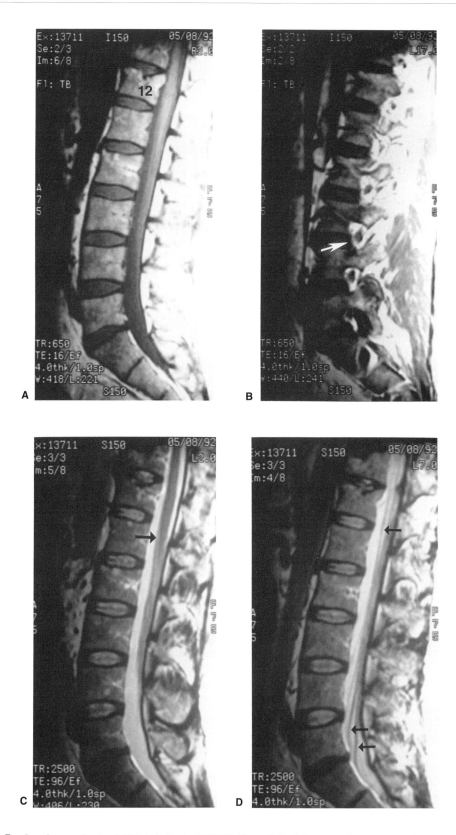

Figure 2–7. Lumbosacral spine MRI. (**A**). Sagittal T1WI. Note slight deformity of posterosuperior aspect of T12 due to old healed fracture. (**B**). Parasagittal T1WI. The dorsal root ganglia (arrow) are well demonstrated within the neural foramina on far lateral images. (**C**). Midline sagittal fast-spin echo T2WI obtained in less than 3 minutes. Note excellent contrast between cerebrospinal fluid and neural elements. The conus medullaris ends at L1 (arrow). (**D**). Adjacent parasagittal image is able to show individual nerve roots of the cauda equina (arrows) because the speed of acquisition helps reduce motion artifact.

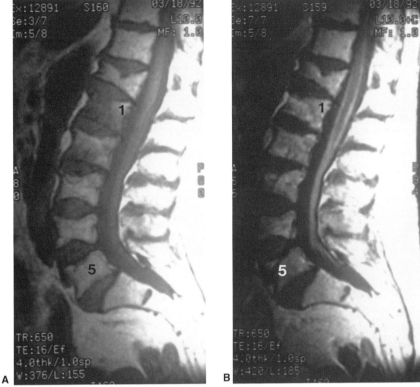

Figure 2–8. MRI of vertebral and leptomeningeal metastasis. (**A**). Sagittal T1WI shows hypointensity of L1 and L2 due to infiltration by metastatic tumor. T12 is compressed but has normal marrow signal consistent with a nonmalignant process at this level. (**B**). T1WI following intravenous paramagnetic contrast shows remarkable abnormal enhancement of the conus and nerve roots due to leptomeningeal metastasis (pathologically proven). Note that the vertebral body tumor enhances as well, becoming isointense with and difficult to distinguish from the normal marrow.

whether pathology is found and on a necessary amount of clinical judgment. The trauma series may be all that is required if the patient has only neck pain and initial evaluation is negative. If there is some question of ligamentous injury, active range-of-motion flexion and extension views may reveal signs of injury. Because instability may be masked by muscle spasm shortly after injury, a follow-up examination with flexion and extension views after muscle spasm has subsided is preferable. A neutral lateral view should be repeated first at follow-up for the same reason. In a patient with subjective neurological complaints (eg, referred pain, dysesthesias, or paresthesias suggestive of radiculopathy or myelopathy), the clinical suspicion may be higher. If radiographs are of high quality and are unrevealing, conventional tomography or CT may sometimes reveal a radiographically occult fracture. CT can only be performed with high resolution over a limited area, so the ability of MRI to image over a large area in the parasagittal plane makes it a useful technique. MRI also has the advantage of directly imaging the spinal contents. A negative MRI in the patient with subjective complaints may reassure by excluding such pathology as ligamentous injury, herniated disk, and epidural hematoma. MRI appears to be more sensitive than CT to ligamentous injury.[15] The patient who is unconscious or intoxicated, but who has no obvious neuro-

logic deficit, may be considered cleared of significant injury if the trauma series is of high quality and is negative.

The patient with a definite neurologic deficit should be evaluated initially with the trauma series. Often the diagnosis is obvious (Figs. 2–1 to 2–3). If the diagnosis is not obvious and there are suspicious areas on radiographs or inadequate coverage is provided, guided CT examination is often the most practical next step. Often patients with a deficit are multiply injured and require CT of the brain or abdomen, so it is usually effective and convenient to perform a limited supplemental CT examination of the spine. Figure 2–11 illustrates this strategy. In this figure, the lateral projection showed the vertebrae adequately only down to the C5 level, and multiple attempts at swimmer's views were unsuccessful. Limited CT of the lower cervical levels and cervicothoracic junction revealed a burst fracture of C6.

The patient with a neurologic deficit should be evaluated exhaustively. This principle is also illustrated by Figure 2–11. Although abnormalities were revealed with CT, this patient had complete quadriplegia, and the severity of injury seemed somewhat inconsistent with his deficit. MRI was obtained, and this revealed evidence of intramedullary hemorrhage consistent with the clinical deficit[16] as well as ligamentous injury. It is the rate and degree of maximal displacement at the time of injury that relates most closely to

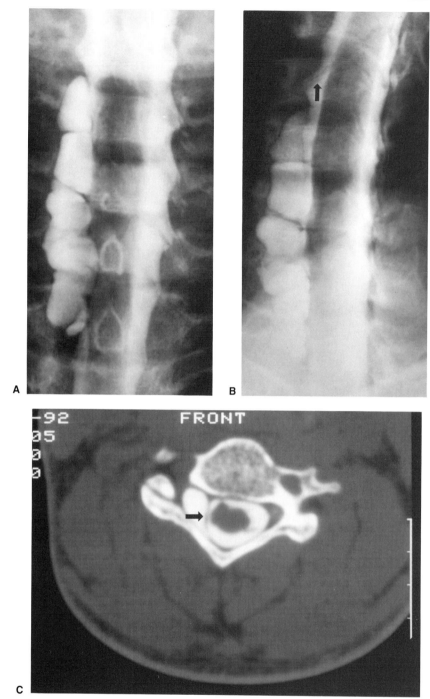

Figure 2–9. Nerve root avulsion with chronic pseudomeningoceles. Young man with flaccid paralysis of right arm 3 months following all-terrain vehicle accident. (**A**). AP myelogram shows multiple septated pseudomeningoceles on the right. (**B**). Oblique view shows normal nerve roots (arrow) with absence of normal roots more caudally on the right. (**C**). Axial CT shows smoothly marginated pseudomeningocele on the right outside the dura (arrow).

the degree of neurologic injury, and this may not necessarily relate to the severity of fracture or the degree of malalignment at the time of imaging.

Conventional tomography remains a useful supplemental technique, especially for the detection and delineation of posterior element injury. Conventional tomography has to some degree been displaced by CT due to convenience rather than any deficiency of the conventional technique.

MRI is becoming increasingly significant in the clinical evaluation of patients with spinal cord injury. The ability to image the spinal cord directly with emphasis on different intrinsic tissue parameters is a powerful tool for diagnosis. MRI provides an ability to image the contents of the spinal conduit, which complements the abilities of radiography and CT. Spinal cord edema is demonstrated as increased signal intensity on T2-weighted images (T2WI) with or with-

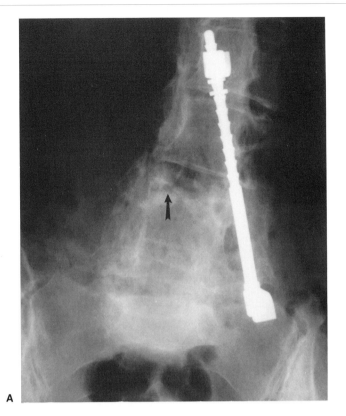

A

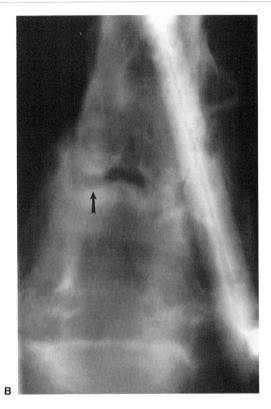

B

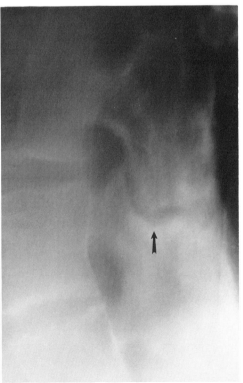

C

Figure 2–10. Pseudarthrosis of fusion mass. Forty-eight-year-old woman had extensive posterior fusion 30 years previously for neurogenic scoliosis. (**A**). AP radiograph shows lucency at L3 to L4 level on the right. (**B**) and (**C**). Coronal and parasagittal tomograms demonstrate pseudarthrosis of the fusion mass.

out cord swelling. Spinal cord hemorrhage that is evident on MRI is manifest most often as focal hypointensity within an area of hyperintensity (edema) on T2WI[16,17] (Fig. 2–11). The hypointensity is due to the presence of intracellular deoxyhemoglobin, which causes preferential T2 shortening locally, resulting in low signal on T2WI.[17,18] This appear-

ance is seen most commonly within 8 days of injury. Later than this, the predominant evidence of hemorrhage will be intramedullary hyperintensity on T1-weighted images due to further oxidation to methemoglobin.[16]

The MRI appearance of the injured spinal cord carries important prognostic information. Spinal cord edema is

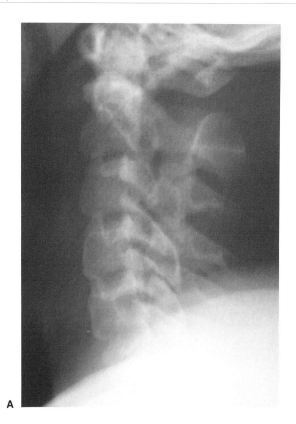

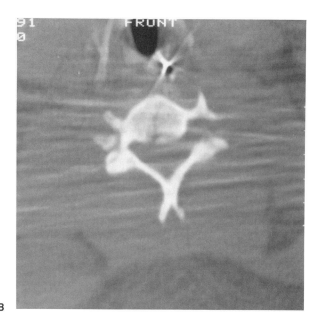

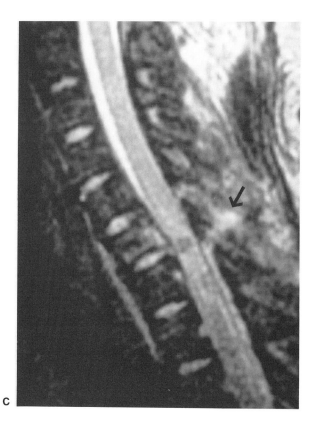

Figure 2–11.   Minimal fracture with cord hemorrhage on MRI. This 21-year-old man was quadriplegic after being thrown from a car at 65 mph. (**A**). Lateral radiograph barely shows C6 vertebra. A swimmer's view was unrevealing. (**B**). Axial CT shows sagittal fracture of C6 as well as rotatory subluxation not evident on the radiographs. (**C**). Parasagittal T2WI shows hyperintensity of the fractured body of C6 and interspinous ligamentous disruption (arrow). Most importantly, there is diffuse hyperintense signal in the spinal cord consistent with edema and a focal area of dark intramedullary hemorrhage at the level of the C6 to C7 disk space.

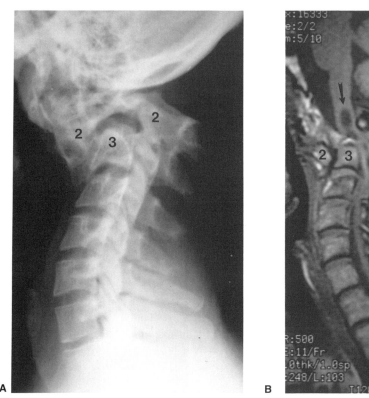

Figure 2–12. Untreated hangman's fracture (traumatic spondylolisthesis of the axis). This man presented 24 years after a motorcycle accident with progressive left upper extremity numbness and weakness. (**A**). Lateral radiograph shows complete spondylolisthesis of the body of C2 on C3. (**B**). Parasagittal T1-weighted MR image obtained after partial decompression via transoral odontoidectomy shows the upper cord compressed between the posterior arch of C1 and body of C3. A syrinx extends the length of the cervical cord and into the medulla (arrow). (2 = C2, 3 = C3).

associated with a wide range in the degree of clinical deficit. Hemorrhage correlates with the more severe clinical deficits, especially complete injury, and the presence of hemorrhage further indicates that the likelihood of recovery is remote.[16,17] Although MRI may be poor at characterizing posterior element fracture, its high soft-tissue contrast resolution makes it ideal for delineating ligamentous injury[15] (Figs. 2–5 and 2–11) and epidural hematoma. In addition, MRI is superior to CT in the detection of traumatic herniated disk, which appears to be a relatively common entity.[15,19,20] In the evaluation of long-term complications of trauma, MRI is excellent at detecting and defining syringohydromyelia, arachnoid cysts, cord atrophy, and myelomalacia.

Traumatic Cervical Instability

The cervical spine must support the head while allowing a wide range of motion to orient the eyes to the environment. This mobility makes the cervical spine vulnerable to a variety of force vectors in trauma, largely acting as moments due to forces applied to the head.

A clinical determination of instability depends on knowledge of the lore associated with each injury type and on some knowledge of injury mechanisms. For the cervical spine, numerous classification schemes have been proposed.

The scheme described by Harris and Edeiken-Monroe[21] has the advantage of simplicity and is based on standard terminology, with each entity being subsumed under a predominant force vector to classify the injury. The predominant force vectors include hyperflexion, hyperflexion and rotation, hyperextension and rotation, vertical compression, hyperextension, lateral flexion (bending), and "diverse or imprecisely understood mechanisms."[21]

White and Panjabi have proposed a checklist approach for the evaluation of instability in the cervical spine, which is based on static or dynamic angular and translational radiographic abnormalities at a given motion segment along with various clinical factors.[11] For example, fixed anteroposterior translation of 3.5 mm or greater or fixed relative angulation of 11 degrees or more would each earn points toward the diagnosis of instability.

Although Denis described the three-column concept of spinal instability in association with thoracolumbar fractures,[22] this is conceptually useful in the cervical spine as well.[21] Holdsworth[23] had defined the anterior column as consisting of anterior vertebral bodies, the anterior longitudinal ligament (ALL), the disk, and the posterior longitudinal ligament (PLL). The posterior column consisted of everything posterior the PLL: the capsular ligaments and facets, the ligamenta flava, the interspinous and supraspinous ligaments. Denis observed that in the thoracolumbar spine disruption of the posterior column alone rarely led to clinical instability; and so proposed that the anterior column be redivided into anterior and middle columns, with the anterior disk and annulus and ALL constituting the former and the posterior disk and annulus and PLL the latter. The resulting three columns seemed to correlate better with instability in Denis's clinical series, with instability being defined as disruption of the middle column. Note that because the middle column is between the other two, middle-column disruption implies that at least one other column is disrupted. The flexion teardrop fracture and bilateral interfacetal dislocation (Fig. 2–1) could both be thought of as three-column (anterior, middle, and posterior) and hence unstable injuries of the cervical spine secondary to hyperflexion forces, although they differ morphologically in that the former has a fracture of the centrum of the involved vertebra and the latter is mostly ligamentous.

Figure 2–12 illustrates the importance of a knowledge of mechanisms of injury. This patient had suffered traumatic spondylolisthesis of the axis 24 years previously in a motorcycle accident but had left the hospital against medical advice. This is often a relatively stable injury. However, associated injury to the disk at C2 and C3 (Effendi Type II or III traumatic spondylolisthesis[24]) in this case led to instability, with eventual total spondylolisthesis of C2 anterior to C3.

Thoracic and Lumbar Trauma: Approach

The imaging workup of suspected thoracolumbar trauma follows the same logic based on a priori likelihood of injury as was outlined for the cervical spine. The major differences are that the screening radiographic study is simpler to perform, and the consequences of a missed injury are perhaps less grave. Because of the long distances involved, the use of CT to evaluate a fracture must be as focused as possible. High-quality radiographs and a good corroborative physical examination are the key to ruling out thoracolumbar trauma efficiently.

Thoracic and Lumbar Trauma: Biomechanics and Mechanisms

Compared to the cervical spine, the thoracic and lumbar spine are relatively more constrained in physiologic motion and in the moments applied during trauma. This is especially true of the thoracic spine, where the rib cage acts as an outrigger to stabilize segmental motion and the costovertebral articulations directly stabilize each motion segment. The structure of the upper thoracic spine and rib cage emphasizes rigidity to allow respiration. The structure of the lower thoracic and lumbar spine emphasizes support of the trunk, with more flexibility than the upper thoracic but less than the cervical spine. These differences in support function and mobility are reflected in anatomic differences such as the changing orientation of the apophyseal joints as one progresses caudally. Axial rotation is progressively more

limited proceeding from the upper thoracic to the midlumbar spine by the change in orientation of the apophyseal joints toward the sagittal plane (compare the change in facet orientation from T10 in Fig. 2–2C to L2 in Fig. 2–4B).

With thoracolumbar fractures as a whole, there is a predominance of injury at the thoracolumbar junction. This probably relates to the change in stiffness from the relatively more mobile lumbar to the thoracic spine, as well as the transition from lumbar lordosis to thoracic kyphosis.

Specific Thoracolumbar Fractures

COMPRESSION FRACTURE

The compression fracture can be thought of as due to hyperflexion, with an axis of rotation corresponding to the middle column. This causes disruption of the anterior column, with the middle and posterior columns intact. The most common location is at the thoracolumbar junction, with some occurring at the midthoracic region. There is a lateral compression variety that is most common at L3.[22] The most common configuration is deformity of the superior endplate with loss of anterior vertebral body height (Fig. 2–2). Buckling of the anterior cortical surface on the lateral radiograph helps distinguish it from nontraumatic wedging of the vertebra (Fig. 2–2B). Because the middle column is by definition intact, there is usually no neurologic deficit. The interpediculate distance is normal on radiographs because the neural arch is not interrupted. CT is the modality of choice for distinguishing compression from burst fractures. One simply follows the contours of the neural arch from slice to slice to see that it is intact (Fig. 2–2). There may be considerable comminution of the anterior vertebral body, but as long as the middle column is intact, this is a single-column and hence stable injury.

BURST FRACTURE

The burst fracture affects the upper lumbar and, less often, the midthoracic vertebrae. The burst fracture is due to loading of the spine such that the disk herniates axially, "exploding" the vertebral body and disrupting both anterior and middle columns. The neural arch is disrupted, accounting for the radiographic sign of increased interpediculate distance (Fig. 2–4). There may be a vertical fracture of the lamina (Fig. 2–4). Computed tomography distinguishes the burst from the compression fracture by showing disruption of the middle column and evidence of neural arch disruption. A laminar fracture is usually detected by CT if not already seen on the radiograph (Fig. 2–4). A fragment of the posterior vertebral body is usually retropulsed into the canal[22] (Fig. 2–4).

Denis considered the burst fracture to be a two-column injury, even with these signs of disruption of the neural arch.[22] McAfee has divided burst fractures into stable and unstable types, with the former defined as a two-column injury with anterior and middle-column disruption and the latter as a three-column injury having, in addition, evidence of disruption of the posterior neural arch (lamina, facets, etc).[25] The cases described by Denis would fit McAfee's definition of the unstable burst fracture.

Except in the thoracic region, where there is little available space for the spinal cord, there is rarely complete neurologic injury. If reduction and internal fixation are performed with a posterolateral or transpedicular approach, intraoperative sonography can confirm reduction of fracture fragments. CT can also confirm reduction, despite some limitation from artifact due to hardware (Fig. 2–4).

SEATBELT-TYPE FRACTURE

The seatbelt-type fracture may be conceptualized as due to hyperflexion, with the axis of rotation located at or anterior to the anterior column. This results in distraction and disruption of the middle and posterior columns, with variable injury to the anterior column. The name *seatbelt* comes from the association with lapbelt restraint injuries in motor vehicle passengers. The association is logical because a decelerating body restrained by an anteriorly located obstruction (the belt) will flex with an axis of rotation that is anteriorly located. Denis described various configurations, some involving one vertebral level and some involving two. The Chance fracture[26] is the classic seatbelt-type fracture (Fig. 2–5). It is a one-level fracture through bone and was the most common type in Denis's series.[22] Note the classic horizontal splitting of the pedicles in Figure 2–5. Because the plane of separation is axial, these fractures are best

demonstrated by radiography and conventional tomography. Reformatted images in the sagittal plane are necessary with CT (Fig. 2–5). MRI demonstrates the ligamentous disruption. Note that there is evidence of partial anterior column disruption in Figure 2–5 in the form of stripping of the ALL along with the anterosuperior endplate fracture. This allows forward subluxation of T12 on L1.

FRACTURE DISLOCATION

The fracture dislocation can be thought of as due to any force vector or combination of force vectors that results in total failure of all three columns.[22] Some of the subtypes are extreme forms of the aforementioned entities. For instance, if there is hyperflexion with axis of rotation similar to a seatbelt-type fracture but there is complete failure of the anterior column in addition to the other two, this will result in the flexion distraction subtype. Addition of a significant vector causing axial rotation to a burst fracture might cause the posterior column, in addition to anterior and middle, to fail. This would result in the flexion rotation subtype. The third subtype is the shear subtype. This is due to a primary force vector not typical of the compression, burst, or seatbelt-type fractures. This is a shear force relatively perpendicular to the spinal axis, often due to a severe blow directly to the spine. Figure 2–13 illustrates such a case. Fracture dislocations commonly result in complete paraplegia, especially the shear and flexion distraction subtypes.

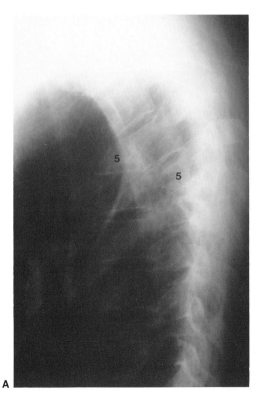
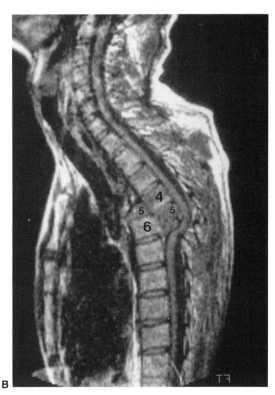

Figure 2–13. Shear type fracture dislocation. Fifty-seven-year-old man run over by another motorcycle during a motorcycle race with complete neurologic injury at T6 (**A**). Lateral radiograph shows posterior dislocation with fracture plane running obliquely through T5. (**B**). T1-weighted MR image shows the cord stretched and deformed but not severed.

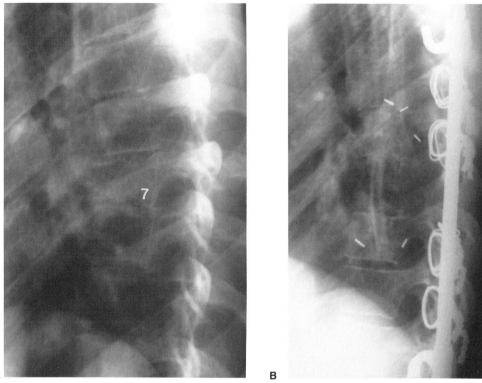

Figure 2–14.   Vertebral metastasis. (**A**). Metastatic renal cell carcinoma involving T7. Note irregular and indistinct cortical margins. (**B**). Vertebrectomy with Harrington rod and sublaminar wire instrumentation for stabilization. Note rib graft.

Nontraumatic Instability

Although not always unstable in the true mechanical sense, there are a number of conditions that are characterized by abnormal motion or displacement and that certainly fit White and Panjabi's definition of clinical instability, with emphasis on the function of the spine as a neural conduit.[11]

NEOPLASTIC INSTABILITY

The spine may be structurally weakened by primary or metastatic neoplasms. MRI is the modality of choice for detecting neoplasms. Often, leptomeningeal metastasis or growth of tumor into the epidural space is responsible for neurological deficit, and in these cases it is not an issue of mechanical instability (Fig. 2–8). If there is leptomeningeal metastasis, this is not a surgical problem. If there is metastatic destruction of a vertebra, this may be ameliorated with surgery, and in this case the instability to be addressed is primarily iatrogenic. The stabilization in Figure 2–14 with rib graft and Harrington rods is necessitated more by the vertebrectomy performed to remove the tumor than by the tumor itself.

INFLAMMATORY INSTABILITY

Rheumatoid arthritis is the classic example of inflammatory disease leading to clinical instability. Figure 2–15 shows erosion of the dens and ligamentous laxity secondary to pannus. There is abnormally increased AP translation with flexion and extension. The MRI here demonstrates the quantity of pannus encroaching on the neural canal even with extension and emphasizes that abnormal translation may be made more clinically significant by concomitant mass effect from the pannus.

INFECTIOUS INSTABILITY

Infection of the vertebra and adjacent disk space may destroy the integrity of the anterior and middle columns. Healing may result in natural stabilization through bony ankylosis or fibrosis, or surgery may be required for stabilization. MRI is the technique of choice to evaluate for spinal infection. MRI with intravenous paramagnetic contrast agents may aid in delineating epidural abscess. Flexion and extension lateral radiographs can be used to assess abnormal motion behavior.

DEGENERATIVE INSTABILITY

Segmental spinal instability or segmental hypermobility is a controversial entity and is difficult to identify.[10,27,28] There is little doubt that abnormal patterns of motion are a consequence of, if not causal in, the process of disk degeneration. It is unclear, however, to what degree abnormal motion per se can be implicated in chronic back pain. There are cases in which there is clearly abnormal displacement as the end result of disk and apophyseal joint degeneration. These probably represent the most clear-cut examples of

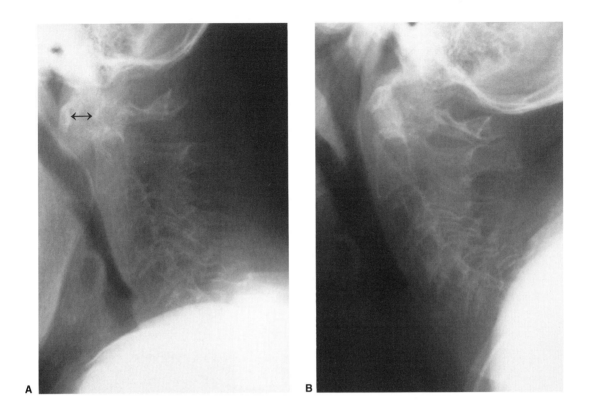

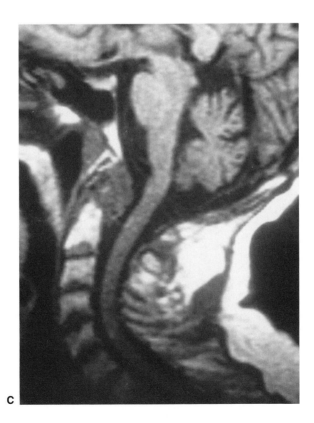

Figure 2–15.   Instability due to rheumatoid arthritis. (**A**). Flexion lateral radiograph. (**B**). Extension lateral radiograph. Both show abnormal C1 to C2 translation in flexion (arrows), which reduces in extension. Note severe osteopenia. (**C**). Sagittal T1-weighted MRI reveals large mass of pannus eroding the dens.

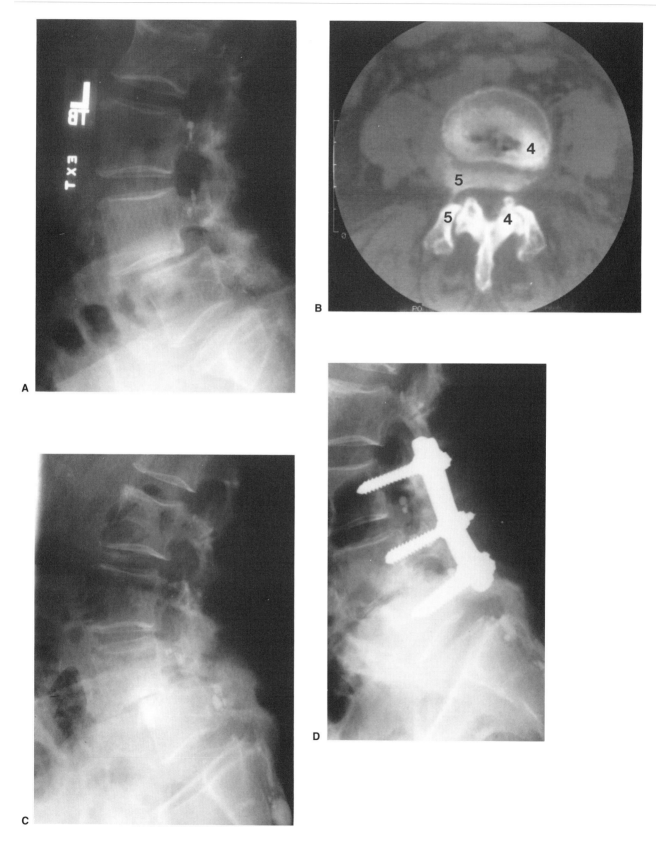

Figure 2–16. Degenerative and iatrogenic instability. Elderly woman with right foot drop. (**A**). L4 to L5 degenerative spondylolisthesis of about 30%. Note residual droplets of iophendylate from previous myelogram. (**B**). Axial CT shows pinching of central canal and neural foramina between posterior elements of L4 and body of L5. (**C**). A lateral radiograph 3 years after decompressive laminectomy shows the spondylolisthesis increased to about 50% and increased loss of disk space. (**D**). Pedicle screw and plate fixation with good reduction of spondylolisthesis.

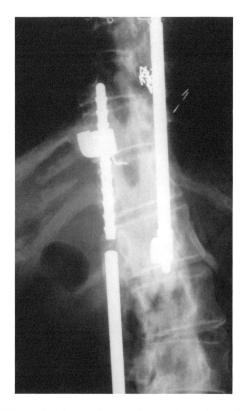

Figure 2–17.   Broken Harrington distraction rod.

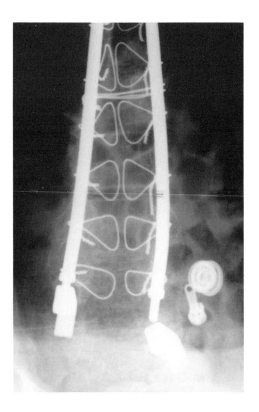

Figure 2–18.   Dislodged Harrington rod. Lower left hook has detached from rod.

degenerative clinical instability, but these cases are rarely mechanically unstable. That is, the deformity and fixed displacement is the primary cause of symptoms rather than decreased mechanical stiffness. An example is illustrated in Figure 2–16.

IATROGENIC INSTABILITY

Figure 2–16 is also an example of postoperative or iatrogenic instability. This patient's abnormal displacement (spondylolisthesis) as well as her neurological deficit were probably exacerbated by the decompressive laminectomy. The displacement was reduced partially, and she improved with transpedicular screw and plate fixation. Other examples of iatrogenic instability include failed fusion or pseudarthrosis (Fig. 2–10) and postlaminectomy kyphosis (swan-neck deformity) in the cervical spine. The latter entity is more common in the skeletally immature and in those where the integrity of the capsular ligaments has been violated.

IMAGING THE COMPLICATIONS OF SPINE FUSION

Radiography is the most useful technique for evaluating hardware complications after spine instrumentation. Broken rods, disconnected hardware components, or dislodged hooks are revealed easily with AP and lateral radiographs (Figs. 2–17 and 2–18).

Complications of cervical diskectomy and fusion include graft extrusion and, if symptomatic, graft collapse and pseudarthrosis. These complications can be evaluated with radiography, plain tomography, and CT. Infection is rare and is best evaluated with MRI. Dural tears may be diagnosed with CT myelography or with MRI if there is a pseudomeningocele. Although not really complications, residual extradural disease at the operated site or disk herniation developing at levels adjacent to the fusion are best evaluated with MRI.

As with the cervical spine, evaluation of dural tears and infection in the lumbar and thoracic spine is best accomplished with MRI. The presence of hardware may sometimes limit image quality, but if nonferromagnetic hardware has been used, the artifact should not be any more limiting than for CT. Residual or recurrent lumbar disk herniation can be diagnosed and differentiated reliably from postoperative scar with paramagnetic contrast enhanced MRI.

Pseudarthrosis following fusion may be considered a complication if it is symptom-producing. The plane of the pseudarthrosis is usually perpendicular to the axis of the spine, so plain tomography in coronal and parasagittal orientations is useful for confirming the lack of bony union (Fig. 2–10).

CONCLUSION

Radiography remains the core technique for evaluating most entities requiring spine fusion and instrumentation. Computed tomography, magnetic resonance imaging, conventional tomography, and CT myelography all have roles in confirming or adding to the information provided by radiography. Knowledge of the strengths and limitations of these techniques will allow complete and efficient diagnostic evaluation.

Acknowledgments.   The assistance of Susan Zollo and Jeanne Cholewa is gratefully acknowledged.

REFERENCES

1. Curry TS, Dowdey JE, Murry RC. *Christensen's Physics of Diagnostic Radiology.* 4th ed. Philadelphia, Pa: Lea and Febiger; 1990.
2. Hounsfield GN. Computerized axial transverse scanning (tomography). *Br J Radiol.* 1973;46:1016.
3. Mitchell DG, Burk DL, Jr, Vinitski S, Rifkin MD. The biophysical basis of tissue contrast in extracranial MR imaging. *AJR.* 1987;149:831–837.
4. Bradley WG. Flow phenomena in MR imaging. *AJR.* 1988;150:983–994.
5. Geisler FH, Mirvis SE, Zrebeet H, Joslyn JN. Titanium wire internal fixation for stabilization of injury of the cervical spine: clinical results and postoperative magnetic resonance imaging of the spinal cord. *Neurosurgery.* 1989;25:356–362.
6. Levit M, Benjamin V, Kricheff II. Potential misinterpretation of cervical spondylosis with cord compression caused by metallic artifacts in magnetic resonance imaging of the postoperative spine. *Neurosurgery.* 1990;27:126–130.
7. Volle E, Assheuer J, Hedde JP, Gustorf-Aeckerle R. Radicular avulsion resulting from spinal injury: assessment of diagnostic modalities. *Neuroradiology.* 1992;34:235–240.
8. Montalvo BM, Quencer RM, Brown, MD. Lumbar disc herniation and canal stenosis: value of intraoperative sonography in diagnosis and surgical management. *AJR.* 1990;154:821–830.
9. Mirvis SE, Geisler FH. Intraoperative sonography of cervical spinal cord injury: results in 30 patients. *AJR.* 1990;155:603–609.
10. Ashton-Miller JA, Schultz AB. Spine instability and segmental hypermobility biomechanics: a call for the definition and standard use of terms. *Sem Spine Surg.* 1991;3:136–148.
11. White AA, Panjabi MM. *Clinical Biomechanics of the Spine.* 2nd ed. Philadelphia, Pa: JB Lippincott; 1990.
12. Shaffer WO, Spratt KF, Weinstein J, Lehmann TR, Goel VK. The consistency and accuracy of roentgenograms for measuring sagittal translation in the lumbar vertebral motion segment: an experimental model. *Spine.* 1990;15:741–750.
13. Mirvis SE, Diaconis JN, Chirico PA, Reiner BI, Joslyn JN, Militello P. Protocol-driven radiologic evaluation of suspected cervical spine injury: efficacy study. *Radiology.* 1989;170:831–834.
14. Berquist TH. Imaging of adult cervical spine trauma. *Radiographics.* 1988;8:667–694.
15. Davis SJ, Teresi LM, Bradley WG, Jr, Ziemba MA, Bloze AE. Cervical spine hyperextension injuries. MR findings. *Radiology.* 1991;180:245–251.
16. Flanders AE, Schaefer DM, Doan HT, Mishkin MM, Gonzalez CF, Northrup BE. Acute cervical spine trauma: correlation of MR imaging findings with degree of neurologic deficit. *Radiology.* 1990;177:25–33.

17. Kulkarni MV, Bondurant FJ, Rose SL, Narayana PA. 1.5 Tesla magnetic resonance imaging of acute spinal trauma. *Radiographics.* 1988;8:1059–1082.

18. Gomori JM, Grossman RI, Yu-Ip C, Asakura T. NMR relaxation times of blood: dependence on field strength, oxidation state, and cell integrity. *JCAT.* 1987;11:684–690.

19. Rizzolo SJ, Piazza MR, Cotler JM, Balderston RA, Schaefer D, Flanders A. Intervertebral disk injury complicating cervical spine trauma. *Spine.* 1991;16:S187–S189.

20. Pratt ES, Green DA, Spengler DM. Herniated intervertebral disks associated with unstable spine injuries. *Spine.* 1990;15:662–666.

21. Harris JH, Edeiken-Monroe B. *The Radiology of Acute Cervical Spine Trauma.* 2nd ed. Baltimore, Md: Williams & Wilkins; 1987.

22. Denis F. The three column spine and its significance in the classification of acute throacolumbar spinal injuries. *Spine.* 1983;8:817–831.

23. Holdsworth FW. Fractures, dislocations and fracture-dislocations of the spine. *JBJS.* 1970;52A:1534–1551.

24. Effendi B, Roy D, Cornish B. Fractures of the ring of the axis. A classification based on the analysis of 131 cases. *JBJS.* 1981;63B:319–327.

25. McAfee PC, Yuan HA, Frederickson BE, Lubicky JP. The value of computed tomography in thoracolumbar fractures. An analysis of one hundred consecutive cases and a new classification. *JBJS.* 1983;65A:461–473.

26. Chance CQ. Note on a type of flexion fracture of the spine. *Br J Radiol.* 1948;21:452.

27. LaRocca H, Macnab I. Value of preemployment radiographic assessment of the lumbar spine. *Ind Med Surg.* 1970;39:31–36.

28. Lehmann TR, Spratt KF, Tozzi JE, et al. Long term follow-up of lower lumbar spine fusion patients. *Spine.* 1987;12:97–104.

3 Biomechanics of the Cervical Spine

Vijay K. Goel, Ph.D., John D. Clausen, B.S., Timothy C. Ryken, M.D., Vincent C. Traynelis, M.D.

INTRODUCTION

The cervical spine is a key component of body mechanics. Not only does it act as a centerpoint for head and upper-body kinematics, but it also serves to protect the pathway for all lower-body communication. Trauma, disease, and the aging process can interfere with the spine's ability to perform these important functions. It is estimated that one out of every two persons will have an attack of severe neck pain sometime during his or her life, and in more than 25% of these cases the pain will be recurrent.[1] Neck pain is often due to muscle or ligament problems, but more serious bone and neural involvement occurs frequently as well. Approximately 100 000 cervical fractures and fracture dislocations occur yearly, and the spinal cord is injured in over half of these cases. Despite the high numbers, these estimates are considered low because many fatal cervical spine injuries are never diagnosed.[1] Neck injuries frequently cause a significant and permanent decrease in quality of life; indeed, injuries of the cervical spine are among the most common causes of severe disability following trauma. The peak incidence of cervical spine injury occurs in adolescence and young adulthood, resulting in a tremendous loss of productivity to society.[2] Wiesel et al showed that although neck cases were only 20% as frequent as low-back cases, the amount of lost time and light-duty time per case was substantially longer for the neck patients, sometimes up to twice that of the lower back.[2] Thus, neck-related disorders are of significant magnitude to warrant multidisciplinary investigations, including thorough biomechanical evaluation of the cervical spine. An understanding of the biomechanics of the cervical spine in conjunction with other related fields not only may increase industrial productivity, but more importantly could significantly improve the quality of life for patients with cervical spine problems.

This chapter outlines the issues of spinal instability that form the basis for a properly designed biomechanical study. Thereafter the biomechanical literature pertaining to the kinematics of the intact/normal, injured, and stabilized ligamentous cervical spine is reviewed. The limitations of the in vitro biomechanical data are presented as a foundation for future research directions. A summary of recent initiatives from our group is presented in the concluding section.

SPINAL INSTABILITY

The human cervical spine has seven vertebrae (C1 to C7) stacked one above the other with the intervertebral disks in between at each level except between C1 and C2. The relative motion between the vertebrae is controlled by the muscles but governed by the ligaments, facets, and disks. The literature is full of controversy as to what constitutes instability across a motion segment, and numerous general definitions of spinal instability have been proposed. Kirkaldy-Willis and Farfan define instability as a precarious clinical status in which a small perturbation of the spinal joint can result in a catastrophic change in the patient's symptoms (ie, pain, ability to function, etc).[3] Nachemson stated that the typical symptoms of segmental instability are not yet defined, but abnormal motion is certainly one of the signs.[4] Lee stated that "in the healthy vertebral segment, horizontal translation does not normally take place. The presence of horizontal translation in the lumbar segment has been claimed to be one of the first signs of disk degeneration."[5] White and Panjabi define the term *clinical instability* as "the loss of the ability of the spine under physiologic loads to maintain relationships between vertebrae in such a way that there is neither damage nor subsequent irritation to the spinal cord or nerve roots and, in addition, there is no development of incapacitating deformity or pain due to structural changes."[6]

Based on these concepts, the underlying biomechanical principle for the term *instability* can be defined. An abnormal motion across a motion segment may activate nociceptors that trigger pain stimuli to the brain. Abnormal motion is most likely to occur as a result of the changes in the spinal structures of a motion segment. Fusion of the spine with or without an internal fixation device to restore stability is indicated in primary or iatrogenic instability.

BIOMECHANICS OF THE CERVICAL SPINE

Determining whether a spine is stable is extremely difficult. Knowledge of normal kinematics (load-displacement characteristics) of the cervical spine in various loading modalities and the changes that occur after injury and/or surgical procedures is necessary to gain an understanding of spinal stability and instability. Both in vivo investigations on humans and animals and in vitro investigations of ligamentous spinal segments have been undertaken to accumulate biomechanical data of clinical significance. The primary advantages of the in vitro studies are that these can be performed under controlled conditions and provide a comparative database for a surgeon's interpretation and decision making.

Biomechanical Tests: Types, Specimen Preparation, and Testing Protocols

There are three basic biomechanical tests: stability, strength, and fatigue.[7,8] Stability testing involves applying a physiological load on the motion segment (one or more than one) and measuring the resultant displacement. Physiological loading represents the load a spine would experience during normal activity. Determination of stability may involve testing of normal, traumatized/injured, and stabilized cervical spines. Physiological loads do not produce damage to the spinal tissue and produce physiological vertebral movements. The loads applied to produce physiological movements should create pure moments about and forces collinear to a principal axis. This type of testing is generally done on ligamentous cervical spines void of gross musculature. Determination of stability or instability is accomplished by comparing the motion of the spine before and after the spine is injured or injured and stabilized. Stability testing forms one basis for determining the effectiveness of a device or procedure.

Strength testing can be carried out on the cervical spine with or without a surgical construct. Strength tests have been performed on the cervical spine to determine the load at which failure occurs. Failure can be defined as the point at which the spine exhibits nonphysiological displacement or motion, or as the complete disruption of a motion segment.

The goal of fatigue (or cyclic) testing is to determine the effectiveness of a surgical construct over a period of time. This can be accomplished using a servo-hydraulic materials testing machine (MTS) with which the spine can be loaded in a cyclic manner to produce the motion desired, such as flexion/extension. Spinal stability can be reassessed following cyclic loading as just described. The results can be compared to the stability of the intact spine and to the stability present immediately after fixation. The number of cycles and the rate of application are extremely important. If the number of cycles is too low, the effect of prolonged fatigue may not be determined. Most importantly, the rate of application cannot be too fast or too slow. Choosing inappropriate rates may adversely affect the data. Throughout all three of these tests (stability, strength, and fatigue), the specimen must be allowed to move freely in response to loading. Any restriction in normal motion produces inaccurate results.

Testing standards for spinal motion segments do not exist, as they do for materials and other mechanical structures. The methods used for biomechanical evaluation are typically determined by the data that are needed to characterize

motion sufficiently as described by the goals of each individual study. Most studies deal with motion and forces in at least two dimensions, typically the sagittal plane. Three-dimensional description of motion fully describes the characteristics of a motion segment. The technique used by the authors is described next as an example to illustrate this point.[9]

For in vitro biomechanical studies, fresh ligamentous spine specimens (one or multiple segments) are prepared by securing the inferiormost end to a testing rig and applying clinically relevant loads at the superiormost end. Clinically relevant loads are those that create physiological flexion, extension, lateral bending, or axial rotation. Although different techniques may be used to apply flexion, extension, and axial rotation loads, the majority of researchers agree that the most physiologically correct method of producing such motions is by a pure moment utilizing a fixture that will allow the full 6 degrees of freedom for the vertebra in response to the applied moment.[7,8] The three-dimensional motion of a vertebra, in response to an applied load with respect to the fixed vertebra, can be described in terms of six components: three rotations about and three translations of a point on the vertebra along the three Cartesian coordinate axes. The six motion components, flexion/extension rotation (R_X), axial rotation (R_Y), lateral bending rotation (R_Z), and translation along each axis (T_{XH}, T_{YH}, and T_{ZH}), are illustrated in Figure 3–1. A number of elegant techniques have been developed to apply loads and measure the resulting motion components, the first of which was developed by Panjabi et al.[10] Subsequent studies and their techniques are described in the literature.[8] In most of these studies, the specimen is allowed to undergo unrestrained motion. The major component of motion occurs in the direction implied by the applied load vector; as a result, some of the six motion components (normally one rotation and one translation) are preferentially larger than the others. For example, in response to pure moment flexion/extension loading, the flexion/extension rotation is the major rotational component of the motion. The remaining components are termed the coupled motions and are usually of lower magnitude.

The three-dimensional motion of the specimen can be monitored using the Selspot II system (Inovision Systems, Warren, Mich). This device is an optoelectronic system based on the principles of stereophotogrammetry. A set of three infrared light-emitting diodes (LEDs) is rigidly fixed to each of the vertebral bodies to serve as definable points. The LEDs, under the control of an LED control unit, are fired sequentially. The emitted light is detected by two infrared cameras and translated into x and y voltage data. Through proper calibration, the spatial position of an LED can be defined in terms of its x and y voltage data.

This protocol can be used to determine the load-displacement characteristics of single- or multilevel cervical motion segments. The data generated from single motion segment studies need to be viewed carefully and not extrapolated

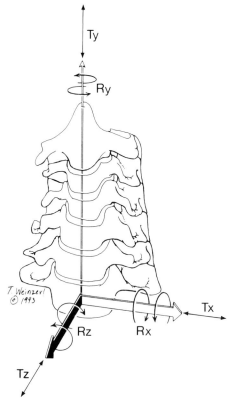

Figure 3–1. Schematic of Cartesian coordinate axes.

beyond what they were intended to show. When evaluating surgical techniques that span more than one motion segment, multilevel specimens are required.[12] Multilevel studies have the advantage of providing a more objective assessment of the effects a surgical procedure has on the motion behavior of not only the involved vertebrae but adjacent vertebrae as well.[12–15]

Occipitoatlantoaxial Complex Motion Data

Normal motion of the cervical spine is difficult to determine with any degree of reproducibility. The size, weight, anatomy, amount of degeneration, bone quality, and age of each person and specimen vary significantly. Nonetheless, some understanding of physiological motion is necessary to determine if abnormal motion is present. Knowledge of load-displacement behavior of normal spines helps improve clinical judgment regarding stability.[16–18] The presence of preload is known to alter the load-displacement characteristics of the spine. Increasing preload alters the force required to create a given displacement. The issue of preload due to head weight and muscle contraction tends to make in vitro models overestimate true in vivo motion to an applied load.[9,12,13,19] Previous investigators have attempted to characterize normal motion in several ways. The majority describe the relative motion of each vertebra with respect to the motion of the spine as a whole. Normalizing data in this manner makes the data more applicable to spines of all sizes and relevant for different load magnitudes. Alternatively, motion may be described as an absolute number; however, this method is highly dependent on the maximum load applied and the specimen used.

Panjabi et al[20] were able to average the three-dimensional motion characteristics of 10 fresh cadaveric whole cervical spines (occiput to C7) with mean age and disk degeneration of 46.7 years (range 29 to 59) and 3.1 (range 2 to 4), respectively. Pure moments were applied (maximum of 1.5 Nm) producing flexion, extension, left and right lateral bending, and left and right axial rotation. The motion of each vertebra was monitored using stereophotogrammetry and analyzed using the principles of rigid body kinematics.

When this study is compared to other recent studies, the results are in relative agreement (Tables 3–1 and 3–2) with the following exceptions. Penning and Wilmink showed less axial rotation across the occipitoatlanto complex than other investigators.[21] The maximum moment applied to the specimens determines, in part, the amount of rotation obtained. For example, Panjabi et al[20] applied 1.5 Nm maximum load to obtain these values, whereas Goel et al[12] applied maximum moments of 0.3 Nm. Goel et al[12] determined that the ratio of extension to flexion in the occipitoatlanto complex was 2.5:1. In this study, relatively small loads were all that was necessary to create motion across the occipitoatlantoaxial complex. Eighty-five to ninety percent of all axial rotation in the occipitoatlantoaxial complex comes from the atlantoaxial complex. There is little lateral bending across the craniovertebral junction, and the occipitoatlantal and atlantoaxial motion segments contribute almost equally to this motion.[12,20]

Penning and Wilmink found that the skull rotated axially an average 72.2° with respect to the first thoracic vertebra, and the atlantoaxial complex accounted for 56% of this rotation.[21] Goel et al,[22] in a study of 12 occipitoatlantoaxial specimens, determined that the average values for axial rotation and torque at the point of maximum resistance were 68.1° and 13.6 Nm, respectively. The specimens offered minimal resistance to axial rotations up to 21° across the complex. They also observed that the value of axial rotation at which complete bilateral rotary dislocation occurred was approximately the point of maximal resistance.

The contribution of stabilization by the alar ligament of the upper cervical spine is of particular interest when evaluating the effects of trauma. The rotation-limiting ability of the alar ligament was investigated by Dvorak et al[23] using 12 cervical spines. A mean increase of 10.8° or 30% divided equally between the occipitoatlantal and atlantoaxial complexes in axial rotation was observed in response to an alar lesion on the opposite side. Dvorak et al[24] verified their laboratory findings with a clinical study of 9 healthy adults and 43 patients with cervical spine instability and concluded that axial rotation of the occipitoatlantoaxial complex can increase after trauma-induced lesions of the alar ligaments.

Grob et al[25] determined the three-dimensional motions of 10 cervical vertebrae (0 to C3) in response to four different posterior atlantoaxial fixation techniques: (1) wire fixation with one median graft (Gallie type)[26]; (2) wire fixation with two bilateral grafts (Brooks type)[27]; (3) transarticular screw fixation (Magerl)[28]; and (4) two bilateral posterior clamps

Table 3–1. C0 to C1 Motion Results Compiled from Several Resources.

OCCIPITOATLANTO COMPLEX (C0-C1)	FLEXION/ EXTENSION	LATERAL BENDING	AXIAL ROTATION	TYPE OF STUDY	TYPE OF LOADING
Dvorak et al (1985)[73]	—	—	5.2	In vivo (CT)	Max. rotation
Dvorak et al (1987)[24]	—	—	4.0	In vivo (CT)	Max. rotation
Penning and Wilmink (1987)[21]	—	—	1.0	In vivo (CT)	Max. rotation
Panjabi et al (1988)[20]	3.5/21.0	5.5	7.2	In vitro	1.5 Nm
Goel et al (1988)[12]	6.5/16.5	3.4	2.4	In vitro	0.3 Nm

Table 3–2. C1 to C2 Motion Results Compiled from Several Resources.

ATLANTOAXIAL COMPLEX (C1-C2)	FLEXION/ EXTENSION	LATERAL BENDING	AXIAL ROTATION	TYPE OF STUDY	TYPE OF LOADING
Dvorak et al (1985)[73]	—	—	32.2	In vivo (CT)	Max. rotation
Dvorak et al (1987)[24]	—	—	43.1	In vivo (CT)	Max. rotation
Penning and Wilmink (1987)[21]	—	—	40.5	In vivo (CT)	Max. rotation
Panjabi et al (1988)[20]	11.5/10.9	6.7	38.9	In vitro	1.5 Nm
Goel et al (1988)[12]	4.9/5.2	4.2	23.3	In vitro	0.3 Nm

(Halifax clamps, American Medical Electronics, Inc., Richardson, Tex). The induced injury consisted of severe soft-tissue injury with transection of the alar, transverse, and capsular ligaments. Loads were applied in the form of pure moments (maximum moment of 1.5 Nm) to produce flexion, extension, lateral bending, and axial rotation. The authors concluded that the Gallie-type fixation was the least stable, allowing significantly greater motion than the other types. In lateral bending and axial rotation, the Magerl C1 to C2 screw technique provided the most stability. The Halifax clamp, Brooks fixation, and Magerl technique were approximately equal in flexion and extension. The Magerl technique allowed significantly less translation than the Gallie procedure. Overall, the Gallie technique was least effective in stabilizing the injured atlantoaxial complex, whereas the Brooks fusion, the Halifax clamp, and the Magerl technique produced comparable biomechanical results. Similar results were obtained by Harvell et al,[29] who compared a simple midline fusion with the Brooks and Gallie techniques. Hanson et al[30] tested the Gallie and Magerl techniques and essentially agreed with the conclusions of Grob et al[25]; however, when the advantages and disadvantages were considered by the authors, they concluded that the Magerl technique was superior. Montesano et al[31] recommended that the Magerl technique not be used unless standard procedures have failed or cannot be performed because of the extensive dissection that this technique requires.

Lower Cervical Motion Data

There have been several studies on the normal motion of the subaxial cervical spine. Tables 3–3 to 3–7 list some of these studies and their results. In addition, numerous studies have been performed to determine the effectiveness of fixation devices or surgical constructs that reported the motion of the lower cervical spine in its intact state. The data for complex loads are described in the following paragraphs.

Coupled motions in the cervical spine due to the complex bony architecture always occur in conjunction with a primary motion. Panjabi et al[32] studied 18 motion segments from four cervical spines (C2 to T1) and found that for anterior and posterior shear loading, primary motions were in the direction of the load (1.6 mm and 1.9 mm, respectively), and the major coupled motions were flexion and extension (3.6° and 6.3°, respectively). The primary motions with right and left lateral shear loading were translations laterally (1.4 mm and 1.6 mm, respectively) with the major coupled motions being flexion and extension (2.0° and 2.8°, respectively) and right and left lateral bending (1.4° and 1.9°, respectively).

The contributions of each component to the overall motion of a motion segment or segments can be valuable in determining whether stability has been compromised. Cervical spine stability is maintained primarily by ligaments joining adjacent vertebrae. Ligaments and other soft tissues appear invisible on roentgenograms, making it difficult to detect ligamentous injury. Ligamentous injury can be inferred by determining abnormal spacing between vertebrae. Knowing the role of each component provides a basis for determining what structures have been compromised and to what degree.

Panjabi et al[33] determined the sagittal displacement and rotation of 17 cervical motion segments in response to a combined load of shear and flexion/extension. The motion segments tested were C2 to C3, C4 to C5, and C6 to C7. Motion was measured in response to anterior shear/flexion as a function of transection of components approached posteriorly. The study was repeated for posterior shear/extension as a function of transection of components approached anteriorly. After each transection, 25% of the body weight was applied as described previously. When all components were intact, no motion segment experienced displacements greater than 2.7 mm or rotations greater than 11°. Failure

Table 3–3. C2 to C3 Motion Results Compiled from Several Resources.

MOTION SEGMENT C2-C3	FLEXION/ EXTENSION	LATERAL BENDING	AXIAL ROTATION	TYPE OF STUDY	TYPE OF LOADING
Penning and Wilmink (1987)[21]	—	—	3.0	In vivo (CT)	Max. rotation
Penning (1978)[74]	12	—	—	In vivo (x-ray)	Max. rotation
White and Panjabi (1978)[75]	8	10	9	Review	Review

Table 3–4. C3 to C4 Motion Results Compiled from Several Resources.

MOTION SEGMENT C3-C4	FLEXION/ EXTENSION	LATERAL BENDING	AXIAL ROTATION	TYPE OF STUDY	TYPE OF LOADING
Penning and Wilmink (1987)[21]	6.5	—	—	In vivo (CT)	Max. rotation
Penning (1978)[74]	18	—	—	In vivo (x-ray)	Max. rotation
Goel et al (1988)[40]	3.5/2.9	3.2	2.3	In vitro	0.3 Nm
White and Panjabi (1978)[75]	13	11	11	Review	Review

Table 3–5. C4 to C5 Motion Results Compiled from Several Resources.

MOTION SEGMENT C4-C5	FLEXION/ EXTENSION	LATERAL BENDING	AXIAL ROTATION	TYPE OF STUDY	TYPE OF LOADING
Penning and Wilmink (1987)[21]	6.8	—	—	In vivo (CT)	Max. rotation
Penning (1978)[74]	20	—	—	In vivo (x-ray)	Max. rotation
Goel et al (1984)[13]	5.9/1.4	2.7	1.8	In vitro	0.3 Nm
	3.7/2.8	3.0	2.5	In vitro	0.45 Nm
White and Panjabi (1978)[75]	12	11	12	Review	Review

Table 3–6. C5 to C6 Motion Results Compiled from Several Resources.

MOTION SEGMENT C5-C6	FLEXION/ EXTENSION	LATERAL BENDING	AXIAL ROTATION	TYPE OF STUDY	TYPE OF LOADING
Penning and Wilmink (1987)[21]	6.9	—	—	In vivo (CT)	Max. rotation
Penning (1978)[74]	20	—	—	In vivo (x-ray)	Max. rotation
Goel et al (1984)[13]	8.7/1.4	2.3	1.4	In vitro	0.3 Nm
White and Panjabi (1978)[75]	17	8	10	Review	Review

Table 3–7. C6 to C7 Motion Results Compiled from Several Resources.

MOTION SEGMENT C6-C7	FLEXION/ EXTENSION	LATERAL BENDING	AXIAL ROTATION	TYPE OF STUDY	TYPE OF LOADING
Penning and Wilmink (1987)[21]	5.4	—	—	In vivo (CT)	Max. rotation
Penning (1978)[74]	15	—	—	In vivo (x-ray)	Max. rotation
Goel et al (1988)[40]	2.9/2.8	1.8	1.7	In vitro	0.3 Nm
White and Panjabi (1978)[75]	16	7	9	Review	Review

resulted in anterior shear, with transection of components approached anteriorly when the ligamentum flavum was cut. With posterior shear load and transection of components anteiorly, failure resulted when all the anterior ligaments were transected. Failure resulted in anterior shear, with transection of components approached posteriorly when the posterior longitudinal ligament was cut. With posterior shear load and transection of components anteriorly, failure resulted when all the components were transected except the anterior longitudinal ligament.

A similar test was performed by Moroney et al[34] in which the three-dimensional motion of 35 fresh adult cervical spine motion segments (C2 to C3, C3 to C4, C4 to C5, C5 to C6, C6 to C7, and C7 to T1 with a mean disk grade of 2.5) was measured. Pure moments were applied through a loading frame attached to the superior vertebra producing flexion, extension, right and left lateral bending, and right and left axial rotation. Anterior and posterior shear was created in a manner that created zero moments about the center of the intervertebral disk. A preload of 49 N was applied to the specimens to simulate the in vivo weight of the head. The authors concluded that cervical motion as tested was not dependent on disk level. Upon removal of the posterior elements, cervical stiffness decreased as much as 50% in all motions compared to the intact specimen. Motion segments with severely degenerated disks were 50% less stiff in compression and 300% more stiff in shear when compared to less-degenerated motion segments. Specimens with bony fusion of the facet joints were significantly stiffer in all loading modalities than those without fusion.

In a study by Goel et al,[13] the three-dimensional load-displacement motion of C4 to C5 and C5 to C6 as a function of transection of C5 to C6 components was determined. Six specimens (C2 to T2) were loaded with pure moments (maximum 0.3 Nm) producing flexion, extension, right and left lateral bending, and right and left axial rotation. Transection was carried out posteriorly, starting with the supraspinous and interspinous ligaments followed by the ligamentum flavum and the capsular ligaments. The C5 to C6 motion segment (injured level) showed a significant increase of motion in extension, lateral bending, and axial rotation with the transection of the capsular ligaments. A significant increase in flexion resulted when the ligamentum flavum was transected. The C4 to C5 motion segment (level above the injured level) did not show a significant increase in motion with extension or axial rotation loading. A significant increase in flexion resulted when the supraspinous ligament was transected, and lateral bending significantly increased with transection of the capsular ligaments. This study also demonstrated increased motion in the segment immediately superior to the level of injury with flexion and lateral bending loading.

In vitro studies to determine the feasibility of the stretch test were carried out by Panjabi et al.[35] Four cervical spines (C1 to T1), ages 25 to 29, were loaded in axial tension in increments of 5 kg to a maximum of one third of the specimen's body weight. Motion segments C2 to C3 through C5 to C6 were tested with anterior-posterior transection and C2 to C3 through C6 to C7 with posterior-anterior transection. The authors concluded that the intact cervical spine goes into flexion under axial tension. Anterior transection produced extension with an increase in anterior displacement and a decrease in posterior displacement. Posterior transection produced the opposite results. Anterior injuries creating displacements of 3.3 mm at the disk space (with a force equal to one third of body weight) and extension changes of approximately 3.8° were felt to be precursors to failure. Likewise, posterior injuries resulting in 27-mm separation at the tips of the spinous process and an angular increase of 30° with loading were felt to be unstable. This work supports the concept that spinal failure results from transection of either all the anterior elements or all the posterior plus at least two additional elements. (Anterior elements were defined as the posterior longitudinal ligaments and all ligaments anterior to it, and posterior ligaments were defined as all ligaments posterior to the posterior longitudinal ligament.)

A major path of loading in the cervical spine is through the vertebral bodies, which are separated by the intervertebral disk. The role of the cervical intervertebral disk has received little attention. In vivo injuries result in disk degeneration and may produce osteophytes, ankylosed vertebrae, and changes in the apophyseal joints.[36] Total discectomy is of interest in investigation of the role of the intervertebral disk in cervical motion. Schulte et al[37] reported a significant increase in motion with 10 specimens (C2 to T2) following C5 to C6 discectomy. Motion between C5 and C6 increased in flexion (66.6%), extension (69.5%), lateral bending (41.4%), and axial rotation (37.9%). Previous studies by Martins[38] and Wilson and Campbell[39] were unable to detect increases in motion roentgenographically, and the spines were deemed functionally stable.

Cervical vertebral laminae join the spinous process to the vertebral body, supplying a path by which loads may be transmitted. Laminectomies result in the removal of part of this loading path and the attachment points for the ligamentum flavum, interspinous ligament, and the supraspinous ligament. It is not surprising that total laminectomy results in significant modifications in the motion characteristics of the cervical spine. Goel et al[40] removed the lamina of nine multisegmental cervical spines (C2 to T2) at the level of C5 and C6. In response to pure moments (maximum of 0.3 Nm) of flexion/extension, an increase in motion of about 10% was observed. The use of older spines significantly decreased the mean percent increase in motion. Specimens were tested intact in flexion, extension, left and right lateral bending, and left and right axial rotation produced by pure moments applied in four equal steps with a maximum of 0.3 Nm. A total laminectomy of C5 was performed, and the load tests were repeated. The supraspinous, interspinous, and flavum ligaments were cut between C4 to C5 and C5 to C6 motion segments, and the vertebral arches were removed. The testing was resumed after inducing injury at C6 in a similar fashion. The specimens were stabilized using a facet wiring construct across the C4 to C7 segment and then tested a final time. The authors concluded that facet wiring is an effective technique to stabilize this type of injured spine. A significant decrease in motion at the injured levels was seen (−80%, P < .02) compared with the motion of the intact spine, and motion of the adjacent segments was not altered.

Facet joints play an integral part in the biomechanical stability of the cervical spine. Total bilateral and unilateral facetectomy significantly decreases the strength of a motion segment in compression flexion. Cusick et al[41] showed, with 12 specimens comprised of C3 to C4 and C6 to C7 motion segments (mean age 71.7, range 65 to 84 years), that unilateral and bilateral facetectomy decreased compression-flexion strength by 31.6% and 53.1%, respectively. Facetectomy resulted in an anterior shift of the instantaneous axis of rotation (IAR), thereby resulting in increased compression of the vertebral body and disk. This work confirmed the findings of Raynor et al,[42] who found that up to a 50% bilateral facetectomy did not significantly decrease shear strength; however, with a 75% bilateral facetectomy, a significant decrease in shear strength was noted. These studies suggest that sheer strength is decreased with total bilateral facetectomies.

In a subsequent study, Raynor et al[43] investigated the role of facet joints in three dimensions and determined that strength and motion are altered after a 50% bilateral facetectomy. Seven specimens comprised of C3 to C4 and C6 to C7 motion segments were loaded with 89 N about the three principal axes with torsion equal to 3.4 Nm. The coupled motions and the primary rotations and displacements were not significantly affected, with the following exceptions: Motion was decreased in lateral bending and lateral translation, and corresponding primary loading modalities and axial displacements were increased in response to axial tension.

Cusick et al[41] investigated two stabilization techniques for bilateral facet disruption: facet-to-facet and facet-to-spinous process fixation. Facet-to-facet fixation was accomplished by drilling holes through the inferior facet of the motion segment and the lower facet segment, securing the joint with either 20-gauge stainless steel or 24-gauge braided wire. Facet-to-spinous process fixation utilized the same wire passed through the inferior facet and looped about the spinous process or the inferior vertebra. Both of the fixation techniques increased the strength of the motion segment with respect to the injured strength. Although the strength was increased in the stabilized specimens, it was not restored to the levels of the intact specimens. The authors concluded that the two stabilization techniques gave essentially the same levels of restoration. Excessive motion was noted, suggesting that wire fatigue may be a factor in fusion failure.

The effects of interspinous wiring and acrylic cement (polymethylmethacrylate [PMMA]) on the motion behavior of C5 to C6 and adjacent segments after injury were determined by Goel et al.[13] The load-displacement data for six cervical spines (C2 to T2) were determined for flexion, extension, left and right lateral bending, and left and right axial rotation as produced by pure moments with a maximum of 0.3 Nm. The testing procedure was performed on the intact specimen and after sequential injuries and stabilization procedures: transection of the supraspinous and interspinous ligaments, ligamentum flavum, and capsular ligaments, and interspinous wiring as per the Rogers technique[44] with the application of PMMA. Holes were drilled in the laminae of C5, C6, and C7 using a drill bit of $1/_8$-in diameter. The wires were passed through the holes between C5 and C6, C6 and C7, and between C5 and C7 and twisted to themselves tightly, and finally a bolus of acrylic cement was placed, incorporating the interspinous wires to stabilize further the specimen at the injured level. Following analysis of the three-dimensional load-displacement data for each vertebra, it was concluded that this stabilization technique was effective in restoring stability across the injured segment. The use of interspinous wiring did not significantly increase the motion at the segment immediately superior (C4 to C5) to the stabilized levels when compared to injury

of the capsular ligament, except in extension. The higher the tension in the wires of the interspinous wiring, the greater the compensation for the damage produced by the transection of the capsular ligaments. The use of PMMA in conjunction with interspinous wiring significantly reduced the relative motion at the motion segment immediately superior (C4 to C5) to the stabilized levels.

Two methods of screw placement for attaching posterior plates to the cervical spine after distractive flexion injuries were studied by Montesano et al.[31] With technique I, the screw was placed in a straight sagittal direction and angled laterally 10 to 20°. Technique II involved placing the screws in a cephalad direction with the screw parallel to the facet joint and angled outward 30 to 40°. Based on the data from six spine tests, technique II was found to be biomechanically superior. The first technique failed by screw pullout whereas the second technique had such a strong screw purchase that failure occurred through the plate. The results may be due in part to the fact that the longer screws used in technique II may have achieved bicortical fixation more often than the shorter screws used in technique I. Similar methods of screw placement have been used clinically with satisfactory results.[45–47]

A biomechanical comparison of posterior fusion techniques was studied by Gill et al[48] in seven cervical spines (C2 to C7). Four types of posterior constructs were tested: (1) modified Rogers interspinous wiring with 18-gauge wire, (2) Halifax laminar clamps, (3) bilateral posterolateral one-third tubular plates secured with unicortical screws, and (4) bilateral posterolateral one-third tubular plates secured with bicortical screws. A prescribed displacement was given to the motion segments to simulate flexion and extension, and the resultant anterior displacement was measured. The authors concluded that the two-hole one-third tubular plates using bicortical screws had the highest mean stiffness, whereas the same plates with unicortical screws showed consistently lower stiffness. The Halifax clamps or interspinous wiring were nearly as stiff as those segments instrumented with plates and cortical screws. There was, however, no statistical difference between any of the fixation techniques.

Fusion of facets through spine-plate application can be detrimental to the stability of the cervical spine under certain conditions. When more than 75% of the facet is destroyed bilaterally, the motion segment suffers a severe decrease in strength.[42] Raynor et al[49] tested the shear of the Roy-Camille plate (Benoist-Girard et Compagnie, Bagneux, France) secured with 3.5-mm-diameter, 16-mm-long screws using specimens in which approximately 50% of the facets were removed bilaterally. The plates were fastened to each facet by drilling a 2.5-mm hole through the center of the remaining inferosuperior facet complex and the facet joint below. The authors concluded that in a severely damaged facet, the drill hole necessary for the screw insertion further weakens the remaining bone, which then fractures easily under stress. They recommended careful evaluation in selecting the treatment modality when facet destruction is present.

The kinematics of the 10 cervical spines (C2 to T2) for the intact spine, after discectomy at the C5 to C6 level, following insertion of a bone graft in the intervertebral space and following the application of an anterior metal plate, was studied by Schulte et al.[37] The load-deformation data were acquired by a Selspot II system, and the motions produced (flexion, extension, left and right lateral bending, and left and right axial rotation) were applied in four equal steps with pure moments up to a maximum of 0.3 Nm. The data showed an immediate increase in motion at the injured level of approximately 70% compared to the intact specimen. Changes in motion adjacent to the stabilized level were insignificant for all states of loading. It was found that use of the anterior metal plate in addition to the bone graft at the injured level provided significant stabilization in all load modalities.

Montesano et al[31] compared anterior cervical plates and Rogers's wiring method after complete transection of all posterior ligaments, including the posterior longitudinal ligament and the intervertebral disk, to allow bilateral facet dislocation. Using five spines (C2 to C7) and measuring the relative anteroposterior translation as well as flexion/extension angulation, the authors concluded that Rogers's wiring method provided more stability than anterior plating. Furthermore, they concluded that in distraction-flexion injuries, anterior plate fixation should not be used alone but should be used in conjunction with posterior instrumentation or rigid external immobilization.

Ulrich et al examined various stabilization procedures applied to the C5 to C6 segment and concluded that bicortical anterior H-plate fixation for complete "discoligamentous" instability required postoperative external immobilization to prevent abnormal flexion.[50,51] There was, however, no statistical difference in the stability provided by anterior fixation as compared to posterior constructs in their model.

The effectiveness of seven separate posterior and anterior constructs on simulated distractive-flexion injuries of the C5 to C6 motion segment was investigated by Coe et al.[52] Six human cadaveric cervical spines were tested with complete disruption of the supraspinous and interspinous ligaments, ligamentum flavum, posterior longitudinal ligament, and facet joint capsules. There was sufficient disruption of the intervertebral disk to allow bilateral C5 to C6 facet dislocation. The specimens were mounted in the testing frame so that the C5 to C6 motion segment was the only movable joint. The constructs were applied and tested in the following order: First the intact spine was tested, followed by testing of sublaminar wire (20-gauge stainless steel wire) construct (after creation of the distractive-flexion lesion at the C5 to C6 level); next the Rogers's wiring (using 20-gauge stainless steel wire) was tested, followed by the Bohlman triple wiring using human corticocancellous bone graft struts wired in with 22-gauge stainless steel wire after tethering the spinous processes with the 20-gauge wires; then the Roy-Camille plate construct was tested, after which AO hook plates (Synthes Spine, Paoli, Pa) were applied and tested; then the Caspar anterior plate (Aesculap, Inc., South San Francisco, Calif) was applied and the AO hook plate left in place (with all screws checked for tightness and retightened as necessary); and finally the AO hook plate was removed and the Caspar anterior plate alone was tested. Each of the constructs was tested in axial compression, axial rotation, flexion, and extension followed by a fatigue test of 100 cycles.

From this work, Coe et al concluded that reconstruction with the anterior Caspar plate provided less stiffness than the other constructs and the intact spine. Posterior strain values were greater for the anterior Caspar plate for both flexion and axial loading tests. There were no significant differences in the static or cyclic loading between the posterior plating and wiring techniques, however, the posterior plating technique was stiffer in torsion. There was no biomechanical advantage to sublaminar wiring over the interspinous techniques. The Roy-Camille plate and AO hook plate created no significant biomechanical increase in stability over the traditional posterior wiring techniques. The authors, based on their study, recommended the Bohlman triple-wiring technique for most distractive flexion injuries. In contrast, Aebi et al[53] reviewed patients with posterior element damage that had anterior plating procedures and found the anterior approach and plating procedure to be atraumatic and clinically effective. Aebi et al criticized Coe et al for failure to place a bone graft, which, they felt, adversely affected the results. The clinical study of Aebi et al was supported by Ripa et al[54] in a separate review of 92 patients.

Traynelis et al simulated a C5 teardrop fracture with posterior ligamentous instability in human cadaveric spines.[55] Using this model, the immediate biomechanical stability of anterior cervical plating from C4 to C6 was compared to the stability provided by a posterior wiring construct over the same levels. Stability was tested in six modes of motion: flexion, extension, right and left axial rotation, and right and left lateral bending. The injured/plate-stabilized spines were more stable than the intact specimens in all modes of testing, and the injured/posterior wired specimens were more stable than the intact spines in axial rotation and flexion. The injured/plate stabilized specimens were not as stable as the intact specimens in the lateral bending or extension testing modes. The injured/stabilized data were normalized with respect to the motion of the intact spines and compared using repeated measures of analysis of variance (ANOVA). ANOVA results indicated that anterior plating provided significantly more stability in extension and lateral bending than did posterior wiring in this model. The plate was more stable than the posterior construct in flexion loading, although the difference was not statistically significant. The two constructs provided similar stability in axial rotation.

IN VIVO MOTION ANALYSIS

In the past, finding an effective way to evaluate cervical spine mechanics in vivo has presented almost as much of a challenge as creating the perfect arthrodesis technique. Conventional radiography has been relied on to provide a two-dimensional representation of a three-dimensional problem. This has greatly limited the accuracy of follow-up assessments. Weinstein et al stated that "surgeons cannot be expected to improve with experience when their tools (roentgenograms) do not allow accurate evaluation of their performance. However, significant improvement in success rate can be expected when accurate evaluation is provided."[56] Dynamic (flexion-extension) lateral radiographs are often used to assess the relative motion across fused and adjacent levels. Based on the magnitude of the relative motions, decisions regarding bone-graft healing are made. Because the displacements in an actual spine are three-dimensional and their quantification from plain radiographs, as stated earlier, is error-prone, surgeons tend to be conservative using orthotics for a prolonged period of time postoperatively. Postoperative orthotics are not without morbidity. For a more accurate assessment of in vivo spinal kinematics, one needs to use an in vivo three-dimensional motion-measuring technique.

Several methods have been developed to analyze the spine in a three-dimensional context. Computed tomographic (CT) scans used for this purpose are tremendously expensive and are associated with large errors when the vertebrae are tilted with respect to the scanning plane. Although Penning and Wilmink[21] stated that in 70% of all measurements the results could be reproduced within 2°, this technique is prone to error when the vertebra is rotated, making it difficult to determine accurately the location of bony landmarks. These set-ups also limit the flexion/extension angles and loading of the spine that can be achieved when the patient is in the standing position.[57] The electrogoniometer technique provides good evaluation of many motion parameters in three-dimensional space; however, the data are only applicable to the spine as a unit and are incapable of providing motion assessment of each intervertebral joint.[58] The biplanar radiographic technique has been used to address some of these problems. Suh[59] performed some of the early work in this area. Many other researchers then began to utilize and improve on this technique, in particular Pearcy et al, who in the early 1980s combined simultaneous roentgen stereophotogrammetry, a variation of biplanar radiography, with the method of direct linear transformation (DLT).[57,60–63] Although much progress has been made by these researchers, they all have relied on anatomic landmarks as reference points on the radiographs. A problem arises in that locating the exact landmark in different radiographs can be difficult and error-prone.[64] It has also been shown that bone healing and growth over time significantly affect the location of true anatomic landmarks. These factors contribute greatly to measurement error and decrease the accuracy of the results.

Selvik[65] and Selvik et al[66] developed a technique that avoids the inaccuracies inherent with the use of bony landmarks by implanting biocompatible metallic markers into the patient's bone and then using simultaneous roentgen stereophotogrammetry to study the longitudinal growth of that bone. Since then, radiopaque markers have been used extensively in many fields from orthopedics to dentistry. Olsson et al[67] applied this technique to study fusion in the lumbosacral region, and Johnson et al[68] used it to determine the timetable for intervertebral stabilization after posterolateral fusion of the lower lumbar spine. These studies and similar ones undertaken by others have established the great variety of applications for this technique.[69] Adaptation of this procedure to the cervical spine allows for the study of in vivo biomechanics as a function of time. We have developed an in vivo protocol to study the kinematics of the cervical spine in patients following surgery. The protocol is based on the simultaneous roentgen stereophotogrammetric (SRS) technique.[70] Two patients undergoing different cervical fusion procedures were initially selected for this study. At the time of their elective surgery, the patients were implanted with vitallium beads in anatomically appropriate positions readily accessible at surgery. Roentgen stereo pairs of a patient in neutral, maximum voluntary flexion and extension were obtained at various time intervals following surgery. The results of two patients are described next.

The first patient had severe atlantoaxial subluxation due to rheumatoid arthritis and was treated with a posterior C1 to C2 fusion and wiring using autogenous bone graft. Metallic beads were implanted from the occiput to C2 during the surgery. Data on the three-dimensional mobility of the operated segment (C1 to C2) as well as adjacent segment (C0 to C1) were obtained. Figure 3–2 shows the range of primary motion during flexion and extension (ie, active range of motion in the sagittal plane from flexion to extension). Preliminary results illustrate a decrease in range of motion over time as the fusion process progressed. At the C1 to C2 level where fusion was performed, the rotational angle decreased from 17° to 6° from 6 weeks to 3 months postoperatively. Ongoing studies will further elucidate the observed decrease in motion.

The second patient had a preoperative diagnosis of cervical spondylosis with stenosis and early myelopathy. He had cervical laminoplasty from C3 to C6 and partial laminectomy at C7. Stereoradiograph pairs in flexion/extension were obtained at 6 weeks and 3 and 6 months postoperatively. The rotation (primary and coupled) data for the three time intervals are listed in Table 3–8 and illustrated in Figure 3–2. The SRS technique made it easy to identify the characteristics of the coupling pattern. The rotational angles across various levels changed with time, as was expected. The flexion-extension range of motion, however, did not change significantly between the 3- and 6-month time intervals. The coupled motions stabilized at 3 months.

Figure 3–3 also provides a comparison of the flexion-extension range of rotation data, at various levels as a function of time, computed using (1) the SRS technique (3D-SRS, data taken from Table 3–8), and (2) only the lateral radiographs (2D technique). At 6 weeks and 3 months postoperatively, the predictions based on these two approaches differed significantly. The trends are similar, however, at 6 months postoperatively.

Although the information collected so far is limited, it appears that the healing process has stabilized 3 months postoperatively, based on the SRS technique predictions. Using the 2D technique, it may be possible to make a similar statement at 6 months following surgery.

The long-term aim of the biomechanical studies undertaken by our group is to develop an analytical finite-element model of the cervical spine for a patient that will enable us to predict the effects of a surgical procedure over time. The model will include the effect of muscles on the mechanics as well the adaptive bone-remodeling concepts. We have already developed a number studies in this direction.[70–72] We have a biomechanical model of the lumbar spine that can predict forces in various structures across a motion segment during lifting.[71] The predictions are then incorporated into a finite-element model of a lumbar motion segment to predict the effects of muscles on the lumbar spine mechanics.[70] We have also developed a protocol to include the adaptive bone-remodeling concepts into the finite-element model of a lumbar motion segment.[72] Once these models are developed fully and reworked for applications in the cervical spine region, the effects of surgery on the spine in conjunction with the in vivo kinematics data collected from studies like the one described earlier can be investigated.

In conclusion, it must be recognized that although a vast amount of literature is presently available, an equally large amount of research is warranted to gain further understanding of cervical biomechanics.

Acknowledgment.   This work was supported in part by an NIH grant (AR40166-02).

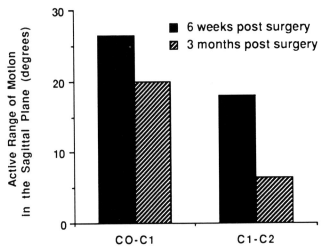

Figure 3–2.   Range of motion in the sagittal plane 6 weeks and 3 months following C1 to C2 fusion determined using the simultaneous roentgen stereophotogrammetric technique.

REFERENCES

1. Balderston RA, An HS. *Complications in Spinal Surgery.* Philadelphia, Pa: WB Saunders; 1991.
2. The Cervical Spine Research Society Editorial Committee. *The Cervical Spine.* 2nd ed. Philadelphia, Pa: JB Lippincott; 1989.
3. Kirkaldy-Willis WH, Farfan HF. Instability of the lumbar spine. *Clin Orthop.* 1982;165:110–123.
4. Nachemson A. The role of spine fusion. *Spine.* 1981;6:306–307.
5. Lee CK. Lumbar spinal instability (olisthesis) after extensive posterior spinal instability. *Spine.* 1983;8:429–433.
6. White AA, Panjabi MM. *Clinical Biomechanics of the Spine I.* Philadelphia, Pa: JB Lippincott; 1978.
7. Panjabi MM. Biomechanical evaluation of spinal fixation devices: I. A conceptual framework. *Spine.* 1988;13:1129–1134.
8. Goel VK, Weinstein JN. *Biomechanics of the Spine: Clinical and Surgical Perspective.* Boca Raton, Fla: CRC Press; 1990.
9. Goel VK, Nye TA, Clark CR, Nishiyama K, Weinstein JN. A technique to evaluate an internal spinal device by the use of Selspot II system—an application to Luque closed loop. *Spine.* 1987;12:150–159.

Table 3–8.   The Primary and Coupled Rotations at the Functional Range of Neck Movement as a Function of Time Following Surgery for a Patient who Underwent a Laminoplasty.

ACTIVE RANGE OF MOTION	6-WEEK POSTOPERATIVE			3-MONTH POSTOPERATIVE			6-MONTH POSTOPERATIVE		
	*Flex-Ext.**	*LAR-RAR*	*RLB-LLB*	*Flex-Ext.**	*LAR-RAR*	*RLB-LLB*	*Flex-Ext.**	*LAR-RAR*	*RLB-LLB*
C3-C4	3.47	0.60	−1.4	8.95	−0.77	−0.08	8.41	−2.37	0.12
C4-C5	2.23	0.45	−2.87	5.13	−0.29	−1.55	5.79	−1.21	0.33
C5-C6	11.32	1.74	−3.49	4.49	−1.08	−0.09	5.95	−1.31	−0.49

*Primary motion; others are coupled motions.

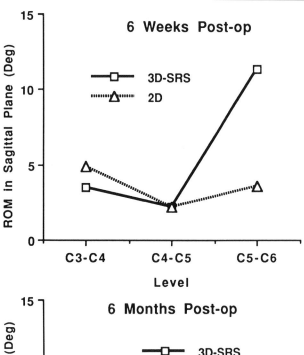

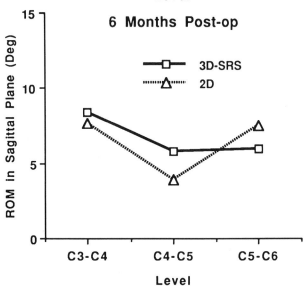

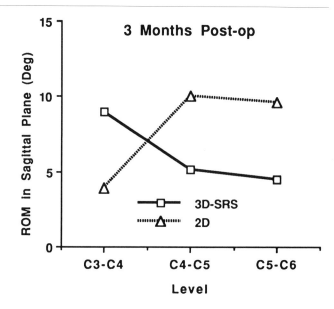

Figure 3–3. Graphic illustration of sagittal plane rotation across C3 to C4, C4 to C5, and C5 to C6 6 weeks, 3 months, and 6 months following surgery. Data obtained using the simultaneous roentgen stereophotogrammetric (SRS) technique and two-dimensional radiographic technique.

10. Panjabi MM, Duranceau JS, Goel VK, Oxland TR, Takata K. Cervical human vertebrae: quantitative three-dimensional anatomy of the middle and lower regions. *Spine.* 1991;16:861–869.

11. Goel VK, Yamanishi TM, Chang H. Development of a computer model to predict strains in the individual fibers of a ligament across the ligamentous occipito-atlanto-axial (C0-C1-C2) complex. *Ann Biomed Eng.* 1992;20:667–686.

12. Goel VK, Clark CR, Gallaes K, Liu YK. Movement-rotation relationships of the ligamentous occipito-atlanto-axial complex. *J. Biomech.* 1988;21:673–680.

13. Goel VK, Clark CR, McGowan D, Goyla S. An in-vitro study of the kinematics of the normal, injured and stabilized cervical spine. *J Biomech.* 1984;17:363–376.

14. Hunter LY, Braunstein EM, Bailey RW. Radiographic changes following anterior cervical fusion. *Spine.* 1980;5:399–401.

15. Fielding JW. Normal and selected abnormal motion of the cervical spine from the second cervical vertebra to the seventh cervical vertebra based on cineroentgenography. *J Bone Joint Surg.* 1964;46A:1779–1781.

16. Jofe MH, White AA, Panjabi MM. Physiology and biomechanics-kinematics. In: Bailey RW, Sherk HH, Dunn EJ, et al, eds. *The Cervical Spine—The Cervical Spine Research Society.* Philadelphia, Pa: JB Lippincott; 1983:23–28.

17. Posner I, White AA, Edwards WT, Hayes WC. A biomechanical analysis of the clinical stability of the lumbar and lumbosacral spine. *Spine.* 1982;7:374–389.

18. Wiesel S, Kraus D, Rothman RH. Atlanto-occipital hypermobility. *Orthop Clin North Am.* 1978;9:969–972.

19. Panjabi MM, Pelker R, Crisco JJ, Phil M, Thibodeau L, Yamamoto I. Biomechanics of healing of posterior cervical spinal injuries in a canine model. *Spine.* 1988;13:803–807.

20. Panjabi M, Dvorak J, Duranceau J, et al. Three-dimensional movements of the upper cervical spine. *Spine.* 1988;13:726–730.

21. Penning L, Wilmink JT. Rotation of the cervical spine: a CT study in normal subjects. *Spine.* 1987;12:732–738.

22. Goel VK, Winterbottom JM, Schulte KR, et al. Ligamentous laxity across C0-C1-C2 complex: axial torque-rotation characteristics until failure. *Spine.* 1990;15:990–996.

23. Dvorak J, Panjabi MM, Gerber M, Wichmann W. CT-functional diagnostics of the rotatory instability of upper cervical spine: 1. An experimental study on cadavers. *Spine.* 1987;12:197–205.

24. Dvorak J, Hayek J, Zehnder R. CT-functional diagnostics of the rotatory instability of the upper cervical spine: Part 2. An evaluation on healthy adults and patients with suspected instability. *Spine.* 1987;12:726–731.

25. Grob D, Crisco JJ III, Panjabi MM, Wang P, Dvorak J. Biomechanical evaluation of four different posterior atlantoaxial fixation techniques. *Spine.* 1992;17:480–490.

26. Gallie WE. Fractures and dislocations of the cervical spine. *Am J Surg.* 1939;46:495–499.

27. Brooks AL, Jenkins EB. Atlanto-axial arthrodesis by the wedge compression method. *J Bone Joint Surg.* 1978;60A:279–284.

28. Magerl F, Seemann P. Stable posterior fusion of the atlas and axis by transarticular screw fixation. In: Kehr P, Weidner A, eds. *Cervical Spine.* New York: Springer-Verlag; 1987:322–327.

29. Harvell JC Jr, Hanley EN Jr. Immediate post-operative stability of the atlanto-axial articulation: a biomechanical study comparing simple midline wiring, the Gallie and the Brooks procedures. Presented at the 16th Annual Cervical Spine Research Society meeting, Key Biscayne, Fla, 1988.

30. Hanson P, Sharkey N, Montesano PX. Anatomic and biomechanical study of C1-C2 posterior arthrodesis techniques. Presented at the 16th Annual Cervical Spine Research Society meeting, Key Biscayne, Fla, 1988.

31. Montesano PX, Juach EC, Anderson PA, Benson DR, Hanson PB. Biomechanics of cervical spine internal fixation. *Spine.* 1991;16:S10–S16.

32. Panjabi MM, Summers DJ, Pelker RR, Videman T, Friedlaender GE, Southwick WO. Three-dimensional load-displacement curves due to forces on the cervical spine. *J Orthop Res.* 1986;4:152–161.

33. Panjabi MM, White AA III, Johnson RM. Cervical spine mechanics as a function of transection of components. *J Biomech.* 1975;8:327–336.

34. Moroney SP, Schultz AB, Miller JA, Andersson GB. Load displacement properties of lower cervical spine motion segments. *J Biomech.* 1988;21:769–779.

35. Panjabi MM, White AA III, Keller D, Southwick WO, Friedlaender G. Stability of the cervical spine under tension. *J Biomech.* 1978;11:189–197.

36. Lipson SJ, Muir H. Proteoglycans in experimental intervertebral disk degeneration. *Spine.* 1981;6:194–210.

37. Schulte K, Clark CR, Goel VK. Kinematics of the cervical spine following discectomy and stabilization. *Spine.* 1989;14:1116–1121.

38. Martins AN. Anterior cervical discectomy with and without interbody bone graft. *J Neurosurg.* 1976;44:290–295.

39. Wilson D, Campbell D. Anterior cervical discectomy without bone graft. *Neurosurgery.* 1977;47:551–555.

40. Goel VK, Clark CR, Harris KG, Schulte KB. Kinematics of the cervical spine: effects of multiple total laminectomy and facet wiring. *J Orthop Res.* 1988;6:611–619.

41. Cusick JF, Yoganandan N, Pintar F, Myklebust J, Hussain H. Biomechanics of cervical spine facetectomy and fixation techniques. *Spine.* 1988;13:808–812.

42. Raynor RB, Pugh J, Shapiro I. Cervical facetectomy and its effect on spine strength. *J Neurosurg.* 1985;63:278–282.

43. Raynor RB, Moskovich R, Zidel P, Pugh J. Alterations in primary and coupled neck motions after facetectomy. *J Neurosurg.* 1987;12:681–687.

44. Rogers WA. Fractures and dislocations of the cervical spine. *J Bone Joint Surg.* 1957;39A:341–376.

45. Grob D, Dvorak J, Panjabi MM, Froelich M, Hayek J. Posterior occipitocervical fusion: a preliminary report of a new technique. *Spine.* 1991;16:S17–S24.

46. Jeanneret B, Magerl F, Ward EH, Ward JC. Posterior stabilization of the cervical spine with hook plates. *Spine.* 1991;16:S56–S63.

47. Anderson PA, Henley MB, Grady MS, Montesano PX, Winn, HR. Posterior cervical arthrodesis with AO reconstruction plates and bone graft. *Spine.* 1991;16:S72–S79.

48. Gill KG, Paschal S, Corin J, Ashman R, Buscholz RW. Posterior plating of the cervical spine: a biomechanical comparison of different posterior fusion techniques. *Spine.* 1988;13:813–816.

49. Raynor RB, Carter FW. Cervical spine strength after facet injury and spine plate application. *Spine.* 1991;16:S558–S560.

50. Ulrich C, Worsdorfer O, Claes L, Magerl F. Comparative study of the stability of anterior and posterior cervical spine fixation procedures. *Arch Orthop Trauma.* 1987;106:226–231.

51. Ulrich C, Worsdorfer O, Kalff R, Claes L, Wilke H. Biomechanics of fixation systems to the cervical spine. *Spine.* 1991;16:S4–S9.

52. Coe JD, Warden KE, Sutterlin CE, McAfee PC. Biomechanical evaluation of cervical spinal stabilization methods in a human cadaveric model. *Spine.* 1989;14:1122–1131.

53. Aebi K, Zuber K, Marchest D. Treatment of cervical spine injuries with anterior plating: indications, techniques, and results. *Spine.* 1991;16:S38–S45.

54. Ripa DR, Kowall MG, Meyer PR, Rusin JJ. Series of ninety-two traumatic cervical spine injuries stabilized with anterior ASIF plate fusion technique. *Spine.* 1991;16:S45–S55.

55. Traynelis VC, Donaher PA, Roach RM, Kojimoto H, Goel VK. Biomechanical comparison of anterior Caspar plate and three-level posterior fixation techniques in a human cadaveric model. *J Neurosurg.* 1993;79:96–103.

56. Weinstein JN, Spratt KF, Spengler D, Brick C, Reid S. Spinal pedicle fixation: reliability and validity of roentgenogram-based assessment and surgical factors on successful screw placement. *Spine.* 1988;13:1012–1018.

57. Pearcy MJ, Whitle MW. Movements of the lumbar spine measured by three-dimensional x-ray analysis. *J Biomed Eng.* 1982;4:107–112.

58. Alund M, Larsson S. Three-dimensional analysis of neck motion—a clinical method. *Spine.* 1990;12:87–91.

59. Suh CH. The fundamentals of computer aided x-ray analysis of the spine. *J Biomech.* 1974;7:161–169.

60. Mimura M, Moriya H, Watanabe T, Takahashi K, Yamagata M, Tamaki T. Three-dimensional motion analysis of the cervical spine with special reference to the axial rotation. *Spine.* 1989;14:1135–1139.

61. Pearcy M, Burrough S. Assessment of bony union after interbody fusion of the lumbar spine using a biplanar radiographic technique. *J Bone Joint Surg.* 1982;64B:228–232.

62. Pearcy M, Portek I, Shepherd J. Three-dimensional x-ray analysis of normal movement in the lumbar spine. *Spine.* 1984;9:294–297.

63. Pearcy M, Portek I, Shepherd J. The effect of low-back pain on lumbar spinal movements measured by three-dimensional x-ray analysis. *Spine.* 1985;10:150–153.

64. Stokes IA, Wilder DG, Frymoyer JW, Pope MH. Assessment of patients with low-back pain by biplanar radiographic measurement of intervertebral motion. *Spine.* 1981;6:233–240.

65. Selvik G. RSA—a method for the study of the kinematics of the skeletal system. *Acta Orthop Scand Suppl.* 1989;232:1–51.

66. Selvik G, Alberius P, Aronson AS. A roentgen stereophotogrammetric system construction, calibration and technical accuracy. *Acta Radiol (Diagn).* 1983;24:343–352.

67. Olsson TH, Selvik G, Willer S. Mobility in the lumbosacral spine after fusion studied with the aid of roentgen stereophotogrammetry. *Clin Orthop.* 1977;129:181–190.

68. Johnson R, Selvik G, Stromquist B, Sunden G. Mobility of the lower lumbar spine after posterolateral fusion determined by roentgen stereophotogrammetric analysis. *Spine.* 1990;15:347–350.

69. Karrholm J. Roentgen stereophotogrammetry—review of orthopedic applications. *Acta Orthop Scand.* 1989;60:491–503.

70. Lee SJ, Harris KG, Nassif J, Goel VK, Clark CR. In vivo kinematics of the cervical spine. Part I: Development of a roentgen

stereophotogrammetric technique using metallic markers and assessment of its accuracy. J Spinal Disord. 1993;6:522–534.

71. Goel VK, Han JS, Ahn JY, et al. Loads in the spinal structures during lifting: development of a three-dimensional comprehensive biomechanical model. European Spine Journal. Provisional acceptance.

72. Seenivasan G. *Application of Shape Optimization Techniques to Spinal Motion Segment.* Iowa City, IA: University of Iowa; 1993. Thesis.

73. Dvorak J. CT-functional diagnostics of the rotatory instability of the upper cervical spine. Presented at the Annual Meeting of the Cervical Spine Research Society, Cambridge, Mass, 1985.

74. Penning L. Normal movements of the cervical spine. *Am J Roentgenol.* 1978;130:317–326.

75. White AA, Panjabi MM. The basic kinematics of the human spine. *Spine.* 1978;3:12–20.

4 Instability of the Thoracic and Lumbar Spine

Patrick W. Hitchon, M.D.

INTRODUCTION

A simplistic definition of spinal instability would be that degree of motion that exceeded normal limits. The extent of motion of the normal spine has been addressed in numerous manuscripts and presented in tabular form.[1–4] A more complete definition is that by White and Panjabi,[1] in which spinal stability is described as that degree of motion that prevents pain, neurological deficit, and abnormal angulation. In an attempt to facilitate conceptualization of stability and instability of the spine, the three-column construct of the spine was advanced.[5] Work by Panjabi et al[6] had shown that instability of the isolated spine can be achieved by sectioning of all ligaments posterior to and including the posterior half of the disk. A similar degree of instability was also achieved by sectioning all ligaments anterior to and including the posterior half of the disk. This work emphasized the role of the posterior half of the disk space and the posterior longitudinal ligament as an important constituent in achieving spinal stability. This recognition led to the three-column construct of the spine, with the anterior half of the bodies and the disks constituting the anterior column; the posterior half of the bodies, disks, and posterior longitudinal ligament composing the middle column; and the neural arches with their facets and attached ligaments comprising the posterior column.[5] This three-column theory has led occasionally to oversimplification in the analysis of spinal fractures. Involvement of two columns subsequent to injury does not equate with spinal instability in all cases. Hence, some have advocated the classification of fractures into stable and unstable. Stable fractures were those with involvement of the anterior column. Instability of the first degree or mechanical instability was exemplified by flexion-distraction injuries or those referred to as Chance fractures or seatbelt-type injuries. Instability of the second degree with or without neurological deficit was exemplified by burst fractures with collapse of both anterior and middle columns. Third-degree instability consisted of those fractures with both mechanical and neurological instability. The latter are represented by fracture dislocations.[5]

In spite of extensive laboratory studies on the functional spinal unit, these studies do not necessarily reflect entirely what is encountered in vivo. In addition to the vertebral bodies and ligaments, muscles contribute significantly to the erect posture and mobility.[7] The thoracic cage increases the buckling load of the thoracolumbar spine by a factor of 3 to 4.[8] Age and gender both influence calcification and strength of bone. In people under the age of 40, cancellous bone bears up to 55% of the load and cortical bone the rest. In those over the age of 40, due to osteoporosis the weight-bearing role of cancellous bone is reduced to 35%, with the remainder being borne by cortical bone.[1] Congenital malformations, such as Klippel-Feil with hemivertebra and failure of segmentation, interfere with mobility and contribute to instability.[9] Degenerative changes of the spine with disk desiccation and facet degeneration also constitute destabilizing factors. Destruction of one or more of the three spinal columns by infection, trauma, neoplasms, or surgery can result in excessive motion and spinal instability.[9] An important factor that is often overlooked in the determination of clinical instability is that of occupation.[1,3] A lytic lesion of a vertebral body may go unnoticed for months in a clerk yet become symptomatic abruptly in a laborer. Thus the factors contributing to spinal stability are numerous. In vitro studies on the denuded spine are indeed helpful, yet do not in themselves reflect the entire spectrum of factors involved in the particular patient.

Once instability has been established based on formulated checklists,[1,3,4] a decision regarding management must be made. The treatment of the unstable spine may require surgery to decompress neural elements, reduce dislocation, or expedite rehabilitation. On the other hand, in the intact patient recumbency may be sufficient until healing occurs and weight bearing can be assumed (see Chapter 34 of this book). Radiological criteria have been advocated to facilitate decisions regarding surgery. Such criteria have consisted of angulation in excess of 30°, vertebral body collapse of more than 50%, or canal compromise exceeding 50%.[10,11] These criteria need to be considered in the clinical context following assessment of the patient with particular emphasis on the neurological condition. It should be kept in mind that it is difficult to improve on the intact patient or to reverse neurological deficit in a patient who is flaccid with total paralysis.

THORACIC SPINE

Mathematical studies on the thoracolumbar spine with and without the attached rib cage have been conducted.[8] These studies based on previous work have shown that the rib cage contributes to an increase of the bending stiffness of the spine in flexion of 27%. In extension the attached rib cage contributes to an increase in stiffness of 132%. This same mathematical model revealed that the rib cage increases the buckling load of the thoracolumbar spine by a factor of 3 to 4. The inherent nature of the thoracic spine with its attached rib cage obviously can be compromised by extensive fractures, surgical resections, or disease. The attached rib cage contributes to fairly rigid immobilization of the thoracic spine, allowing it the least amount of translation (≤2.5 mm) and the least degree of sagittal rotation (≤5°).[1,2,3,6] These values are less than their counterparts in the cervical and lumbar spine.

This stability rendered by the thoracic cage can, however, be compromised under certain clinical conditions, including surgery. Biomechanical studies on the functional spinal unit consisting of two adjacent vertebral bodies have been conducted with and without removal of posterior elements.[12] The posterior elements consisted of the facet joints, the intertransverse ligaments, the ligamenta flava, the inferior half of the laminae, the spinous processes, and intervening interspinous ligaments. This degree of destabilization showed a statistically significant increase in the range of motion of the thoracic spine in flexion, extension, and axial rotation. Similar studies have been conducted on the entire thoracic spine from T1 to L1 without the attached rib cage. Two-level decompressive laminectomies were performed in a random fashion in the lower half of the spinal column.[13] These studies showed that laminectomy resulted in a significant decrease in the overall strength, stiffness, and energy-absorbing capacity of the thoracic spine. These studies emphasize the importance of recognition of associated disease processes involving the thoracic spine when posterior decompression is contemplated. Such decompressive procedures in the face of vertebral body disease may have catastrophic consequences. A checklist for the identification of clinical instability of the thoracic spine has been formulated, similar to that of the cervical spine.[1,3] This checklist includes the following factors: neurological deficit, the integrity of the posterior and anterior spinal columns, disruption of facet joins, motion exceeding normal limits in both translation (>2.5 mm) and angular rotation (>5°), and the

anticipated load bearing by the spine (Table 4–1). Whereas a thoracic spine afflicted with disease may suffice to provide stability in one patient, it may fail when subjected to excessive loading in another. Figures 4–1 and 4–2 are examples of instability arising from metastatic breast cancer and osteomyelitis, respectively. Both examples show evidence of progressive instability brought about by decompressive laminectomy and failure of stabilization. The patient with metastatic cancer underwent Luque rectangle fixation posteriorly. This device had to be removed following wound dehiscence arising from radiation therapy. In the case of infection, stability was finally achieved with a posterolateral bony fusion.

The preceding examples reveal the importance of identification of the site and extent of pathology in selecting the surgical approach. This is further exemplified in the patient shown in Figure 4–3. This patient sustained a slice fracture through the inferior body of T9 with disruption of all three columns. Such a patient would have been ill served by the use of distraction instrumentation. This patient was fused in situ and successfully using Luque rods and sublaminar wires. Regardless of the immediate methods of stabilization, the goal is to achieve a solid bony fusion whenever possible. Such fusion can often be achieved with recumbency and immobilization. This is particularly advantageous in the presence of complicating medical conditions. The patient depicted in Figure 4–4, with a severe burst fracture of T10, failed to heal with bony fusion in spite of 2 months of recumbency. Surgery had been ruled out due to alcoholic hepatitis accompanied by coagulopathy. Although healing and fusion could have resulted in an otherwise healthy patient, this was not achieved due to associated medical factors. Surgical stabilization with instrumentation was eventually undertaken.

LUMBAR SPINE

As in the cervical and thoracic, the range of motion of the lumbar spine has been quantitated and presented.[1,2,4] A checklist for the lumbar spine similar to that of the cervical and thoracic spines has been presented.[1,4] This checklist also emphasizes the importance of neurological deficit, anterior

Table 4–1. Checklist for the Diagnosis of Clinical Instability in the Thoracic and Thoracolumbar Spine.

ELEMENT	POINT VALUE
Anterior elements destroyed or unable to function	2
Posterior elements destroyed or unable to function	2
Relative sagittal plane translation >2.5 mm	2
Relative sagittal plane rotation >5°	2
Spinal cord or canda equina damage	1
Disruptions of costovertebral articulations	1
Dangerous loading anticipated	2

Total of 5 or more = unstable.

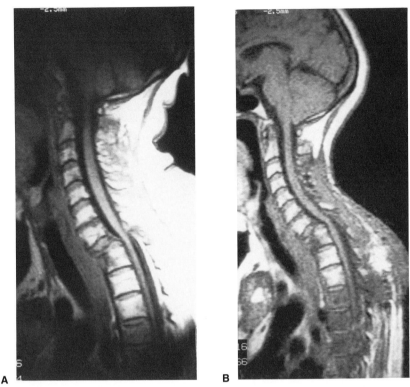

Figure 4–1.   Metastatic breast cancer to T1 resulting in collapse, subluxation, and myelopathy. (**A**). At the time of presentation, compromise of the canal and cord compression are appreciated. (**B**). Subsequent to transpedicular decompression and Luque rectangle stabilization, wound dehiscence occurred related to radiation therapy. The stabilizing device had to be removed and a trapezius flap was rotated for wound closure. Although the patient did not suffer any progression in her myelopathy, her instability is obviously worse.

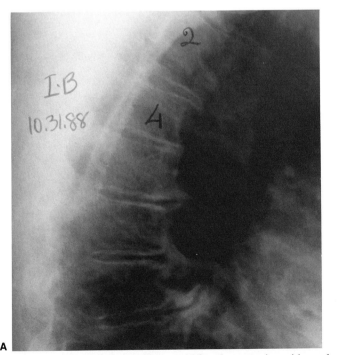

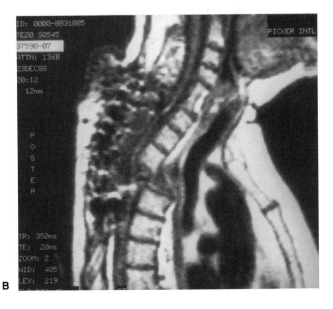

Figure 4–2.   A 64-year-old female presenting with myelopathy secondary to osteomyelitis of the spine at T3. (**A**). Plain roentgenogram upon admission shows total collapse of T3 vertebral body. (**B**). MRI following decompressive laminectomy reveals progressive instability and retrolisthesis of T2 on T4.

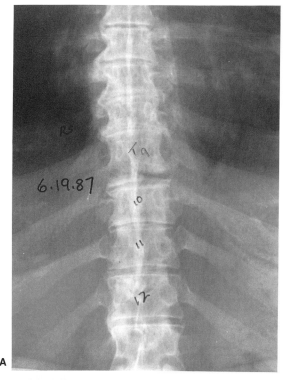

A

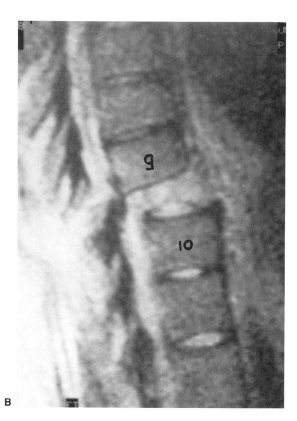

B

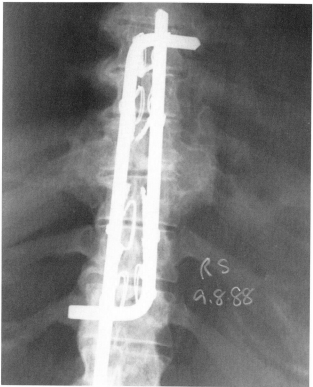

C

Figure 4–3. A 34-year-old female with paraplegia secondary to a slice fracture of T9. (**A**). Anteroposterior projection showing the slice fracture through the inferior body of T9. (**B**). MRI sagittal image reveals the extent of separation between T9 and T10 due to three column disruption. (**C**). Fusion and reduction was achieved with in situ stabilization using Luque rods and sublaminar wires.

and posterior column disruption, sagittal translation (>8%), and forward angulation (>9°) (Table 4–2). As dictated by facet orientation,[1] axial rotation exceeds flexion/extension in the thoracic spine, whereas the reverse is true in the lumbar spine. As noted earlier, instability of the lumbar spine can be encountered with surgical procedures due to their ex-

tent or underlying pathology. Biomechanical studies on the lumbar spine have shown that motion increases subsequent to unilateral or bilateral facetectomy.[14,15] Furthermore, deflection increases significantly when the posterior ligaments (ligamenta flava and interspinous) are excised.[15] Similar studies have been conducted in vitro following lumbar dis-

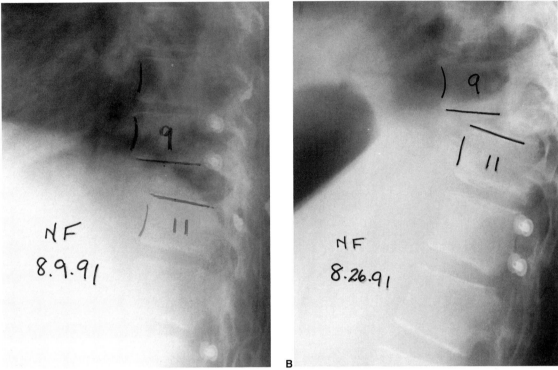

Figure 4–4. A 36-year-old patient with severe burst fracture of T10, dislocation, and paraplegia. (**A**). Cross-table lateral film obtained nearly 2 months following admission shows destruction of T10 with anterior dislocation of T9 on T11. Surgery for stabilization and fusion was contraindicated due to alcoholic hepatitis and coagulopathy. (**B**). Mobilization to the upright position 2.5 months following admission shows the instability at the fracture site with failure to fuse spontaneously with recumbency. Surgery with Harrington rodding and posterolateral bony fusion was eventually performed.

cectomy.[16,17] These studies reveal that total discectomy is associated with a greater degree of motion in all planes (flexion extension, right and left lateral bending, and right and left axial rotation) when compared to partial discectomy, partial laminotomy, or partial facetectomy. These results emphasize the importance of removal of the least amount of disk to minimize instability. These operative procedures are sometimes conducted with impunity and may often be responsible for failure, chronic pain, and destabilization. Some factors that predispose the thoracolumbar spine to injury are anatomic as exemplified by the thoracolumbar junction. This junction is often the site of injury

due to the interface between the thoracic spine stabilized by the rib cage and the lumbar spine, affixed to the pelvis. Nowhere is this elucidated more clearly than in flexion-distraction injuries, clinically referred to as seatbelt-type or Chance fractures, in which the pelvis is immobilized and the torso is thrown forward (Fig. 4–5).

The patient depicted in Figure 4–6 exemplifies instability arising from surgical intervention. Extensive laminectomy for lumbar stenosis was performed on two occasions. This obviously compromised the integrity of the facets, resulting in subluxation 5 months later. Surgery for reduction and stabilization was accomplished using transpedicular screw and

Table 4–2. Checklist for the Diagnosis of Clinical Instability in the Lumbar (L1 to L5) Spine.

ELEMENT	POINT VALUE
Cauda equina damage	3
Relative flexion sagittal plane translation >8% or extension sagittal plane translation >9%	2
Relative flexion sagittal plane rotation >9°	2
Anterior elements destroyed	2
Posterior elements destroyed	2
Dangerous loading anticipated	1

Total of 5 or more = clinically unstable.

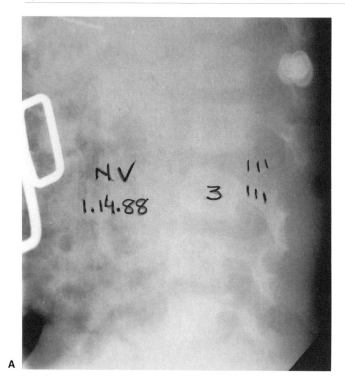

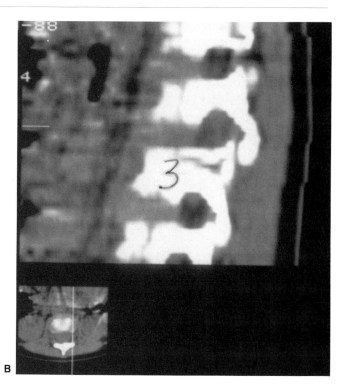

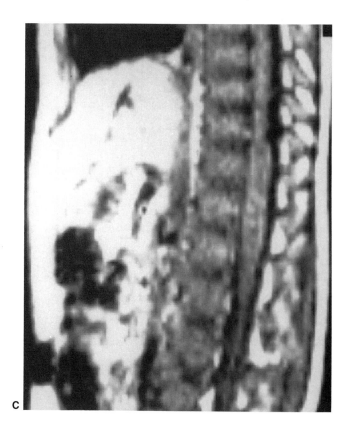

Figure 4–5. Twenty-month-old patient wearing a lap seatbelt involved in a motor vehicle accident. This head-on collision resulted in a flexion-distortion injury with flaccid paraplegia. (**A**). Plain lateral roentgenogram shows the fracture through the neural arch of L3 with the vertebral column hinged on the anterior longitudinal ligament. (**B**). Reformated sagittal computerized axial tomogram further reveals the fracture through the neural arch and pedicle. (**C**). Sagittal T2-weighted MRI image shows increased signal from the conus arising from the contusion complicating the flexion distraction injury. Treatment was provided with recumbency and thoracolumbar bracing.

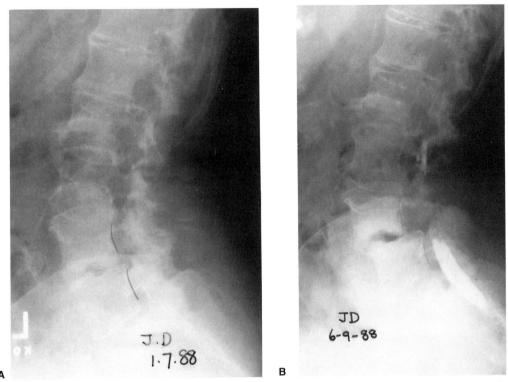

A   B

Figure 4–6.   A 56-year-old female presenting with lumbar stenosis and neurogenic claudication. (**A**). Lateral projection prior to surgery reveals a degenerative disease and facet hypertrophy. (**B**). Subsequent to two operative procedures for laminectomy from L3 to L5, instability develops with anterolisthesis of L4 on L5. Patient required reduction and stabilization with transpedicular screws and plates and a posterolateral bony fusion. Reduction was associated with improvement in her bilateral foot drop.

plate fixation. Although instrumentation as in this case may achieve reduction and stability, this may prove to be temporary and precarious. Experimentally, biomechanical studies have shown that in simulated lumbar fractures, transpedicular and screw fixation reduces motion but does not achieve normal strength.[18] Cases should be studied and scrutinized to avoid the problems that can be worse than the initial ailment.

Acknowledgment.   The authors acknowledge Ms. Judy Rehbehn for the preparation of the manuscript.

REFERENCES

1. White AA, Panjabi MM. *Clinical Biomechanics of the Spine.* Philadelphia, Pa: J B Lippincott; 1978:chaps 1, 2, and 5.
2. White AA, Panjabi MM. The basic kinematics of the human spine. *Spine.* 1978;3:12–20.
3. Panjabi MM, Thibodeau LL, Crisco JJ, White AA. What constitutes spinal instability. *Clin Neurosurg.* Vol. 34, pp. 313–339, 1988 Williams & Wilkins Publishers.
4. Posner I, White AA, Edwards MW, Hayes WC. A biomechanical analysis of the clinical stability of the lumbar and lumbosacral spine. *Spine.* 1982;7:374–389.
5. Denis F. The three column spine and its significance in the classification of acute thoracolumbar spinal injuries. *Spine.* 1983;8:817–831.
6. Panjabi MM, Hausfeld JN, White AA. A biomechanical study of the ligamentous stability of the thoracic spine in man. *Acta Orthop Scand.* 1981;52:315–326.
7. Maiman DJ, Pintar FA. Anatomy and clinical biomechanics of the thoracic spine. *Clin Neurosurg.* 1990;38:296–324.
8. Andriacchi T, Schultz A, Belytschko T, Galante J. A model for studies of mechanical interactions between the human spine and rib cage. J. of Biomechanics 1974, Vol. 7, pp. 497–505.
9. Frymoyer JW, Krag MH. Spinal Stability and Instability: Chapter 1, Definitions, Classification, and General Principles of Management: The Unstable Spine. Dunsker SB, Schmidek HH, Frymoyer J, Kahn A, eds. pp. 1–16. Grune & Stratton Publishers.
10. Riebel GD, Yoo JU, Fredrickson BE, Yuan HA. Review of Harrington rod treatment of spinal trauma. *Spine.* 1993;184:479–491.
11. Wiberg J, Hauge HN. Neurological outcome after surgery for thoracic and lumbar spine injuries. *ACTA Neurochir (Wien)* 1988;91:106–112.
12. White AA, Hirsch C. The significance of the vertebral posterior elements in the mechanics of the thoracic spine. Clinical Orthopaedics and Related Research. (November–December). 1971;81:2–14.

13. Yoganandan N, Maiman DJ, Pintar FA, et al. Biomechanical effects of laminectomy on thoracic spine stability. *Neurosurg.* 1993;324:604–610.
14. Pintar FA, Cusick JF, Yoganandan N, et al. The biomechanics of lumbar facetectomy under compression-flexion. *Spine.* 1992;177:804–810.
15. Cusick JF, Yoganandan N, Pintar FA, Reinartz JM. Biomechanics of sequential posterior lumbar surgical alterations. *J. Neurosurg.* 1992;76:805–811.
16. Goel VK, Goyal S, Clark C, et al. Kinematics of the whole lumbar spine effect of discectomy. *Spine.* 1985;106:543–554.
17. Goel VK, Nishiyama K, Weinstein JN, Liu YK. Mechanical properties of lumbar spinal motion segments as affected by partial disk removal. *Spine.* 1986;1110:1008–1012.
18. Yoganandan N, Larson SJ, Pintar F, et al. Biomechanics of lumbar pedicle screw/plate fixation in trauma. *Neurosurg.* 1990;27:873–881.

5 Intraoperative Electrophysiological Spinal Cord Monitoring

Richard K. Osenbach, M.D., Thoru Yamada, M.D.

INTRODUCTION

Over the past decade, intraoperative electrophysiological monitoring has come to play an increasingly important role in neurosurgery. The use of intraoperative somatosensory-evoked potentials (SSEPs) for monitoring spinal cord function has become widespread and probably represents the single most important clinical application of evoked potentials in neurosurgery.[1-3] More recently, techniques for eliciting and recording motor-evoked potentials (MEPs) have been employed that complement the traditional SSEPs.[4-10]

This chapter reviews the anatomical and physiological bases of SSEP and MEP monitoring and the techniques employed for the intraoperative use of these modalities. The advantages and limitations of evoked potential monitoring will be discussed. Finally and perhaps most importantly, the clinical correlation of intraoperative monitoring and neurological outcome will be presented.

INDICATIONS FOR INTRAOPERATIVE SPINAL CORD MONITORING

The rationale for performing intraoperative monitoring is based on the premise that evoked potentials can detect dysfunction of neural structures at a point when the processes or events that might result in permanent injury are still reversible such that appropriate corrective measures can be undertaken. As a corollary, in some cases the continued preservation and stability of intraoperative SSEPs and MEPs might occasionally allow one to be more aggressive surgically than would otherwise be possible or justified.

To utilize intraoperative monitoring effectively, one must have an understanding of the indications for monitoring (ie, which patients benefit from monitoring). In the broadest sense, any patient undergoing spinal surgery in which a neural pathway is at risk for injury might benefit from intraoperative monitoring. However, situations exist in which a surgical procedure cannot be altered despite deterioration of evoked responses.

Grundy[11] has proposed several criteria that should be met for intraoperative monitoring to be beneficial: (1) It is technically possible to monitor the neural pathway at risk; (2) appropriate stimulation and recording sites are available

during a given procedure; (3) the proper equipment is available for obtaining technically adequate recordings; (4) personnel skilled in the technical performance and interpretation of the responses are available; and (5) intervention is possible in the event that deterioration of the response occurs.

Currently, there are six basic methods commonly employed for intraoperative spinal cord monitoring.[1] Four of these methods monitor ascending pathways; these include traditional SSEPs, somatosensory spinal-evoked potentials (SSpEPs), spinal-spinal evoked potentials (SpSpEPs), and dermatomal evoked potentials (DEPs). The remaining techniques monitor the descending motor pathways and include MEPs and the wake-up test. Many still consider the wake-up test the standard against which all other monitoring techniques are compared.

SSEPs

SSEPs monitor primarily the ascending sensory pathways. As described earlier, there are a number of methods (SSEP, SSpEP, SpSpEP) by which the somatosensory pathways can be monitored intraoperatively. To understand the use of SSEPs, it is beneficial to review the anatomic pathways involved.

Anatomic Basis of Somatosensory-Evoked Potentials
The somatosensory system is comprised of receptors in the skin, muscles, and joints. These receptors are activated primarily by natural mechanical stimuli that are, in turn, converted into an action potential that is then conducted centrally through a peripheral nerve. The somatosensory system can just as easily be activated by applying an appropriate electrical stimulus to a peripheral nerve, such as the median or posterior tibial nerve (PTN). Regardless of the method of stimulation, the action potential generated is conducted centrally through first-order neurons whose cell bodies are located in the dorsal root ganglion. The central processes of these first-order neurons enter the spinal cord through the dorsal root entry zone and ascend in the ipsilateral dorsal column. Fibers from the leg and trunk travel in the more medial fasiculus gracilis, whereas those from the upper extremity enter the fasiculus cuneatus. Fibers within the

Table 5–1. Stimulation and Recording Parameters for Intraoperative SSEPs.

STIMULUS		
Sites	Unilateral median and/or posterior tibial	
Type	Constant current	
Intensity	3–4 × motor threshold (typically 3–10 mA)	
Duration	200–250 μs	
Rate	<5 Hz	
RECORDING		
Filters	Low frequency < 1–10 Hz	
	High frequency 250–2000*	
Repetitions	125–250	
Sweep	Median nerve, 40 ms	
	Posterior tibial nerve, 75 ms	
	MEDIAN NERVE STIMULUS	**TIBIAL NERVE STIMULUS**
Channels	1: $F_3 = A_2$ or $F_4 = A_1$	$C'_z = F_z$ (F_{pz})
	2: $C'_3 = A_2$ or $C'_4 = A_1$	$C'_z = A_1 + A_2$
	3: Cv5-anterior neck	L1 spine-iliac crest
	4: Lt Erb-Rt Erb	Popliteal fossa

*Depends on whether cortical/dendritic or subcortical/axonal data are being collected.

ing is acceptable and what changes indicate a potential neurological injury? There can be significant variation of the SSEP within a given patient, and it is important to know what changes are acceptable and what changes constitute a warning of impending neurological injury. Owen reviewed the literature regarding the criteria employed for interpreting intraoperative data.[3] In general, amplitude of the evoked responses is considered a more reliable indicator of spinal cord dysfunction than is latency.[1–3,11,20] Based on his review of the literature, Owen developed several criteria for interpreting intraoperative SSEPs.[3] He concurred that amplitude was indeed the most reliable parameter for interpretation of data and that a 60% decrement from baseline value was cause for warning the surgeon. If the signal remains stable, without further decline, no additional warnings are made. However, if amplitude continues to fall and anesthetic and technical problems have been excluded, one should search for a surgically related cause and attempt to alter the procedure in an attempt to restore the SSEPs. Although latency changes in and of themselves are not a primary criteria for interpretation, a latency prolongation of greater than 10% should prompt a warning. Brown has proposed that in addition to the absolute reduction in amplitude, the period of time the recordings remain degraded is also important.[20] Loss of responses for greater than 15 minutes was often associated with new neurological deficits.

If significant changes occur intraoperatively, there are a number of steps that can be taken. Technical problems should be excluded immediately. Physiological effects related to hypotension, hypothermia, and cold irrigation solutions should also be excluded as well as anesthetic effects. Once these problems have been excluded, there are several options. One can wait for several minutes to see if the signal improves in the event that the degradation of the response was valid but due to a transient event. Alternatively, any instrumentation that has been inserted can be removed to see if this was the cause of the abnormality. Another course of action would be to perform a wake-up test. These are all reasonable strategies depending on the given circumstances. Proceeding with surgery and ignoring the changes, however, implies that one has little confidence in the recordings. In such cases, it probably is preferable not to perform intraoperative recordings.

Anesthetic Effects on SSEPs

Of the agents known to alter the SSEP, anesthetics are particularly important.[11,21,22] Anesthetics are especially prone to altering cortical potentials, whereas subcortical potentials are relatively unaffected.[11] Some cortical potentials can be recorded with certain anesthetics but not with others. Many, if not all, of the volatile anesthetics have been shown to degrade cortical potentials. Halogenated agents are particularly prone to altering cortical SSEPs.[23] Ethrane is compatible with obtaining good cortical responses in concentrations under 0.5%; higher concentrations are sometimes tolerated, but this is patient-specific.[1] Forane has an unpredictable effect on cortical SSEPs, whereas halothane almost uniformly abolishes the cortical response and is unsuitable for monitoring.[1] Barbiturates and diazepam, especially in higher doses, reduce amplitudes and prolong latencies, whereas narcotics can have a variable effect. However, neuromuscular blocking agents do not interfere with intraoperative recordings.

The anesthetic technique chosen for a given procedure will depend on a number of factors, including the patient's physiological status, the particular procedure, and the desire for monitoring. The anesthetic employed should provide for maximum patient safety and comfort, facilitation of the operative procedure, and minimal effects on SSEPs.[11] In general, preoperative medications such as diazepam, midazolam, and droperidol should be avoided. Intraoperatively, a balanced anesthetic is preferred, avoiding bolus injections of agents that might alter the SSEP. Likewise, long-lasting agents should also be avoided because of the necessity of clinical assessment in the immediate postoperative period. Grundy has recommended using a combination of narcotics and low-dose thiopental.[11] The protocol employed by Brown utilizes a balanced nitrous oxide and narcotic anesthetic supplemented by low concentrations of Ethrane. It is important that blood pressure remains adequate and normothermia is maintained because hypotension and hypothermia both cause reduction in SSEP amplitude.

Special Techniques of Intraoperative SSEP Monitoring

Techniques for monitoring SSEPs can be divided into invasive and noninvasive methods. Up to this point, the techniques discussed are examples of noninvasive monitoring. Cortical potentials are recorded from scalp electrodes, and subcortical potentials are recorded using a scalp electrode and noncephalic reference. Spinal potentials can also be recorded from surface electrodes placed over the spine. The obvious advantage of noninvasive recording is that it is safe; the disadvantage, particularly of recording spinal cord potentials with surface electrodes, is that the amplitude is significantly less than that recorded using invasive electrodes.

INVASIVE TECHNIQUES FOR INTRAOPERATIVE SSEP MONITORING

Invasive techniques obviously involve more intervention and risk than do surface recordings. Invasive techniques comprise all methods that require placement of electrodes beneath the skin surface (not including subdermal electrodes). There are four basic types of invasive SSEP monitoring that have been described and employed: (1) subarachnoid, (2) epidural, (3) spinous process, and (4) interspinous ligament.[2,24] The main advantage to monitoring invasive spinal cord potentials is that these potentials are more stable than cortical SSEPs and are not degraded by anesthesia. In addition, monitoring more than one type of potential provides data from multiple sites, which assists in differentiating pathological changes from technical problems in the event that the evoked potentials change during surgery.

SUBARACHNOID RECORDING

Of the various invasive methods available, subarachnoid monitoring is the most invasive. Tamaki et al described the technique and used it to monitor spinal cord function in 229 cases.[25,26] This technique involves the introduction of specially designed platinum-tipped electrodes through a Tuohy needle into the subarachnoid space, with the electrodes positioned at the level of the conus. Stimulation is performed with an extradural electrode positioned at the upper thoracic level. Stimulation is carried out using rectangular pulses of 0.3 milliseconds with a presentation rate of 30 to 50 Hz and an intensity of 30 to 120 mV. The potential elicited consists of an initial spike followed by a multiphasic waveform with an amplitude of 100 to 150 μV.[25] Tamaki et al utilized this technique in 229 patients; half of this group underwent surgery for correction of scoliosis. Six patients in this series developed new postoperative deficits that correlated with a greater than 50% reduction of amplitudes in all cases. Although these authors reported no complications related to the monitoring technique, others have been concerned regarding the invasiveness and potential for injury associated with this technique.[2,24]

EPIDURAL RECORDING

The technique of recording spinal-evoked potentials using epidural electrodes was developed and introduced in Japan by Tsuyama and associates in 1978.[27] Since its introduction, a number of authors have employed this technique in their practice of intraoperative monitoring.[28,29] This method is less invasive than subarachnoid recording and has been used widely in countries outside the United States, particularly Japan and England. This method involves the placement of electrodes into the spinal epidural space either percutaneously or directly at the time of surgery. Ideally, electrodes are placed both caudal and rostral to the surgical site; peripheral nerve stimulation is otherwise performed in a fashion similar to routine SSEPs (Fig. 5–1). Dinner and associates reviewed the literature in which epidural electrodes were utilized for monitoring SpSEPs in humans.[24] A total of 294 cases were monitored using this technique. Amplitude changes occurred in 10 patients monitored, and 6 of these patients developed a new neurological deficit.

Epidural monitoring represents an attractive alternative to the more invasive method of subarachnoid monitoring. Technically, intraoperative placement of epidural electrodes rostral and caudal to the surgical site is relatively easy, especially with multilevel exposures. This technique is safe, and specially designed electrodes have been adapted specifically for epidural recording.[30]

SPINOUS PROCESS ELECTRODES

SSpEPs can also be monitored using Kirschner wires placed into the spinous processes. This method was initially described in cats by Nordwall and associates[31] and later applied in humans.[32–34] This technique at first might appear attractive because it is less invasive than the previously described methods. Additionally, because the electrodes are fixed in the spinous processes, they should remain stable throughout the procedure. The disadvantages of this technique are that placement of the wires into the high thoracic and cervical spinous processes can be difficult and time-consuming. However, the most important drawback is that the response amplitude is substantially less than that obtained with epidural recording, making interpretation more difficult. For this reason alone, spinous process electrodes are not widely accepted.

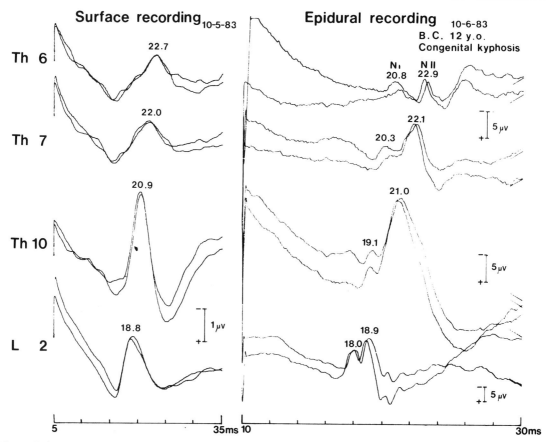

Figure 5–1. Spinal evoked potentials resulting from stimulation of the posterior tibial nerve recorded preoperatively from surface electrodes over the spine (left) and intraoperatively from epidural electrodes placed at corresponding spinal levels (right). Both recording methods demonstrate a major peak that increases in latency in a caudal-to-rostral direction. The epidural recordings also demonstrate an additional smaller negative peak (N1) that precedes the major negative peak. Note that the amplitude of the epidural recordings is substantially greater than that from surface recordings.

INTERSPINOUS LIGAMENT RECORDING

The last method for invasive recording of SSpEPs involves placement of needle-recording electrodes into the interspinous ligament both rostral and caudal to the operative field.[35] Dinner and colleagues reviewed their overall experience with spinal cord monitoring in 220 patients using both noninvasive and invasive techniques.[36] Interspinous recordings were performed in 100 of these patients and obtained reproducible, stable, high-amplitude recordings.

Generator Sites of SSEPs

Although SSEPs were first described in 1947, there remains considerable debate on the putative generator sites of the various evoked potential peaks. Much of the knowledge regarding generators in humans has been inferred from indirect evidence.[37] This includes analysis of surface waveforms, calculation of conduction velocities made in peripheral nerves and extrapolated to the central nervous system (allowing adjustments for fiber size and length), transmission across synapses, and the effects of various lesions on specific evoked potential peaks.

The potentials recorded using standard techniques are of two basic types: near-field and far-field potentials. Near-field potentials are recorded from electrodes in close proximity to the generator source of the potential, whereas far-field potentials are recorded from electrodes relatively remote from the potential source. Near-field potentials have an amplitude that is maximal near the generator site and attenuates as the electrode is moved farther from the source. In contrast, far-field potentials have an amplitude and morphology that remains relatively constant regardless of electrode position.[38]

COMPONENTS OF THE MEDIAN NERVE SSEP

Following electrical stimulation of the median nerve at the wrist, widely distributed scalp electrodes record a series of peaks for approximately 18 milliseconds. These peaks represent far-field potentials generated from remote sites within the nervous system.

With the use of noncephalic reference, the initial scalp recorded positive peak (P9) is the far-field representation of the afferent volley traversing the brachial plexus.[37,39] Immediately following P9, Emerson and Pedley noted that two negative peaks can be detected, N10 and N12.[37] The scalp N10 far-field potential coincides with a traveling wave that can be recorded simultaneously from a series of electrodes placed over the anterior border of the sternocleido-

Rt median N. Stimulation

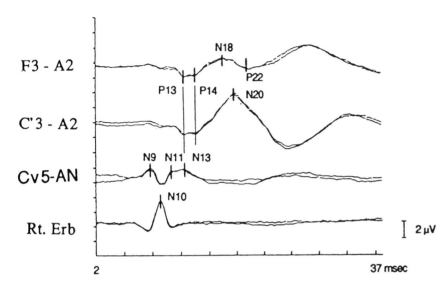

Figure 5–2. The recommended four-channel SEP recording following stimulation of the right median nerve at the wrist. P13 and P14 are present in both the F_3 and C'_3 electrodes. F_3 also registers N18. N20 from C'_3 peaks slightly later than N18 recorded from F_3. N9, N11, and N13 are recorded from Cv5-AN. Although P13 from F_3 or C'_3 and N13 from Cv5-AN may represent slightly different generators, their latencies are very close. N10 from right Erb's point occurs between N9 and N11 of the Cv5-AN recording.

mastoid muscle. This traveling wave or proximal plexus volley represents passage of the impulse through either the plexus or cervical roots proximal to Erb's point.[37] Approximately 2 milliseconds following N10, a second negative deflection, N12, is recorded from the scalp electrodes. This peak corresponds to a second traveling wave that can be recorded simultaneously from another series of electrodes placed in a caudal-to-rostral direction over the cervical spinous processes. This traveling wave is the dorsal column volley (DCV). Because the far-field N12 coincides with the arrival of the DCV at C1, it is believed that N12 represents a presynaptic potential prior to the DCV terminating in the nucleus cuneatus.[37]

The peaks just described are all derived from passage of the volley through white-matter pathways. Following these waves, a small positive deflection (P13) can be recorded. This peak corresponds to a fixed or stationary potential (P13–N13) that can be recorded from a ring of electrodes placed around the neck. This potential is believed to be generated by postsynaptic activity in the nucleus cuneatus.[37,40]

The next peak is a clear-cut positive potential (P14) that is recorded at all scalp locations. This peak is believed to correspond to the rostral passage of the afferent volley through the medial lemniscus.[37] Following P14, a negative peak, N18, can be recorded from all scalp electrodes, although N18 is best delineated at the frontal and ipsilateral central electrode positions. The widespread distribution of N18 is characteristic of a far-field potential. Lesions of the thalamus that have resulted in preservation of N18 with loss of subsequent components support the belief that N18 is generated rostral to the thalamus (Fig 5–2).

The earliest localized scalp potential is N20, which is recorded from a relatively restricted area from the parietal region contralateral to the stimulated side.[37] Most investigators favor a cortical origin for this potential. Recording elec-

trodes placed anterior and posterior to the central sulcus have demonstrated that this peak behaves as an electrical dipole, with the negative peak oriented posteriorly on the Rolandic sulcus corresponding to Brodman's area 3.[41]

COMPONENTS OF POSTERIOR TIBIAL NERVE SSEPS

Following stimulation of the PTN at the ankle, a series of waveforms can be recorded from electrodes placed over the spine. These waves can be identified based on their spatial, temporal, and physiological characteristics as follows: (1) N22, lumbar potential; (2) traveling negative wave, plexus volley; (3) dorsal column volley (DCV); and (4) N29 cervical potential.[42]

The first negative peak, N22, has a relatively restricted spatial distribution. Its amplitude is maximal between 5 and 15 cm rostral to the L4 spinous process; this region corresponds to the dorsal root entry zone for the roots subserving the PTN. This potential is believed to be generated by interneuron activity in the dorsal gray horn of the cord based on studies of the refractory period of this peak using a paired stimulus paradigm with various interstimulus intervals.[42] The second negative peak recorded over the spine is the DCV. This potential is a traveling wave similar to that recorded from median nerve stimulation. Using sequential electrodes, it can be traced from the sacral to cervical region and is of constant conduction velocity.[42] At recording sites over the sacral spine, this wave and N22 are distinguished as separate peaks. At sacral levels, this traveling wave corresponds to the proximal plexus volley being conducted through the lumbosacral plexus and nerve roots. This traveling wave merges into N22 in the lumbar region and subsequently reemerges as a distinct wave over the thoracic spine, which represents the continuing DCV.

At cervical levels, the DCV from PTN stimulation merges into a fixed negative potential, the cervical N29 potential,

4 Ch. Tibial SEP Recording

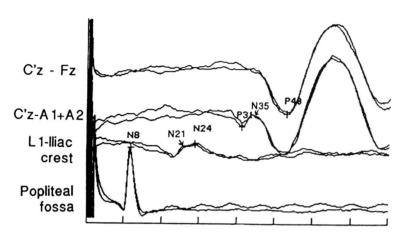

C'z - Fz

C'z-A 1+A 2

L 1-Iliac crest

Popliteal fossa

N8   N21   N24   P31   N35   P40

Figure 5–3. The recommended four-channel tibial SEP recording with the electrode derivations shown to the left. $C'_z = A_1 + A_2$ demonstrates the P31 and P40 peaks. P31 is equivalent to the median P14, and is thought to be generated in the brainstem. P31 is not seen in the $C'_z = F_z$ derivation because of the equipotential between the C'_z and F_z electrodes. The interpeak latency between the N24 peak recorded from the L1 spine and P31 represents a close approximation of the spinal cord conduction time.

which has a maximal amplitude over the second cervical spine.[42] The long refractory period of N29, limited distribution, and location support the belief that this peak is generated from synaptic activity in the nucleus gracilis.[42] Following synapse in the nucleus gracilis, the volley continues rostrally in the medial lemniscus to the cortex with an intervening synapse in the thalamus. Cortical potentials are generally recorded approximately 37 and 45 milliseconds following PTN stimulation. A typical four-channel tibial nerve SSEP is shown in Figure 5–3. The various evoked potential peaks and their generators are summarized in Table 5–2.

Clinical Correlations of Intraoperative Monitoring
The utility of intraoperative monitoring is grounded in the belief that irreversible changes in SSEPs are predictive of new postoperative neurological deficits, whereas lack of change correlates with a good neurological outcome. Various studies, both experimental and clinical, have confirmed this belief.[20,33,43–52]

Koht et al successfully monitored SSEPs in 381 (97%) of 395 patients undergoing surgery for a variety of spinal

pathologies. Acute SSEP alterations were detected in 124 (33%) patients.[47] Just over one third (34%) of these events were causally related to technical, anesthetic, or physiological factors and in all instances were reversible and not associated with new deficits. The remaining 82 events were related to surgical manipulation such as passage of sublaminar wires, spinal distraction, and graft insertion. Seventy-four of the surgically related alterations resolved and resulted in no additional neurological deficits. However, all eight patients in whom there were irreversible SSEP changes developed new neurological deficits. There were no false-negative cases in this series.

Dinner and coworkers monitored intraoperative SSEPs in 220 patients and correlated SSEP alterations with postoperative outcome.[46] The authors found a true negative correlation between SSEPs and outcome in 209 (95%) patients (ie, SSEPs were unchanged and there was no change in neurological status). Significant SSEP deterioration occurred in seven (3%) patients; in four of these individuals, there was no change in neurological status (false-positive), whereas in three patients irreversible SSEP alterations were associated

Table 5–2. Generator Sites of SSEP Peaks.

PEAK	GENERATOR
Median	
P9	Brachial plexus
N13	Cervical cord
P14	Brainstem
N18	Rostral to thalamus
N20	Primary somatosensory cortex
Posterior tibial	
N22	Dorsal root entry zone
N24	Conus medullaris
P31	Brainstem
P37 (P40)	Primary somatosensory cortex

with new motor deficits (true-positive). Significantly, four (2%) patients suffered new postoperative deficits despite preservation of intraoperative SSEPs (false-negative). In this series of 220 patients, significant SSEP alterations were associated with a high incidence of neurological deficit (three of seven patients, 43%). On the other hand, in patients without SSEP changes, the risk of neurological deficit was less than 2% (4 of 213 patients, 1.8%).

Jones et al retrospectively analyzed the results of epidural spinal cord monitoring in 410 unselected patients who underwent posterior instrumentation and fusion.[45] Twenty-four (6%) developed significant SSEP alterations; one quarter of these patients suffered a new neurological deficit. There were no instances of false-positive recordings in this series.

Brown and Nash analyzed the monitoring change and postoperative status of 137 consecutive cases of posterior spinal fusion and instrumentation.[20] In 79 (58%) patients, intraoperative recordings were completely unchanged. Of this group, 75 (95%) were neurologically unchanged and 4 (5%) suffered transient sensory deficits that resolved within 2 weeks in all cases. Transient amplitude deterioration (40 patients, 29%) and transient latency increases (14 patients, 10%) were associated with short-lived new sensory problems postoperatively in three and two patients, respectively. In four patients, SSEPs demonstrated a greater than 50% decrease in amplitude and–or 3-millisecond increase in latency that persisted until the end of the procedure; all of these patients awoke with a new major neurological deficit. From these data Brown and colleagues drew the following conclusions: (1) Significant irreversible alterations of intraoperative SSEPs are uniformly associated with major neurological deficits; (2) there is a low incidence (3.7%) of false-negative intraoperative recordings; and (3) there exists a "gray zone" in which intraoperative SSEP changes occur but are resolving toward baseline by the end of the procedure. In these instances, there may be a higher incidence of postoperative deficits that tend to be minor and transient.

Although it would appear that SSEPs are indeed reliable indicators of spinal cord function, it is apparent from the foregoing discussion that problems do exist. False-positive alterations are not uncommon. Although the majority of these changes can usually be related to a nonsurgical problem and corrected, the occasional persistence of an SSEP abnormality is unsettling, especially when nonsurgical causes have been eliminated. In such cases it may be appropriate to perform a wake-up test to ensure that the patient is neurologically unchanged. Even more concerning is the occurrence of false-negative recordings.[20,46,53,54] This is one of the major criticisms of using SSEP to monitor motor function. Because SSEPs are primarily conducted through ascending sensory pathways, there is a belief that simultaneous monitoring of descending motor pathways should also be performed. However, many (if not most) of the surgical manipulations that cause significant SSEP deterioration result in global spinal cord dysfunction rather than selective injury to either motor or sensory pathways.

MOTOR EVOKED POTENTIALS

Over the past decade, there has been considerable interest in developing and implementing a technique for monitoring, the motor pathways of the spinal cord. A large measure of credit goes to Levy and colleagues for providing both experimental and clinical investigation into the use of MEPs.[4–6] Subsequently other investigators have provided experimental evidence that MEPs are indeed valuable in predicting motor function and recovery following spinal cord injury.[8,9,55–58]

Techniques of MEP Monitoring

There are three basic techniques of eliciting MEPs in humans; one involves direct stimulation of descending pathways whereas the other two utilize noninvasive stimulation of the motor cortex through the intact scalp.

DIRECT STIMULATION OF MOTOR PATHWAYS

The descending pathways can be stimulated directly using a number of invasive techniques. Levy et al described a method of direct stimulation of the spinal cord between the dentate ligament and the intermediolateral sulcus.[4] This technique is obviously invasive, requiring exposure of the spinal cord. Although this technique may be useful in cases such as intradural tumors, it is not practical or suitable for the majority of surgical procedures in which MEP monitoring is desirable.

Alternatively, the descending pathways can be activated indirectly using epidural stimulation rostral to the surgical site[57,59] (Fig. 5–4). Although reproducible reliable MEPs can be obtained in this manner, there are a number of limitations with this technique. First, stimulating electrodes must be placed rostral to the surgical site; although many procedures provide adequate exposure for this maneuver, in some instances an additional laminotomy may be required. Second, electromyographic responses may be difficult to record in the presence of muscle relaxants. Although muscle relaxants can be titrated such that MEPs can be recorded, the amplitude and morphology of the responses are variable and alterations may be difficult to interpret. This limits the sensitivity of this technique in detecting significant changes. Alternatively, MEPs can be recorded from peripheral nerves although so-called neurogenic MEPs are also not without problems.[3]

TRANSCRANIAL STIMULATION OF THE MOTOR CORTEX

MEPs can also be elicited through noninvasive stimulation of the motor cortex. This can be performed using either electrical[4,60] or magnetic stimulation.[61–63] Although electrical stimulation is technically feasible and produces reliable MEPs, it is painful and is therefore not suitable in awake patients.

Transcranial magnetic stimulation (TMS) is a relatively new technique capable of providing information regarding

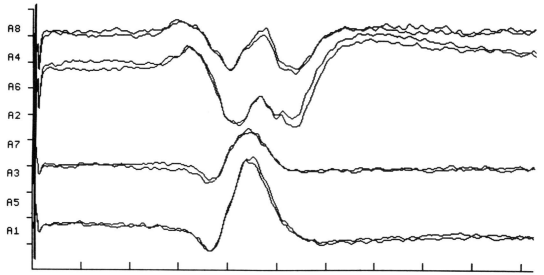

Figure 5–4. Intraoperative MEPs recorded from the quadriceps (upper tracings) and tibialis anterior (lower tracings) following midline epidural stimulation.

the integrity of the descending motor pathways. TMS is performed using a magnetic stimulator. The basic stimulator consists of a high-voltage power source, a storage capacitor, and an electromagnetic coil. The power source charges the storage capacitor; the capacitor is connected to the magnetic coil through a low-resistance circuit. When the circuit between the capacitor and the coil is completed, current flows into the coil and this current produces a time-varying magnetic field. This magnetic field, in turn, generates an induced electrical field. Because the induced electrical field is generated in the brain, which is a conductive medium, current flows within the brain. If the induced current is of sufficient amplitude and–or duration, neuronal depolarization occurs.[64,65]

Following TMS, compound muscle action potentials (CMAPs) or magnetic MEPs can be recorded from electrodes placed over various muscles (Fig. 5–5). Several types of stimulating coils are available; however, for most clinical applications of TMS, a circular or figure-eight coil is used. The typical CMAP typically consists of a triphasic wave between 100 µV and 20 mV. Motor maps depicting optimal stimulation sites for producing responses in individual muscles have been produced, although most often optimal stimulation sites must be determined on an individual basis.[66] However, in normal individuals, response latency to distal upper limb muscles ranges from 19 to 25 milliseconds, with proximal muscles being 5 to 8 milliseconds shorter.

Intraoperative Monitoring Using Magnetic Stimulation

On the surface TMS would appear to be an ideal tool that would complement intraoperative SSEPs. It has the advantage of producing high-amplitude responses that, unlike SSEP, do not require time for signal averaging. Therefore, data are obtained instantaneously. Despite its attractiveness,

there has been relatively little experience to date with this technique for intraoperative monitoring.

Shields and coworkers performed both SSEPs and TMS in 36 patients undergoing surgery for a variety of spinal pathologies, including correction of scoliosis, tumor resection, and intervertebral disk excision.[66] These authors initially noted some difficulty in obtaining reproducible responses intraoperatively. With increasing experience and refinement of the technique, this has become less of a problem.

Zentner performed intraoperative TMS in 50 patients during neurosurgical operations on the spinal cord.[10] During neuroleptanesthesia, reliable responses were obtained from the tibialis anterior in 43 (86%) patients; good responses were also obtained from the thenar muscles in 21 of 24 (88%) patients. Similar to SSEPs, amplitude was found superior to latency as a evaluation criterion for significant intraoperative changes. Intraoperative magnetic MEPs recorded from the tibialis anterior and thenar muscles correctly correlated with postoperative neurological status in 81% and 76% of patients, respectively. Of significance is the lack of any false negative tracings. In every instance the occurrence of a new neurological deficit was associated with a greater than 50% reduction in CMAP amplitude.

Although the experiences of Shields and Zentner are encouraging, they do not yet provide sufficient data to draw meaningful comparisons between the sensitivity and specificity of SSEPs and transcranial magnetic MEPs. They do, however, provide a significant groundwork on which future studies should be based.

SUMMARY AND CONCLUSIONS

Clearly, intraoperative monitoring with somatosensory and motor evoked potentials is an important adjunct for the safe

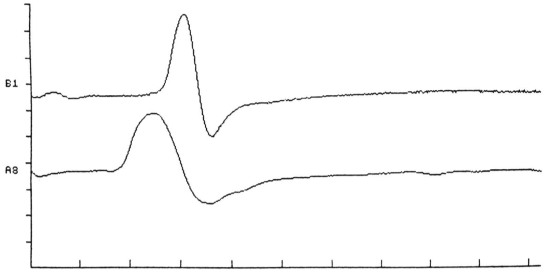

Figure 5–5. Transcranial magnetic motor evoked potentials recorded from the abductor pollicis brevis (upper tracing) and biceps (lower tracing) in a normal awake volunteer.

performance of many neurosurgical procedures involving the spine and spinal cord. An understanding on the part of the surgeon of the indications for monitoring, the electrophysiology of evoked potentials, the techniques involved in the production and interpretation of evoked potentials as well as their limitations is important in optimizing the benefit of both SSEPs and MEPs for intraoperative spinal cord monitoring. SSEPs have been criticized for not providing data regarding motor function; however, this criticism in many instances seems unfounded based on review of the available literature. Indeed, there are rare instances of false-negative SSEP recordings. It is in these cases in particular where MEPs will be helpful in detecting potential spinal cord injury that might otherwise escape detection. As techniques for recording MEPs evolve and improve (especially transcranial magnetic stimulation), intraoperative MEPs will play an increasingly important role in intraoperative monitoring.

REFERENCES

1. Brown RH, Nash CL. Intra-operative spinal cord monitoring. In: Frymoyer JW, ed. *The Adult Spine: Principles and Practice.* New York, NY: Raven Press; 1991:549–563.
2. Dinner DS, Shields RW, Leuders H. Intraoperative Spinal Cord Monitoring. In: Rothman RH, Simeone FA, eds. *The Spine.* Philadelphia, Pa: WB Saunders; 1992:1801–1814.
3. Owen JH. Evoked potential monitoring during spinal surgery. In: Bridwell, KH, DeWald J, eds. *Textbook of Spinal Surgery.* Philadelphia, Pa: JB Lippincott; 1991:31–64.
4. Levy WJ, York DH. Evoked potentials from the motor tract in humans. *Neurosurgery.* 1983;12:422–429.
5. Levy W. The electrophysiological monitoring of motor pathways. *Clin Neurosurg.* 1988;34:239–260.
6. Levy W. Clinical experience with motor and cerebellar evoked potential monitoring. *Neurosurgery.* 1987;20:169–182.
7. Owen JH, Laschinger J, Bridwell K, et al. Sensitivity and specificity of somatosensory and neurogenic-motor evoked potentials in animals and humans. *Spine.* 1988;13:1111–1118.
8. Boyd SG, et al. Monitoring spinal motor tract function using cortical stimulation: A preliminary report. In: Schramm J, Jones SJ, eds. *Spinal Cord Monitoring.* Heidelberg: Springer-Verlag; 1985;227–230.
9. Boyd SG, et al. A method of monitoring function in corticospinal pathways during scoliosis surgery with a note on motor conduction velocities. *J Neurol Neurosurg Psychiatr.* 1986;49:251–257.
10. Zentner J. Noninvasive motor evoked potential monitoring during neurosurgical operations on the spinal cord. *Neurosurgery.* 1989;24:709–712.
11. Grundy BL. Monitoring of sensory evoked potentials during neurosurgical operations: methods and applications. *Neurosurgery.* 1982;11:556–575.
12. Giblin DR. Somatosensory evoked potentials in healthy subjects and in patients with lesions of the central nervous system. *Ann NY Acad Sci.* 1964;112:93–142.
13. Halliday AM, Wakefield GS. Cerebral evoked potentials in patients with dissociated sensory loss. *J Neurol Neurosurg Psychiatr.* 1963;26:211–219.
14. Powers SK, Bolger CA, Edwards MS. Spinal cord pathways mediating somatosensory evoked potentials. *J Neurosurg.* 1982;57:472–482.
15. Ducati A, Schiepatti M. Spinal pathways mediating somatosensory evoked potentials from cutaneous and muscle nerves in the cat. *Acta Neurochir.* 1980;52:99–104.
16. Schiepatti M, Ducati A. Effects of stimulus intensity, cervical cord tractotomies, and cerebellectomy on somatosensory evoked potentials from skin and muscle afferents in the cat hind limb. *Electroencephalogr Clin Neurophysiol.* 1981;51:363–372.
17. Tsuji S, et al. Effect of stimulus intensity on subcortical and cortical somatosensory evoked potentials by posterior tibial nerve stimulation. *Electroencephalogr Clin Neurophysiol.* 1984;59:229–237.
18. Kellway P. An orderly approach to visual analysis. Parameters of normal EEG in adults and children. In: Klass D, Daley DD, eds. *Current Practice of Clinical Electroencephalography.* New York: Raven Press; 1979:73.
19. Jasper HH. Report of Committee on Methods of Clinical Examination in EEG. Appendix: the ten-twenty electrode sys-

quires autogeneic bone marrow before bone forms around the demineralized or undemineralized implants. The argument that demineralized bone is osteoinductive in humans comes by extrapolation from studies on rabbits and rodents.[20,21] Whereas demineralized bone has not been proven osteoinductive in the dog and monkey,[22,23] Ripamonti has demonstrated that it is inductive in the baboon.[24–26] Credible scientific evidence that demineralized powders are osteoinductive in humans has not been presented. Aspenberg injected himself intramuscularly with demineralized powder, and the implant resorbed.[22]

MORPHOLOGICAL ASPECTS OF BONE-GRAFT REPAIR

Autografts

Autogeneic cancellous and cortical bone heal with similar histological transformations during the first 2 weeks after grafting.[2,12] A blood clot initially surrounds the graft, following which an inflammatory response occurs and vascular buds penetrate through existing Volkmann's or haversian canals of the graft. Mesenchymal cells accompany the vessels. Vascularization is complete within 2 weeks in cancellous bone and in 1 to 2 months in autogeneic cortical bone. In cancellous bone, osteoblasts deposit osteoid over existing trabeculae and strengthen the necrotic central core, which is later remodeled. In cortical bone, the devitalized matrix releases BMP. First, blood-borne, marrow-derived monocytoid cells (homing action) become osteoclasts that cause resorption of necrotic bone. After this, appositional new bone forms on the margins of the resorption cavities.[4] Strength of human cortical bone through resorption is reduced by 50% during the first 6 months and is regained gradually over the next 1 to 2 years. In cortical bone, 50% to 60% of the original donor bone remains and is as strong as viable new bone.

Allografts

Unprocessed fresh allografts are never transplanted in humans in that contained cells and matrix proteins would provoke a severe immunogenic response by the host. Removal of cells followed by freezing or freeze drying reduces the antigenicity of the graft.

Incorporation of a processed allograft initially follows that of an autograft. By the end of the first week, an inflammatory response occurs, peaks in the second week, and continues for 2 months.[2,12] Chronic inflammation can ensue for several months, interfering with revascularization. The allograft subsequently remodels or, in the presence of greater genetic dissimilarity, is surrounded by fibrous tissue or resorbs.

Whereas the autograft most likely remodels through both osteoinductive and osteoconductive mechanisms, the allograft heals most likely in dogs, monkeys (including baboons), and humans primarily by osteoconduction.[4,22–24] Through the years, efforts have been made to improve the incorporation of an allograft. Freezing and freeze-drying

techniques arrest enzymatic digestion of the graft and reduce immunogenicity. Cells are removed mechanically and/or killed by freezing. The bone matrix has further been demineralized partially or in total to expose BMP. Whereas demineralized bone powder is osteoinductive in heterotopic sites in the rodent model, osteoinduction in dogs, monkeys, and humans requires BMP and autogeneic bone marrow.[4] Demineralization results in greater elasticity of bone matrix but also promotes greater resorption in primates.

Choice of a Graft

The fresh autograft is superior to all others because it contains viable cells and undenatured matrix, is genetically identical with the recipient, and retains its biomechanical properties. It will most likely be remodeled and thereby achieve the osteosynthetic goals of the surgeon. It should be used where the recipient site lacks corticocancellous surfaces rich in osteogenic cells, where the blood supply is sparse, and where tensile strain predominates.[27,28] Fresh autogeneic corticocancellous bone must be the primary graft for posteolateral spinal applications. Allogeneic cancellous bone may be used to augment the supply of fresh autograft.

Satisfactory quantity and quality of autogeneic bone may be lacking in children, patients with multiple operations, or in the older, osteopenic adult. Moreover, there are consequences the patient must accept in opting for an autograft: donor site pain and the possibility of wound hernia, pelvic fracture, instability, nerve damage, hemorrhage, etc.

Under such circumstances allograft or bank bone may be preferable. Although there is a 1- to 2-month delay in incorporation, properly processed allogeneic bone may be used in cervical, thoracic, and lumbar interbody applications where compressive loading of the allograft results in an identical fusion rate with that attained with autogeneic bone.[29–31] The cancellous bone of the vertebrae provides an optimal source of vessels and osteogenic bone marrow components to remodel the allograft with a fusion rate comparable to the autograft. Even in posterolateral fusions with internal fixation in scoliosis surgery and in bone cysts, allografts have been used successfully.[32–39]

SAFETY OF ALLOGENEIC BONE

Although the efficacy of allografts has been demonstrated consistently, their safety has been questioned mostly since the advent of AIDS. Bacterial infection due to transplantation of contaminated bone is uncommon. Tomford et al reported an infection rate of 5% in 324 culture-negative, aseptically procured unsterilized allografts.[40] One case of hepatitis from frozen bone was reported in 1954 in a Yale medical student.[41] Another case of frozen-bone–transmitted hepatitis C virus has been well documented in 1992.[42] Tuberculosis was transmitted from infected rib allografts about 40 years ago.[43]

HIV-1 can be recovered from bone, bone marrow, and

7 Cervical Spine Stabilization with Flexible, Multistrand Cable System

Setti S. Rengachary, M.D., Derek A. Duke, M.D.

INTRODUCTION

Internal stabilization utilizing heavy-gauge monofilament wire and bone has been one of the oldest techniques used in the management of the unstable spine, especially the cervical spine. This technique has been a time-tested and simple procedure offering good results. However, monofilament wire has several disadvantages.[1–3] First, the wires tend to break over time. Generally, this occurs at a point near the base of the wire twist. It is believed that during the twisting of the wire, a stress riser is created immediately below the twist. This is confirmed by the fact that wire breaks occur virtually invariably at this point. Second, because heavy-gauge monofilament wires (16- or 18-gauge wires) are stiff; there is a risk of canal intrusion with the possibility of dural tears and injury to the neural structures during sublaminar passage. When the wires are left in over time, they may cause pressure necrosis of the dura and can exert pressure on the spinal cord itself. During removal of the broken wires or during the removal of hardware that was held by wires, there is additional risk of damage to the dura by the cut or broken ends of the wire.

The introduction of a highly flexible, multistrand, stainless steel cable system by Songer and associates represents a significant advance in the use of the wire fusion technique.[4] The major advantage of the multistrand cable over the monofilament wire is the higher strength. Biomechanical testing has shown that the static strength of stainless steel cable loop was 2.85 times greater than a steel monofilament wire loop. Fatigue testing has shown that the stainless steel cables require anywhere from 6 to 22 times more cycles before failure than the steel wire. Thus, when implanted, the cable system is likely to last much longer under greater loads than monofilament wire. Flexibility is another major advantage of cable over monofilament wire. The multistrand cables are much softer and highly flexible. This advantage is particularly felt during sublaminar passage. Because of the pliability, there is less risk of injury to the dura and the spinal cord. In addition, when the sublaminar construct has been completed, the wire tends to follow the contour of the inner surface of the lamina rather than forming a convex loop under it. Thus, canal intrusion is minimal with sublaminar cable. Because the cable surface is smooth and the cable

end has only a single, soft, pliable lead wire, there is less risk of damage to the gloves and fingers by the sharp end of the wire. Because the cable system is designed to be tightened and anchored with a crimp system, no twisting of the cable is required, unlike monofilament wire; thus, there are no stress risers. The stress is distributed uniformly throughout the cable in the construct. In addition, the cable system has been designed in a manner in which one can obtain a reproducible, known tension within the cable. Thus, one can tailor the tension depending on the quality of the bone and the type of construct.

INSTRUMENTATION

Cables

DOUBLE CABLE

The double cable is meant primarily for sublaminar constructs. It consists of two 49-strand 316L stainless steel cables welded to a single, flexible, 3-in leader. Titanium cables have been introduced recently. The leader portion is passed underneath the laminae by utilizing one of the several standard techniques. Generally, it consists of either passing the lead wire in the shape of a C or L curve under the laminae or in the shape of an L curve. The loop of the leader is then drawn out with a nerve hook and pulled through. An alternative technique is to pass a guide suture utilizing an aneurysm needle or a suture needle passed in the reverse. The guide suture is then pulled under the laminae and the leader loop is tied to the guide suture and pulled under the laminae. Regardless of the technique used, once the sublaminar passage has been completed, the tip of the leader is cut, separating the two cables, one under each lamina. The leader is then passed through the loop or eyelet, thus forming a noose. The noose can be placed around either a bone graft or a Luque rod. A crimp is then threaded into the free end of the cable. Using the tensioner crimper, the crimp is compressed and the excess cable is cut.

SINGLE CABLE WITH BAR OR SINGLE CABLE WITH CRIMP

The single cable is designed primarily to form a cerclage around a flat surface. It is generally used with a bar. The leader wire is passed through the bar to the end of the cable. The cable is then wrapped around the bony construct and tightened with the tensioner crimper. A crimp is applied in the manner described earlier and the excess cable is cut off. A minor variation of the single cable is a new single cable with an eyelet leader.

Tensioner Crimper

The tensioner crimper is a device that holds a crimp between its jaws. The lead wire is then threaded through the crimp and drawn back through an opening in the tensioner and secured with a set screw. A torque wrench is attached to the hexnut of the tensioner and the torque is increased until the desired level is reached (generally, 8 to 12 inch pounds). Once the appropriate tension has been achieved, the crimp is compressed and the excess cable is cut off with the cutter. The cutter is designed such that it will cut either on the end or on the side.

The crimp inserter is a pencil-shaped instrument that helps to hold the crimp and load it into the tensioner crimper.

CONSTRUCTS

High Cervical Constructs

High cervical constructs are generally utilized to correct upper-cervical spine instability, such as unstable fractures of the odontoid or atlantoaxial subluxation. The most popular construct is a modified Gallie construct (Fig. 7–1). For this technique, a single cable or one arm of a double cable can be used. The cable is folded in half gently and the cable loop is then passed under the lamina of C1. The loop of the cable that appears in the top of the C1 laminae is then pulled through and folded under the spinous process of C2. The inferior cortical surface of C1 and the superior surface of C2 laminae are then decorticated. A form-fitting bone graft is then impacted between the C1 arch and C2 posterior elements. The ends of the cable are then brought around under

the spinous process once again and, depending on whether a single cable or one arm of a double cable is used, either a bar or top hat is applied and tensioning and crimping are performed. Excess cable is cut off. Additional cancellous bone can be packed around the posterior arch of C1 and posterior elements of C2.

In an alternate technique, sublaminar cable passage under the laminae of C2 and C1 is carried out starting at the inferior border of the laminae of C2 (Fig. 7–2). This is done in two stages. A guide suture is pulled under the lamina of C2 and brought out in the space between C1 and C2. It is then passed again under the lamina of C1 and brought out at the superior border of C1. The leader cable, which has been bent to conform to the undersurface of the laminae, is secured to the guide suture. The cable is passed under the laminae, maintaining tension with the guide suture at all times. The tip of the double cable leader is sectioned, separating the double cable into individual half strands. Decortication of the inferior border of C1 and the superior border of C2 laminae is completed. Two triangular pieces of bone grafts are wedged between C1 and C2 laminae bilaterally (Brooks technique). Each cable is tightened by passing the leader wire through the ipsilateral eyelet, and then the cable is cinched down and crimped. Similar maneuvers are carried out on the opposite cable. Excess cable is cut off.

Mid and Lower Cervical Constructs

A representative example of this construct is triple-cable spinous process fixation. For this procedure, one single cable and one double cable are used. We will assume that the spinous process of C5, C6, and C7 requires stabilization. Holes are created at the bases of the spinous processes of the identified vertebrae. A single cable leader is passed through the midspinous process, namely the spinous process of C6,

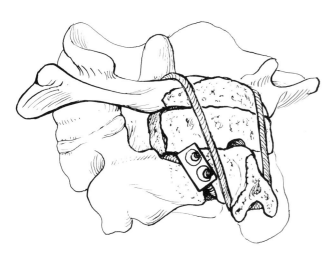

Figure 7–1. C1 to C2 fusion (modified Gallie technique) using the multistrand steel cable/crimp system.

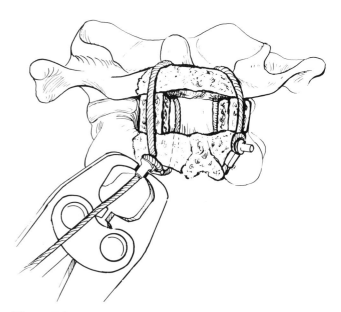

Figure 7–2. C1 to C2 fusion—an alternate technique (Brooks fusion).

and looped under the spinous process of C7. The leader wire is brought through the cross bar and cinched down; a top hat is applied and crimped. This initial single cable fixates C6 and C7. After completion of this wire loop, the C5 and C7 cables are introduced in an opposing fashion. The leader of the individual half of the double cable is passed sequentially through bone graft, spinous process hole, and then bone graft again in that order. The leader is passed through the ipsilateral eyelet. A top hat is applied to one side and crimped. Another top hat is applied to the opposite side and crimped after final cinching is completed (Fig. 7–3).

Total Cervical Constructs

A total cervical spine construct is best exemplified by the application of Luque loops to stabilize the cervical spine after extensive decompressive laminectomy (Fig. 7–4). This procedure involves a laminectomy from C3 to C7 for the treatment of cervical spondylitic myelopathy. After the laminectomy is completed, a Luque loop is placed over the laminae of C2 and between the spinous processes of T2 and T3. The Songer cables are then passed sublaminarly under C2 at the superior end and under T1 and T2 at the inferior end and anchored to the Luque loop. This offers a rigid construct that immobilizes the spine from C2 to T2.

PRECAUTIONS

The crimp can be applied only in one direction. The hat should be pointed inferiorly toward the construct. It cannot be applied backward. The leader wire is strictly used as a leader and should not be used as part of the construct. The tension in the cable should be optimum depending on the

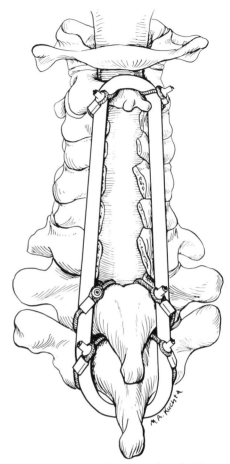

Figure 7–4. Extensive stabilization using the Luque loop and sublaminar cables.

strength of the bone. Excessive tension in an osteoporotic bone will risk cutting through the bone. In the cervical spine, 8 to 12 inch pounds is recommended. Premature compression of the top hat will make it difficult to slide the crimp along the wire and thus should be avoided. A badly kinked leader wire will make crimp passage difficult as well, so the leader wire should be kept as nonkinked as possible. The leader wire should not be cut off flush with the cable before applying the crimp. This will make the application of the crimp impossible.

REFERENCES

1. Schrader WC, Bethem D, Scerbin V. The chronic local effects of sublaminar wires. An animal model. *Spine.* 1988;13:499–502.
2. Johnston CE, Happel LT, Norris R, et al. Delayed paraplegia complicating sublaminar segmental spinal instrumentation. *J Bone Joint Surg.* 1986;68A:556–1209.
3. Bernard TN, Johnston CE, Roberts JM, et al. Late complications due to wire breakage in segmental spinal instrumentation. Report of two cases. *J Bone and Joint Surg.* 1983;65A:-1339–1345.
4. Songer MN, Spencer DL, Meyer PR, et al. The use of sublaminar cables to replace Luque wires. *Spine.* 1991;16-(suppl):S418–S421.

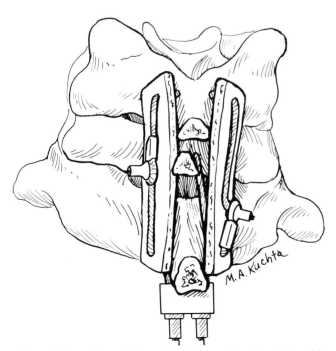

Figure 7–3. C5 to C6 to C7 fusion using the triple-cable technique.

8 Occipitocervical Fusions: Indications, Technique, and Avoidance of Complication

Arnold H. Menezes, M.D.

INTRODUCTION

The craniovertebral junction (CVJ) is structurally a composite of many bony and ligamentous structures; yet functionally, it is a stable, interlocking unit that acts as a transition between the skull and the spine. It allows for extension, flexion, and lateral rotation of the head. The geometry of the articular surfaces provides for mobility, and stability is provided for by the muscular and ligamentous attachments that span the skull and the cervical spine.[1] This versatile function necessitates numerous synovial joints; and this, together with the complex mobility of the region, makes the occipitoatlantoaxial complex vulnerable to traumatic injury as well as diseases affecting the synovial joints, such as rheumatoid arthritis and the vast number of vasculitides.[2,3]

The early surgical treatment of pathology at the cranioverteb ral junction was via posterior decompression and, at times, an occipitocervical or atlantoaxial fusion.[4,5] Thus, posterior cervical and high cervical fusions were attempted because of the ease of operative exposure and large bony recipient surface areas that could be spanned.

TYPES OF OCCIPITOCERVICAL FUSION

A number of innovations have been described subsequent to the initial description by Foerster in 1927 of the use of fibu-lar graft for occipitocervical fusion in the management of trauma (see Table 8–1). The modifications to the original technique involve the choice of grafting material, placement of stabilizing wires, use of methyl methacrylate, and craniocervical instrumentation.[7–13]

Incorporation of the occiput in a craniocervical fusion has serious implications because of the loss of motion segments, which interferes with a patient's ability to handle everyday life. The occipitoatlantoaxial dorsal fixation eliminates 25° of flexion and extension and the first 40° of lateral rotation, which normally occurs between the atlas and the axis.[1,14] Occipitoatlantoaxial instability may be more common than generally recognized within certain patient populations, such as the patient with rheumatoid arthritis, ankylosing spondylitis, or congenital and developmental abnormalities.

Occipitocervical fusions may be categorized into the anterior and posterior varieties. In the anterior approach, the most promising technique appears to be bone grafting between the clivus, the anterior arch of the atlas, and the axis body after a transoral surgical procedure or after a lateral extrapharyngeal approach to the anterior craniocervical border.[15,16] However, this procedure, unless accompanied by a dorsal fixation, would still allow a toggle effect to take place between the clivus and the upper cervical spine bridged by the bone graft. In addition, unpublished reports substantiate a significant incidence of abscess formation and infection

Table 8–1. Types of Occipitocervical Fusion.

I. Anterior	A. Bone graft between clivus, the anterior arch of the atlas, and the axis body (eg, after transoral surgery)
	B. Wire fixation of clivus to C1 anterior arch and C2 body; embedded in methyl methacrylate
II. Posterior	A. Bone grafts
	1. Dorsal occipitointerlaminar C1 to C2 fusion
	2. Dorsal lateral occiput/C1 to C2 facet fusion
	3. Methyl methacrylate in addition to A1 and A2
	4. Midline occiput to C2 spinous process bone strut fusion
	B. Instrumentation
	1. Contoured loop fixation between occiput-posterior C1 arch and C2 to C3 with bone supplement
	2. Plate fixation with occipital midline screws and C1, C2 facet screws with inverted Y plate

with the free bone graft, although this is surprising considering that maxillofacial surgical procedures are carried out through a contaminated area without any problems.

Wire fixation of the clivus to the anterior arch of C1 and C2 has been utilized via the extrapharyngeal route, embedding the wire mesh in methyl methacrylate.[17] The posterior route of dorsal occipitocervical fixation employing bone grafts and methyl methacrylate, as well as contoured loop instrumentation, appears to be the most tried and successful.[6,12,18,19] This chapter will deal with dorsal occipitocervical fusion utilizing bone grafts and wire and supplemented in specific conditions with methyl methacrylate, and at times with a threaded contoured loop custom fitted between the occiput and the posterior arches of C1, C2, and C3.

Between 1977 and 1982, 716 patients underwent surgical treatment for osseous pathology at the craniocervical border (surgery performed by the author). Of these, 256 had irreducible ventral pathology that led to an anterior transpharyngeal or transmaxillary decompression and 218 patients were felt to be unstable. These underwent dorsal occipitocervical fixation. Sixty-nine other patients had an unstable craniocervical junction that required dorsal occipitocervical fixation after a posterior fossa and upper cervical decompression. Two hundred and four other individuals had a reducible basilar invagination or cranial settling that was treated with dorsal occipitocervical fixation. These 491 patients form the basis of the discussion in this chapter.

INDICATIONS FOR OCCIPITOCERVICAL FUSION

The complex pathology requiring occipitocervical fixation makes enumeration of each individual entity impossible.[20] The 491 patients who underwent dorsal occipitocervical fu-

sion by the author at the University of Iowa hospitals and clinics over a 14-year period form the basis of Table 8–2. This is divided into the congenital, the developmental, and the acquired lesions. The most common indication for dorsal occipitocervical fixation was rheumatoid cranial settling, followed closely by primary basilar invagination and congenital and developmental phenomena. The author believes that traumatic occipitocervical dislocation in the adult (past the age of 12) should undergo occipitocervical fixation with relative urgency, especially in the vertical and posterior occipitocervical dislocations. Complex craniovertebral junction fractures involving the atlas and the axis may require spanning of these by incorporating the occiput in the fixation. Approximately 80% of individuals undergoing a transoral operation for irreducible ventral craniocervical junction pathology will require dorsal occipitocervical fixation. The inflammatory states such as psoriasis, pseudogout, inflammatory ileitis, and Grisel's syndrome may cause gross ligamentous destruction and laxity, and immobilization alone for 8 to 12 weeks will not allow for bony or ligamentous reconstitution; thus, an early fusion should be undertaken.

The primary malignancies affecting the craniovertebral junction, such as chordomas of the clivus, invariably have involvement of the occipital condyles leading to severe occipital headaches. Plasmacytomas and osteoblastomas likewise have been recognized in this region, and a fusion procedure is essential. Our experience with metastatic breast disease to the atlas and the axis vertebrae has led us to believe that these individuals lead a precarious life. In the majority of circumstances, the patient has already undergone focal radiation therapy to this area or will require it after the fixation. Thus, it is essential that these individuals be stabilized using a custom-built contoured loop device to anchor

Table 8–2. Indications for Occipitocervical Fusion.

A. Congenital:	1. Anterior and posterior bifid arches of C1
	2. Absent occipital condyles
B. Developmental:	1. Severe reducible basilar invagination
	2. Unstable dystopic os odontoideum
	3. Unilateral atlas assimilation with chronic rotary C0 to C1 to C2 luxation
C. Acquired:	1. Traumatic C0 to C1 dislocation (especially vertical and posterior occipitocervical)
	2. Complex CVJ fractures of C1 to C2
	3. Reducible rheumatoid cranial settling
	4. After transoral CVJ decompression
	5. Cranial settling in ankylosing spondylitis, psoriasis, pseudogout, Down's syndrome, inflammatory ileitis
	6. Inflammatory disease—chronic Grisel's syndrome
	7. Primary malignancies affecting the craniovertebral junction (CVJ) (eg, chordoma of clivus and occipital bone, plasmacytoma, osteoblastoma, chondroma, neurofibromatosis)
	8. Secondary metastatic disease affecting the CVJ (eg, breast metastasis)

and stabilize the occiput to the upper cervical spine. This is described in greater detail in Chapter 10.

The failure to incorporate the occiput in the rheumatoid cranial settling, as well as in the unstable dystopic os odontoideum, has led to disasters. This is because the actual pathology involves an occipitocervical dislocation, and a less than adequate operation is performed in an attempt to limit the fusion to the atlantoaxial joint.

PREOPERATIVE MANAGEMENT

The primary treatment for reducible craniocervical junction lesions is stabilization.[21] Surgical decompression is performed on patients with irreducible pathology. When irreducible lesions are encountered, the decompression is performed in the manner in which encroachment occurs. If a ventral encroachment is present, an anterior decompression is mandated. With dorsal compression, a posterior approach is advisable; and if instability exists following either situation, a posterior fixation is essential.

The diagnostic procedures performed for evaluating lesions of the craniocervical junction are governed by the factors that will influence treatment. Hence, imaging of the craniocervical junction should first start out with plain anteroposterior and lateral radiographs of the craniocervical border. Imaging of the craniocervical junction is then performed with magnetic resonance imaging (MRI) in the axial, coronal, and sagittal planes. Flexion-extension dynamic views are then obtained in the midsagittal and parasagittal planes. Cervical traction via an MRI-compatible halo is used subsequently to determine the reducibility of the lesion. Detailed imaging of the osseous pathology is best delineated with pleuridirectional tomography or thin, sectioned high-resolution computerized tomography (CT). In selected individuals, vertebral angiography has been utilized to locate abnormal vessels and see the effect of head position on the vasculature. In rare situations, opacification of the subarachnoid space with iohexol and thin-section CT scanning may be essential to identify and locate abnormalities.

It is imperative that the nutritional status of individuals be accessed prior to embarking on surgical treatment. This is especially important in frail, rheumatoid patients who have cranial settling and end-stage disease. Preoperative attention to the nutritional state will help avoid wound complications as well as the occurrence of laryngeal edema and pulmonary problems.

OPERATIVE TECHNIQUE

Preoperative cervical traction is obtained using a Crown halo, with traction utilized at 7 lb to support the head. However, with reducible lesions the traction is maintained at the level at which reduction has been obtained and should not exceed 15 lb in the adult.[2,20]

An awake fiberoptic oral endotracheal intubation is performed by a skilled anesthesiologist utilizing regional block

anesthesia as well as topical anesthesia. Following this, the patient is positioned awake on the operating table, in a prone position with traction maintained. The halo ring rests on a modified Mayfield horseshoe headrest, with traction maintained over a pulley bar to allow for dynamic motion during the operative procedure (Fig. 8–1). A fixation of the halo is to be avoided. This procedure may not be possible in the young individual, and careful positioning during intubation and in turning to a prone position mandates placement in a cervical collar and then positioning. Unfortunately, there has been a trend toward placing these children in a halo vest with the idea that this would protect the patient while both in the prone and supine positions. This is false.

Neurophysiological monitoring, such as utilizing the median nerve evoked responses and recording brainstem latencies, has been tried by the author in over 300 individuals. It has not been useful and is now not performed during craniovertebral junction procedures.

The position of the head and neck is dictated by the preoperative studies that show the last neural compression. The chest is elevated on laminectomy rolls or on a Vince Wilson frame. The neurological status is accessed. After radiographic studies have been performed and positioning adjustments made, general anesthesia ensues. Cervical traction is maintained to allow for the dynamic changes during the operation. A constantly moving mobile traction, which adapts to the patient's position during the operation, is essential.

The posterior cervical region and the scalp are prepared, as is the area for harvesting of donor bone (which is usually the posterior inferior rib cage or the iliac crest). Cephalothin sodium, 1 g every 6 hours, is administered intravenously 12

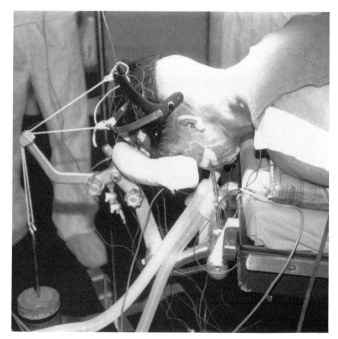

Figure 8–1. Patient positioned for dorsal occipitocervical fusion. The chest is elevated on rolls and the crown halo rests on the horseshoe with traction over a pulley.

hours prior to the start of the operation and maintained for 48 hours after the procedure.

A midline incision from the external occipital protuberance to the spinous process of the fifth cervical vertebra is made. A subperiosteal exposure is obtained of the squamous occipital bone and the posterior arches of the upper three cervical vertebrae. If gross instability is present, a towel clip fixates the spinous process of the axis. This is likewise done to the posterior arch of the atlas when muscle dissection is performed. Stabilization of the operative exposure can be obtained by placing the D'Errico or Miskimon retractors at 90° to each other. This placement stretches and fixates the bone-muscle relationship to prevent motion of the occiput, cervical, and atlantoaxial joints.

It is important that paralyzing agents not be utilized during the operative procedure, especially in unstable situations. This would lead to gross instability and an adverse outcome.

The posterior rim of the foramen magnum is excised using Kerrison-punch rongeurs or a high-speed drill.[22] The decompression is carried upward for about 1.5 cm to remove the exoccipital bony ridge and is carried out laterally for 1 cm. This facilitates the passage of braided wire or soft cable from the laterally placed trephines toward the midline in the occiput (Fig. 8–2A). These trephines are placed 2.5 cm on either side of the midline in the squamous occipital bone, about 1.5 to 2 cm above the foramen magnum. Epidural braided number 22 wire or soft braided cables are passed from the occipital trephine to the midline craniectomy. Similarly, braided wire cable is passed beneath the laminae of the axis vertebra and the atlas vertebra.[23] An unbraided number 20 wire may be passed beneath the lamina of the atlas to prevent the sawlike cutting of the posterior arch of the atlas. This latter may occur in circumstances such as rheumatoid arthritis or with a dystopic os odontoideum.[24,26]

Donor bone is harvested from the rib utilizing full thickness and removing the rib close to the head of the rib to provide a contour that approximates the dorsal surface of the occiput and the upper cervical spine. Decortication of the spinous processes and laminae is essential to the recipient site and the occiput. The donor bone is secured to the occiput, atlas, and axis vertebrae by passing the wires through the graft and transfixing them to anchor them into position (Fig. 8–2B). Matchstick-sized slivers of bone are then packed into the remaining crevasses of the donor-recipient bone complex. A similar technique is utilized when decompressive laminectomies of the atlas and axis are required (Fig. 8–3A). A lateral facet fusion is accomplished to the atlas and the axis vertebrae (Figs. 8–3B and 8–3C).[18] In these situations, an unbraided wire is preferable to prevent destruction of the facets.[20]

In the severely disabled patient, such as those with rheumatoid arthritis, immediate internal stabilization can be obtained by supplementing the bone construct with wire fixation and acrylic.[24] The wires anchoring the bone grafts are preserved for about 1.5 to 2 cm. These are then converted into hooks to act as pegs for the oncoming methyl methacrylate (Fig. 8–4A). The methyl methacrylate is next fashioned into a cigarlike structure before hardening occurs and is then converted into a horseshoe shape, with the horizontal limbs being molded to the occiput and the vertical limbs cascading over the donor bone (Fig. 8–4B). This then envelopes the wire pegs, staying on the dorsal surface of the bone to provide for anchorage and support of the occiput and upper cervical spine. Care is taken to prevent overflow of the methyl methacrylate onto the lateral surfaces of the bone because this is the portion where contact is made with the cervical musculature that brings in the blood supply (Fig. 8–4C).

When a posterior decompression of the posterior fossa and upper cervical spine is accomplished, the fusion is modified as described previously and the fixation of methyl methacrylate is made over this.[24]

Over the past 6 years, when immediate fixation of the occiput to the upper cervical spine was required and the instability was of a severe magnitude (vertical traumatic occipitocervical dislocation, severe dorsal occipitocervical dislocation with rheumatoid basilar invagination), a threaded contoured loop custom fitted to the occiput and upper cervical spine was made and anchored with the wires or cables, as described previously (Fig. 8–5A). It is imperative that the superior horizontal limb of the contoured instrumentation be fixated and supported by cables superiorly and laterally in the occiput. A transverse cross-bar fixation of the descending limbs at an interspace, usually below C2, is essential to augment the biomechanical strength of the construct.[19,26–28] This is then supplemented with bone (Fig. 8–5B).

The wound closure is made in anatomic layers with an interrupted 1–0 polyglycolic suture. No drainage of the wound is necessary. The patient is maintained in skeletal traction for 3 to 4 days after the operation and then placed in a halo vest. This halo immobilization is required for 6 months after occipitoatlantoaxial arthrodesis.[20] Less prolonged immobilization results in nonunion, union in an abnormal position, or additional cranial settling with subsequent increased neurological deficits.[29]

In the severely disabled patient, such as those who have had internal stabilization with methyl methacrylate or the metallic instrumentation, mobilization is effected with a custom-built extended collar for 3 to 4 months, after which fixation and osseous integration of the graft have been recognized.[24]

RESULTS OF OCCIPITOCERVICAL FIXATION

As with any fusion, long-term stability depends on osseous integration between the donor bone and the recipient bone. Internal stabilization may be provided by the methyl methacrylate or metallic instrumentation, but there is always a race between the incorporation of the bone for permanent fusion and the stress fatigue that occurs progressively with

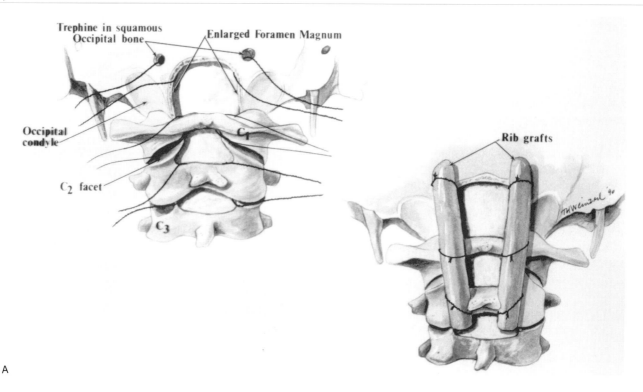

A

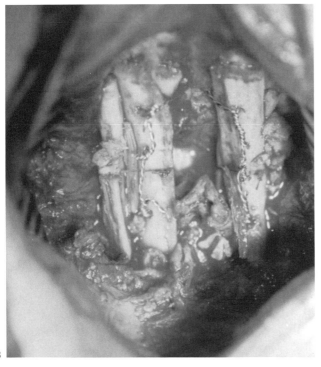

B

Figure 8–2. (**A**). Illustrations on the technique of dorsal occipitocervical fusion. (**B**). Operative photograph of C0 to C2 fusion with braided wire and rib grafts.

time.[30] Thus, both the internal and external stabilization must withstand the stress until complete bony fusion has occurred. Maximum strength of a construct, before complete osseous integration has occurred, is at the time that the construct is placed. Subsequently, there is a loosening and motion of the construct at the fusion site that will increase progressively. Thus, it is common that complications such as pseudoarthrosis, broken wires, graft resorption, nonunion, and loss of alignment can occur when the external immobilization is reduced to 3 months or less.

Ranawat et al reported on 19 individuals who underwent an occipitocervical and atlantoaxial fusion.[31] In their series, there was no improvement in six individuals, and postoperative death occurred in five. Meijers et al performed a fusion in 29 individuals with an operative mortality of 12%.[32] Twenty-one percent showed no improvement. In the series by Conaty and Mongan, 21 individuals underwent an occipitocervical fusion with one perioperative death.[9] A pseudoarthroses occurred in four individuals. A poor result may occur despite "good fusion" as described by Santavirta

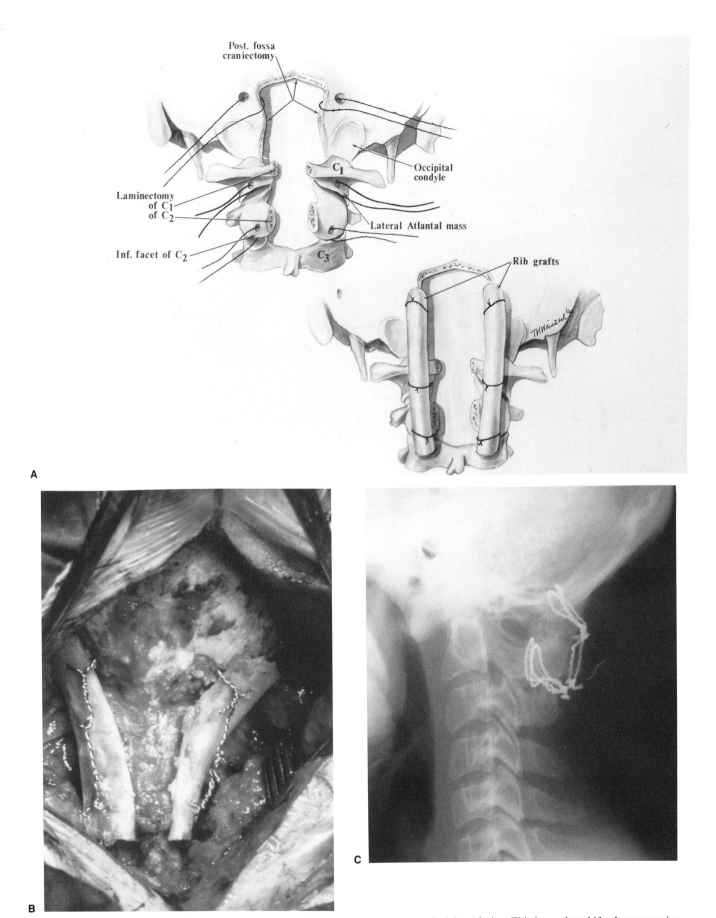

Figure 8–3. (**A**). Illustrations of the author's technique of dorsal occipitolateral cervical facet fusion. This is employed if a decompression laminectomy has to be made. (**B**). Operative photograph of occipitocervical facet fusion. This 16-year-old had previously undergone posterior fossa and upper (C1 to C2) cervical decompression for hindbrain malformation with basilar invagination. Note the lateral position of the rib grafts. (**C**). Lateral radiograph of craniocervical area made 6 months after dorsolateral C0-C1-C2 fusion (same patient as in Fig. 8–3B). The osseous fusion is complete.

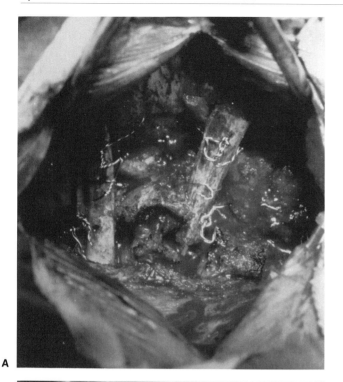

A

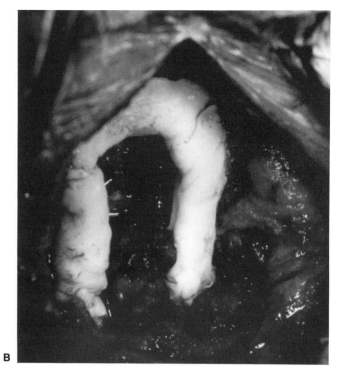

B

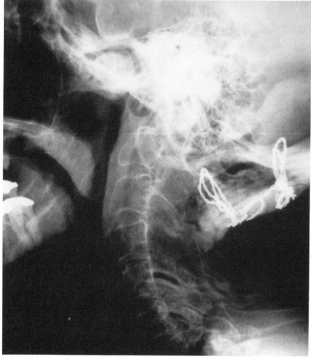

C

Figure 8–4. (**A**). Operative exposure of C0 to C1 to C2 dorsal fusion in a 66-year-old rheumatoid with cranial settling. An anterior odontoid resection was made previously. Note the braided wires twisted into hooks over the rib grafts. (**B**). Operative photograph of patient in (A). The methyl methacrylate is fashioned into a horseshoe to envelope the wires and provides immediate support to the occiput. (**C**). Lateral craniovertebral radiograph made 5 months after dorsal occipitocervical fusion with bone, wire, and methyl methacrylate. There is solid bony fusion evident.

et al.[33] They reported that three of five patients who underwent an occipitocervical fusion had an increase in cranial settling. Unfortunately, similar statements have been made by others. An operative mortality of 8% and a success rate of 57% were reported by Zoma et al in patients who underwent dorsal bony decompression and fusion to relieve irreducible ventral compression with subluxation.[34] The failure rate was 35%. Thus, it is recognized that not only are the operative techniques and postoperative care crucial, but the preoperative indication for the operation provides for the success of the procedure. Hamblen described 13 patients requiring occipitocervical fusion.[12] Twelve of the thirteen had improvement in their neurological condition. All obtained a successful fusion, although three suffered graft fractures. In

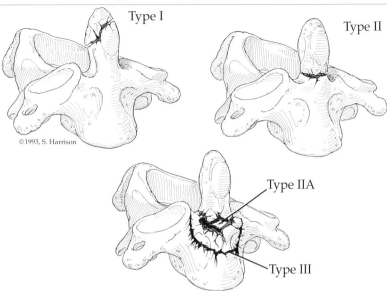

Type I

Type II

Type IIA

Type III

©1993, S. Harrison

Figure 9–2. Common C2 anterior column fracture types treatable by atlantoaxial arthrodesis to reestablish spinal stability. These may occur in combination with C1 and/or posterior arch fractures, adding to instability and complexity of management.

Any of these conditions can result in C1 to C2 instability and dislocation, with cord compression and progressive myelopathy requiring reduction or decompression along with surgical fusion.[33,34]

Rheumatoid Arthritis

Inflammatory dissolution of bone, joint, and ligament occurs at the atlantoaxial joint from rheumatoid arthritis, causing C1 to C2 subluxation and cranial settling. This settling results in upward migration of the odontoid process into the foramen magnum, with variable amounts of brainstem impingement. This can be measured radiographically in relation to McGregor's line, the line of the transverse diameter of the foramen magnum.[35] Radiographic criteria have been developed to determine cranial settling and C1 to C2 instability with rheumatoid arthritis.[36] This is a common process development in patients suffering with rheumatoid arthritis. About 25% of those who develop C1 to C2 subluxation will progress with neuraxis compression.[37] Erosion and osteoporosis of the odontoid process can cause spontaneous odontoid fracture, producing severe neck pain and crepitus on neck movement.[38] Criteria for classification of neurological deficit due to rheumatoid spondylitis help in analyzing the individual patient: (I) no deficit, (II) subjective weakness with hyperreflexia and dysesthesia, (III) objective weakness and long-tract signs, (IIIA) independently ambulatory, and (IIIB) quadriparetic and nonambulatory.[39] Indications for surgical arthrodesis are (1) progressive myelopathy, (2) intractable suboccipital pain, (3) subluxation in young patients of 10 mm or more, (4) transient syncope of nonhemispheric origin, and (5) transient loss of dexterity, gait disturbance, or Lhermitte's phenomenon (electrical shock spinal sensations) with neck flexion.[18] Subluxation can worsen over time, but neurological progression is less severe than might be expected; once myelopathy occurs, the natural history is grave

without effective surgical treatment.[40] However, these are chronically ill patients who are considered poor operative risks with a high rate of fusion failure due to graft lysis and fracture.[41] Although pseudoarthrosis and early postoperative mortality are problems with these patients, early diagnosis, detailed radiographic evaluation, and reduction of subluxation with surgical stabilization can improve neurological function and prevent progressive deterioration.[36,39]

Surgical Treatment of Persistent C1 to C2 Translation Deformity and Instability

Patients who harbor inherently unstable lesions or who have failed to heal after an adequate trial of orthotic immobilization are candidates for atlantoaxial arthrodesis from either an anterior or posterior approach. Skeletal traction applied continuously via halo ring or skull tongs provides security in maintaining safe alignment during patient transport, movement, and positioning. Posterior cervical fusions are performed with the patient prone. The patient is prepared while supine either on a gurney or in the bed that has been used for transport to the surgical suite. Preferably the trachea is intubated via the nasal route under topically applied local anesthesia while the patient is still awake and responsive. The intubation can be facilitated by using a flexible fiberoptic bronchoscope. The table is prepared with blanket rolls or a fabricated bodyrest that relieves abdominal and thoracic compression while the patient is prone. The headrest is also prepared and may be a well-padded horseshoe, a three-pinned skull support, or a clamp designed to engage the halo ring. While supine, intubated, and awake the patient is brought next to the operating table and "log lifted" by four or more attendants standing at the patient's side opposite the table. The surgeon secures the patient's head and neck during the maneuver. The patient is lifted off of the bed and the bed is pulled away from beneath the patient. The attendants

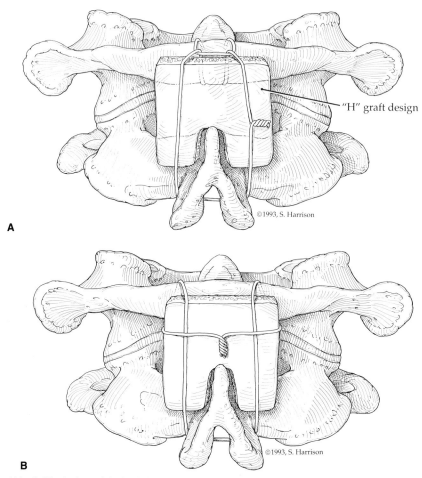

"H" graft design

©1993, S. Harrison

A

©1993, S. Harrison

B

Figure 9–3. (**A**). Gallie fusion with single-loop wire around C1 posterior arch securing the onlay H graft to the posterior arch of C2. (**B**). Gallie fusion with double-loop wire around C1 posterior arch holding the onlay H graft in place. Both wiring methods shown avoid wire loops coursing simultaneously under the C1 and C2 posterior arches.

then carry the supine patient in unison to the table. Then in a carefully coordinated movement the patient is rolled to prone on the table and the head is positioned. After the operative position is achieved, the patient is examined for motor and sensory function. The patient can then be anesthetized for the surgical procedure. If the patient is in a halo-vest orthosis, this can be maintained and the procedure performed keeping the halo vest in place and removing the back part for the procedure. The patient could be anesthetized prior to positioning if secured in a halo-vest orthosis. A lateral projection radiograph is made prior to commencing to verify that the C1 to C2 alignment has not changed significantly during the positioning process.

POSTERIOR ATLANTOAXIAL FUSION TECHNIQUES

Multiple methods for fusing the atlantoaxial joint complex both from the anterior and posterior approach have been described. This discussion will be limited to the posterior approach, which is the most familiar and widely accepted route. Regardless of the method used, the goal of the proce-

dure is to establish a stabilizing tension band against flexion moments between C1 and C2. Biomechanical studies of the more common methods of C1 to C2 fusion have shown them to be generally effective in eliminating significant movement in flexion, anteroposterior translation, lateral bending, extension, and axial rotation, with exception of the Gallie procedure.[42] Most of these procedures are supplemented with external immobilization using an orthotic device such as a collar or halo for several weeks. Most use osseous grafts of onlay morselized bone or solid struts of cortical/medullary bone that is secured in place with wire, with an occasional exception.[43] Rods and plates secured by wire or screws are used in some procedures to establish immediate stability. Some require incorporation of the uninvolved atlantooccipital joint for stability. At times procedures require sublaminar manipulation of the spinal canal. Some use acrylic polymerized in situ to gain immediate fixation. All have advantages and disadvantages. A method is adequate as long as it fulfills the conceptual goal of achieving an effective tension band resisting flexion and rotation moments. A significant rate of fusion failure can occur when this goal is not achieved.[44]

Gallie Type

This is a single median graft situated between the posterior arch of C1 and C2 that is secured by sublaminar wires passed beneath the arches of both C1 and C2. The graft is notched to fit over the C2 spinous process.[45] This is the poorest biomechanical construct that offers little or no fixation against rotation.[42] Spanning more than one segment with sublaminar wire is to be avoided because the severe encroachment of the wire into the canal causes distortion and compression of the cord not only during passage of the sublaminar wire but static encroachment and potential cord compression once the wire is in place. An advantage of this procedure is that it is technically easy to perform. Results are improved if this procedure is supplemented with orthotic immobilization (Figs. 9–3A and B).

Brooks Type

This is a bilateral, interlaminar bone graft construct in which the grafts are secured with bilateral sublaminar wires passed under both the posterior arch of C1 and C2.[46] Using oversized wedges of autogenous ilium bone grafts that are grooved for the wires and double strands of twisted wires are modifications that improve results with this method.[47] This construct resists rotation better than the Gallie. It has the same disadvantage of spanning more than one segment with sublaminar wire, and for this reason it is a dangerous maneuver.[48] Passing a heavy-gauge wire simultaneously under the laminae of both C1 and C2 requires a broad curvature of the wire that encroaches deeply into the canal and that can cause a "clothesline" cord compression. This risk is increased in the presence of persistent anterior dislocation of C1 on C2, which further reduces the cross-sectional diameter of the spinal canal, leaving less room for the cord and anything else. Stabilization using this construct is improved with external immobilization (Fig. 9–4).

Sonntag's Modified Gallie Type

Patients are positioned preoperatively in a halo vest to optimize alignment between C1 and C2 and placed prone, with the halo fixed to the table with a Mayfield fixation device.

The C1 posterior arch and C2 spinous process and laminae are exposed through a midline incision. Pericranium and soft tissue between C1 and the occipital squama are preserved to retard assimilation of the fusion to the occipital bone. The interlaminar space is widened with a drill. The C2 laminae and spinous process are also decorticated. A tricorticate or bicorticate graft from the iliac crest is fashioned with a drill to a curvilinear strut that fits in the interlaminar space and is notched to fit over the proximal superior edge of the C2 spinous process so that the concave cortical surface lies over the dura. The proximal undersurface of the C2 spinous process is notched. A loop of number 24 twisted wire is passed under the posterior arch of C1. This wire requires two-handed control to avoid encroachment of the spinal canal by the wire. This wire loop is then passed over the posterior arch of C2 and secured under the base of the spinous process and into the previously prepared notch. The bone graft is then trapped in the interlaminar space within the wire loop. The lower free ends of the wire are then brought over the dorsal surface of C2 laminae and under the base of the C2 spinous process and twisted tightly to secure the graft between the two lamina.[49] This avoids sublaminar wires under more than one laminar segment. It also avoids simultaneous sublaminar manipulation at C2, which is the risk of the original Gallie procedure, as mentioned earlier. The use of a flexible multistrand cable system, Songer Cable®, for the fixation facilitates this procedure and allows a tighter fit and possibly stronger construct[50,51] (Fig. 9–5).

Acrylic/Pin Type

Polymers such as methyl methacrylate have been advocated for direct application and in situ polymerization to the construct to produce immediate stability. When precise principles of technique are followed, this construct produces an immediate fixation that has not failed in a large series of patients with several years follow-up.[52,53] The acrylic does not bind to bone and there are no anchoring surfaces to grip and hold the polymer, therefore, it must be anchored effectively to the bone surface. The anchor should be of a type that does not erode through bone. Wire used in the construct must be

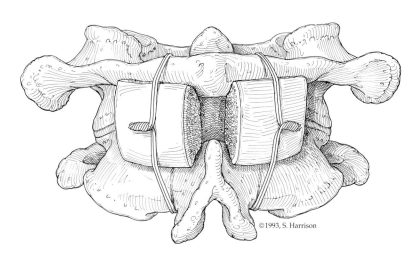

©1993, S. Harrison

Figure 9–4. Brooks fusion method with bilateral grafts interposed between the posterior arches of C1 and C2 secured in place by wires spanning under the arches of both C1 and C2. It is more stable than the Gallie method but involves the hazard of spanning simultaneously more than one sublaminar segment with a wire.

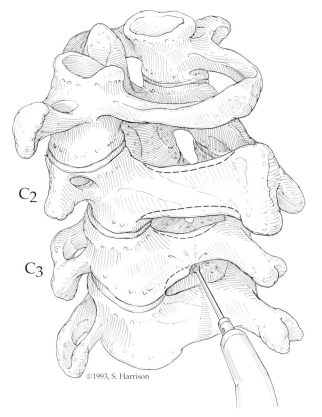

Figure 9–8. The interlaminar space is widened to the medial edge of the facet joint using a high-speed drill. The ligamentum flavum (not shown) is kept intact.

wire (Fig. 9–8). A trochar uterine needle is flattened slightly to reduce the curve toward the point and is grasped by a needle holder, so that the eyed blunt end is passed in a flattened-cephalad direction under each hemilamina and a single strand of number 28 wire is brought out from under the lamina with the eye of the needle separately at each hemilamina, including the C1 posterior arch. Each of these wires is used to pass a pair of doubled, twisted number 28 wires under each hemilamina (Fig. 9–9). The passing single strand is looped twice around the twisted strands, which are bent to form as low a profile as possible. Using two hands and adjusting the curve of the wires as needed with constant ten-

sion on the passing and passed wires, the twisted wire pairs are brought under each hemilamina. The ends of one of the twisted pair are cut flush with the twist, and the other is left long so that each wire can be identified later. A drill hole is made through each hemilamina at the base of the spinous process on each side toward the interlaminar space in a caudal direction. A small dissecting instrument is inserted under the lamina at the spinous process to protect the spinal canal. This leaves an interval of cortical bone at the inferior laminar base of the spinous process. This is a critical difference from anchor holes drilled simply from one side to the other at the base of the spinous process, as described for other methods[52] (Fig. 9–10). The number 20 wire is then passed in a caudal direction and brought out from the undersurface of the lamina at the interlaminar space. It is then back-threaded from the undersurface through the laminar hole on the contralateral side from a ventral-to-dorsal direction. In this manner the heavy wire is passed under the spinous process without encroaching the spinal canal. The wire is apposed to cortical bone at three points, which affords a solid anchoring base to secure the tie bar. The multistrand cable (Songer®) is more flexible and easier to manipulate during the passing maneuvers and has currently supplanted the number 20 wire. Both types of wire produce a comparably stable construct. The paired ends of each wire are secured with clamp hemostats individually and left on tension to prevent any inadvertent wire encroachment into the canal that could cause neural injury. If the drill holes at the spinous process base are too far apart, "clothesline" epidural cord compression can occur from the wire spanning and encroaching the posterior spinal canal (Fig. 9–11).

Autogenous rib graft is harvested in the same surgical field through a separate oblique incision over the rib palpable just caudal to the angle of the scapula, which is usually the seventh rib. The lateral boarder of the trapezius muscle can be dissected longitudinally and retracted medially. The erector spinae muscles are transected over the donor rib so that the costotransverse articulation is exposed. The rib is dissected subperiosteally; care is taken not to violate the parietal pleura. The rib is transected as medial as possible to get the maximum rib curvature for the strut graft. The lateral rib osteotomy is carried as far laterally as is needed to procure a rib

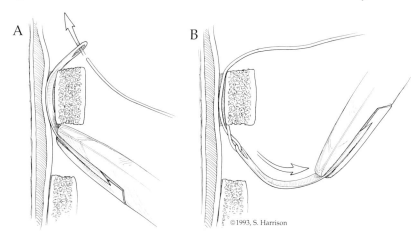

Figure 9–9. (**A**). A partially flattened uterine trochar needle is passed under the partially drilled lamina in a cephalad direction. (**B**). A single-strand number 28 wire is threaded through the needle eye and pulled under the lamina caudally, thus positioning the sublaminar passing wire.

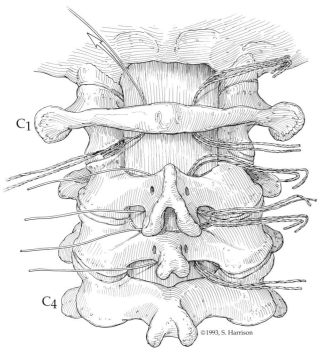

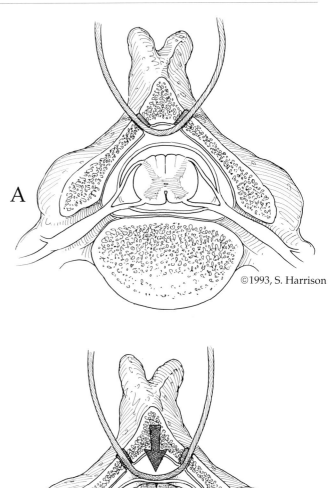

Figure 9–10.   The passing wire is used to pull two doubly twisted number 28 wires under the hemilamina in a caudal to cephalic direction. This is performed separately at each hemilamina bilaterally. Drill holes have been placed through the lamina at the base of the spinous process bilaterally; each hole exits in the interspinous space.

Figure 9–11.   (**A**). The proper position of the drill holes at the base of the spinous process allows passage of the number 20 wire or cable while avoiding neural compression. (**B**). Wider drill hole placement or perpendicular orientation of the drill holes can cause "clothesline" encroachment by the wire/cable to cause neural compression. This is avoided by initiating the hole close to the spinous process base, angling it in a medial and caudal direction.

graft of adequate length. Preferably the rib will be long enough so that bisecting the graft will allow a whole rib segment for each strut. This affords maximum strength for the bone-graft portion of the fusion construct. The chest wound is filled with saline, and a Valsalva maneuver is performed to ensure that there is no air leak or pleural fistula. If a hole is made in the parietal pleura, it should be closed by simple suture. The rib graft is then denuded of soft tissue. It is not necessary to decorticate the graft or the laminar bed to which it is apposed to get bone-growth assimilation of the graft.

The pairs of twisted number 28 wire at each hemilamina are separated, and each twisted strand is identified by the ends left long or short at the twist. The ends are separated at each level one side at a time. The rib strut is laid over the laminar bed, and each twisted wire is crossed over the rib so that each pair of twisted wires encircles the rib in a figure eight at each hemilamina. The wires are twisted loosely until each hemilamina is tied to the rib. Each wire is tightened individually. The second rib strut is secured to the contralateral side in the same manner. The curve of the rib may not make full contact with the laminar surface, but this has not prevented successful fusion (Fig. 9–12).

After the rib struts are secured tightly by the sublaminar wires, the tie bar is placed over the spinous processes. The tips of the spinous processes can be removed or the plate bent to fit the individual anatomy. The heavy wire ends are threaded through the holes of the plate and tightened by twisting until the surface sheen of the wire dulls. If cable is used, care must be taken not to apply excess tension that can

cause pull-through. This is particularly a hazard in rheumatoid arthritis, where even the cortical bone is soft. The method described results in an immediately stable construct. The patient can be mobilized postoperatively without additional support.

Inclusion of C3 does not cause any significant added limitation of movement to a C1 to C2 fusion, but it does strengthen the tension-band resistance of the construct. This can also supplement the extension moment to assist in reduction of persistent anterior C1 translation (Fig. 9–13).

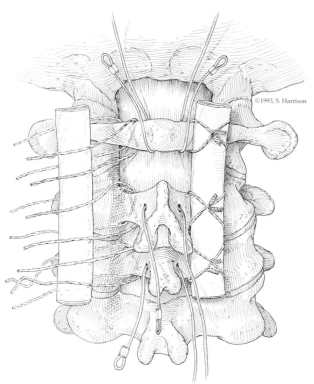

Figure 9–12. Rib grafts are secured to each hemilamina in a figure eight fashion by twist tying the doubled, twisted strand of number 28 wire, which is pared at each level to be fused. The cable is passed through the drill holes at the spinous process base. Two cables are passed under the intact posterior arch of C1.

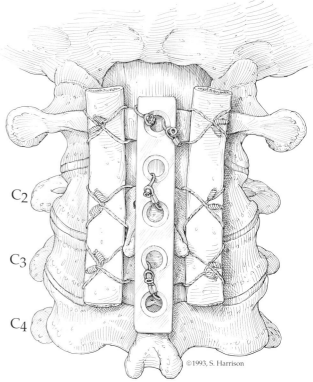

Figure 9–13. After wiring the rib grafts to each hemilamina, the metal tie bar is tightly secured in the midline between the rib grafts to the spinous process by the wire/cable passed previously at the spinous process. This completes the construct.

This procedure avoids excessive C1 to C2 compression, which can result in posterior angulation of a loose odontoid process. It can be adapted to any cervical level. It can substitute for loss of ventral column support, such as loss of one vertebral body. Loss of the posterior C1 arch can be compensated by using a T plate with wires at the laminar/pedicle junction of C1.

CLINICAL SERIES OF ATLANTOAXIAL FUSION VIA THE INTERSEGMENTAL TIE BAR

The author's (McDonnell) experience with this procedure extends from 1969 to the present and comprises 13 patients (30%) who underwent C1 to C2 fusion from the total series of 43 patients. This excludes the occipital-cervical fusion group. The series is listed in Table 9–1. One death occurred in a 60-year-old diabetic rheumatoid arthritic man on chronic steroid therapy with progressive myelopathy. The surgical wound became infected with *staphylococcus aureus,* causing osteomyelitis that required debridment with removal of the fusion construct. The patient was maintained in skeletal traction, but the myelopathy progressed slowly. The patient expired in respiratory arrest 5 months following the attempted arthrodesis of C1, C2, and C3.

A delayed infection occurred in a 46-year-old man who suffered a type II odonotoid fracture from a fall. The fusion

construct healed, but the patient presented with a purulent draining cutaneous sinus in the otherwise healed scar. The initial surgical procedure was performed in September 1972. The wound was debrided so that the plate and heavy wire were removed in January 1976. The arthrodesis was solid, and the wound healed subsequently without further sequelae.

There was one additional infection in this overall series of 43 patients for a 7% infection rate. There have been no infections since December 1979, and 30 patients in the series have undergone the procedure since then. All 13 patients of the C1 to C2 fusion group fused without additional neurological deficit. The alignment was maintained; six patients operated from 1969 to 1980 were treated in a collar, and no external support has been used in the seven patients operated since then.

The more typical experience with the Locksley procedure is exemplified in Figure 9–14. An overview of the series of atlantoaxial fusion using this technique is seen in Table 9–1.

REFERENCES

1. VanGilder JC, Menezes AH, Dolan KD. Embryology and development of the craniovertebral junction. In: *The Craniovertebral Junction and Its Abnormalities.* Mount Kisco, NY: Futura; 1987:1–8.
2. Dvork J, Panjabi MM. Functional anatomy of the alar ligaments. *Spine.* 1987;12:183–189.
3. Panjabi M, Dvorak J, Crisco J III, Oda T, Hilibrand A, Grob D. Flexion, extension and lateral bending of the upper cervical

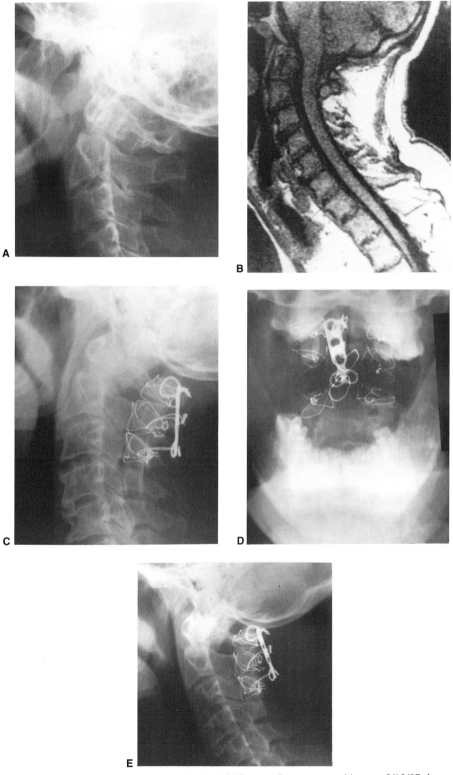

Figure 9–14. A 56-year-old machinist sustained a Type II odontoid fracture in an auto accident on 2/13/87; he complained of neck pain and right arm numbness but was neurologically intact. He was treated for 3 weeks in a halo brace but became noncompliant and took off the halo. A SOMI brace was tried, but he became noncompliant with this as well. His original complaints continued and he remained neurologically intact. An intersegmental tie bar/rib graft atlantoaxial fusion was done on 3/31/87. (**A**). Lateral radiograph 2/14/87 shows odontoid fracture with slight posterior angulation. (**B**). MRI scan on 3/25/87 shows mild ventral cord compression. (**C**). Lateral radiograph on 4/6/87 shows odontoid alignment and position of rib graft/tie bar fusion construct. (**D**). Anterior/posterior radiograph on 7/10/87 shows position of fusion construct. (**E**). Lateral radiograph on 3/4/88 shows 1-year follow-up of fusion. Patient had returned to his work 6 weeks after surgical arthrodesis.

Table 9–1. Atlantoaxial Arthrodesis by Intersegmental Tie Bar/Rib Graft Construct: A Clinical Series, 1969 to 1992.

RACE/SEX	AGE	DIAGNOSIS	PREOPERATIVE NEUROLOGICAL EXAM	DATE OF SURGERY + LEVELS	POSTOPERATIVE NEUROLOGICAL EXAM	EXTERNAL ORTHOSIS	SURGICAL COMPLICATIONS	OUTCOME BONE + NEURAL FUNCTION
W/M	21	Type II Fracture	Intact	7/69 C1, C2, C3	Intact	Collar	None	Fused, intact
W/M	32	Type II nonunion	Intact	5/76 C1 to C2	Intact	Collar	None	Fused, intact
W/M	33	Type II Fracture	Intact	2/77 C1, C2, C3	Intact	Collar	None	Fused, intact
W/M	60	Rheumatoid C1 to C2 Diabetes	Quadriparesis	11/78 C1, C2, C3	Neurological deterioration	Collar + traction	Wound infection quadriplegia	Death 4 months postop
W/M	46	Type II Fracture	Intact	9/72 C1, C2, C3	Intact	Collar	Delayed infection	Fused, intact
W/M	55	Rheumatoid C1-2 to C2	Quadriparesis	2/80 C1, C2, C3	Neurological Deficits Recovered	Collar	None	Fused, Intact
W/M	32	Os odontoideum	Quadriparesis	12/92 C1, C2, C3	Residual	None myelopathy	None	Fused, improved
B/M	21	Type III FX nonunion	Intact pain	5/85 C1, C2, C3	Pain resolved	None	None	Fused, intact
W/F	53	Rheumatoid C1 to C2	Quadriparesis ambulatory	9/85 C1, C2, C3	Residual myelopathy	None	None	Fused, improved
W/M	56	Type II Fracture	Intact	3/87 C1, C2, C3	Preop halo failed	None	None	Fused, intact
W/M	40	Type II FX + facet FX of C3	Intact	11/88 C1, C2, C3	Intact	None	None	Fused, intact
W/M	51	Os odontoideum	Quadriparesis	1/90 C1, C2, C3	Residual mild myelopathy	None	None	Fused, improved
W/M	15	Os odontoideum	Intact	4/92 C1 to C2	Intact	None	None	Fused, intact

spine in response to alar ligament transections. *J. Spinal Disord.* 1991;4:157–167.

4. Pueschel SM, Moon AC, Scola FH. Computerized tomography in persons with Down syndrome and atlantoaxial instability. *Spine.* 1992;17:735–737.

5. Yoshiko H, Kanai H. Atlantoaxial instability in athetoid-dystonic cerebral palsy: a case report. *Spine.* 1992;17:1434–1437.

6. Ehara S, El-Khoury GY, Clark CR. Radiologic evaluation of dens fracture: role of plain radiography and tomography. *Spine.* 1992;17:475–479.

7. Dvorak J, Panjabi M, Gerber M, Wichmann W. CT-functional diagnostics of the rotatory instability of upper cervical spine. 1. An experimental study on cadavers. *Spine.* 1987;12:197–205.

8. Dickman CA, Mamourian A, Sonntag VKH, Drayer BP. Magnetic resonance imaging of the transverse atlantal ligament for the evaluation of atlantoaxial instability. *J Neurosurg.* 1991;75:221–227.

9. Alexander E Jr. Classics in neurosurgery: fractures of the odontoid. *Surg Neurol.* 1977;8:239–242.

10. Anderson LD, D'Alonzo RT. Fractures of the odontoid process of the axis. *J Bone Joint Surg.* 1974;56A:1663–1674.

11. Scott EW, Haid RW Jr, Peace D. Type I fractures of the odontoid process: implications for atlanto-occipital instability. *J Neurosurg.* 1990;72:488–492.

12. Hadley MN, Browner CM, Liu SS, Sonntag VKH. New subtype of acute odontoid fractures (Type IIA). *Neurosurgery.* 1988;22:67–71.

13. Anderson LD, D'Alonzo RT. Fractures of the odontoid process of the axis. *J Bone Joint Surg.* 1974;56A:1663–1674.

14. Schatzker J, Rorabeck CH, Waddell JP. Fractures of the dens (odontoid process): an analysis of 37 cases. *J Bone Joint Surg.* 1971;53B:392–405.

15. Schiff DCM, Parke WW. The arterial supply of the odontoid process. *J Bone Joint Surg.* 1973;55A:1450–1456.

16. Hadley MN, Dickman CA, Browner CM, Sonntag VKH. Acute axis fractures: a review of 229 cases. *J Neurosurg.* 1989;71:642–647.

17. Ekong CEU, Schwartz ML, Tator CH, Rowed DW, Edmonds VE. Odontoid fracture: management with early mobilization using the halo device. *Neurosurgery.* 1981;9:631–637.

18. Dunn ME, Seljeskog EL. Experience in the management of odontoid process injuries: an analysis of 128 cases. *Neurosurgery.* 1986;18:306–310.

19. Paradis GR, Janes JM. Posttraumatic atlantoaxial instability: fate of the odontoid process fracture in 46 cases. *Trauma.* 1973;13:359–367.

20. Hanigan WC, Powell FC, Elwood PW, Henderson JP. Odontoid fractures in elderly patients. *J Neurosurg.* 1993;78:32–35.

21. Appuzo MLJ, Heiden JS, Weiss H, Ackerson TT, Harvey JP, Kurze T. Acute fractures of the odontoid process: an analysis of 45 cases. *J Neurosurg.* 1978;48:85–91.

22. Clark CR, White AA III. Fracture of the dens. *J Bone Joint Surg.* 1985;67A:1340–1348.

23. Dickman CA, Hadley MN, Browner C, Sonntag VKH. Neurosurgical management of acute atlas-axis combination fractures: a review of 25 cases. *J Neurosurg.* 1989;70:45–49.

24. Deen HG, Tolchin S. Combination Jefferson fracture C1 and Type II odontoid fracture requiring surgery: report of two cases. *Neurosurgery.* 1989;25:293–297.

25. Robertson PA, Swan HAP. Traumatic bilateral rotatory facet dislocation of the atlas on the axis. *Spine.* 1992;17:1252–1254.

26. Fielding JW, Hawkins RJ, Hensinger RN, Frances WR. Atlantoaxial rotary deformities. *Orthop Clin N America.* 1978;9:955–967.

27. List CF. Neurologic syndromes accompanying developmental anomalies of the occipital bone, atlas, and axis. *Arch Neurol Psychiat.* 1941;45:577–616.

28. Karlen A. Congential hypoplasia of the odontoid process. *J Bone Joint Surg.* 1962;41A:567–570.

29. Kline DG. Atlanto-axial dislocation simulating a head injury; hypoplasia of the odontoid: case report. *J Neurosurg.* 1966;24:1013–1016.

30. Sherk H, Nicholson JT. Rotatory atlanto-axial dislocation associated with ossiculum terminale and mongolism. *J Bone Joint Surg.* 1969;51A:957–964.

31. Wollin DG. The os odontoideum: separate odontoid process. *J Bone Joint Surg.* 1963;45A:1459–1471.

32. Fielding JW, Hensinger RN, Hawkins RJ. Os odontoideum. *J Bone Joint Surg.* 1980;62A:376–383.

33. Nagashima C. Atlanto-axial dislocation due to agenesis of the os odontoideum or odontoid. *J Neurosurg.* 1970;33:270–280.

34. Dyke P. Os odontoideum in children: neurologic manifestations and surgical management. *Neurosurgery.* 1978;2:93–99.

35. McGregor M. The significance of certain measurements of the skull in the diagnosis of basilar impression. *Br J Radiol.* 1948;21:171–181.

36. Clark CR, Goetz DD, Menezes AH. Arthrodesis of the cervical spine in rheumatoid arthritis. *J Bone Joint Surg.* 1989;71A:381–391.

37. Rana NA. Natural history of atlanto-axial subluxation in rheumatoid arthritis. *Spine.* 1989;14:1054–1056.

38. Toyama Y, Hirabayashi K, Fujimura Y, Satomi K. Spontaneous fracture of the odontoid process in rheumatoid arthritis. *Spine.* 1992;17(suppl):S436–S441.

39. Ranawat CS, O'Leary P, Pellicci P, Tsairis P, Marchisello P, Dorr L. Cervical spine fusion in rheumatoid arthritis. *J Bone Joint Surg.* 1979;61A:1003–1010.

40. Lipson SJ. Rheumatoid arthritis in the cervical spine. *Clin Orthop Related Res.* 1989;239:121–127.

41. Zoma A. Sturrock RD, Fisher WD, Freeman PA, Hamblen DL. Surgical stabilization of the rheumatoid cervical spine. *J Bone Joint Surg.* 1987;69B:8–12.

42. Grob D, Crisco JJ III, Panjabi MM, Wang P, Dvorak J. Biomechanical evaluation of four different posterior atlantoaxial fixation techniques. *Spine.* 1992;17:480–490.

43. McLaurin RL, Vernal R, Salmon JH. Treatment of fractures of the atlas and axis by wiring without fusion. *J Neurosurg.* 1972;36:773–780.

44. Fried LC. Atlanto-axial fracture-dislocations: failure of posterior C1 to C2 fusion. *J Bone Joint Surg.* 1973;55B:490–496.

45. Gallie WE. Fractures and dislocations of the cervical spine. *Am J Surg.* 1939;46:495–499.

46. Brooks AL, Jenkins EB. Atlanto-axial arthrodesis by the wedge compression method. *J Bone Joint Surg.* 1978;60A:279–284.

47. Griswold DM, Albright JA, Schiffman E, Johnson R, Southwick WO. Atlanto-axial fusion for instability. *J Bone Joint Surg.* 1978;60A:285–292.

48. Geremia GK, Kim KS, Cerullo L, Calenoff L. Complications of sublaminar wiring. *Surg Neurol.* 1985;23:629–634.

49. Dickman CA, Sonntag VKH, Papadopoulos SM, Hadley MN. The interspinous method of posterior atlantoaxial arthrodesis. *J Neurosurg.* 1991;74:190–198.

50. Songer MN, Spencer DL, Meyer PR Jr, Jayaraman G. The use of sublaminar cables to replace Luque wires. *Spine.* 1991;16:S418–S421.

51. Huhn SL, Wolf AL, Ecklund J. Posterior spinal osteosynthesis for cervical fracture/dislocation using a flexible multistrand cable system: technical note. *Neurosurgery.* 1991;29:943–946.

52. Six E, Kelly DL Jr. Technique for C-1, C-2, and C-3 fixation in cases of odontoid fracture. *Neurosurgery.* 1981;8:374–377.

53. Duff TA, Khan A, Corbett JE. Surgical stabilization of cervical spine fractures using methyl methacrylate: technical considerations and long term results in 52 patients. *J Neurosurg.* 1992;76:440–443.

54. McAfee PC, Bohman HH, Ducker T, et al. Failure of stabilization with methylmethacrylate. A retrospective analysis of twenty-four cases. *J Bone Joint Surg.* 1986;68A:1145–1157.

55. Duff TA. Surgical stabilization of traumatic cervical spine dislocation using methyl methacrylate. Long-term results in 26 patients. *J Neurosurg.* 1986;64:39–44.

56. Kelly DL Jr, Alexander E Jr, Davis CH Jr, Smith JM. Acrylic fixation of atlanto-axial dislocations: technical note. *J Neurosurg.* 1972;36:366–371.

57. Cybulski GR, Stone JL, Crowell RM, Rifai MHS, Gandhi Y, Glick R. Use of Halifax interlaminar clamps for posterior C1-C2 arthrodesis. *Neurosurgery.* 1988;22:429–431.

58. Holness RO, Huestis WS, Howes WJ, Langille RA. Posterior stabilization with an interlaminar clamp in cervical injuries: technical note and review of the long term experience with the method. *Neurosurgery.* 1984;14:318–322.

59. Duthel R, Brunon J, Jurine N, Giroud C. Utilization of the Knodt's device in atloaxoid instabilities. *Lyon Chir.* 1986;92:52–57.

60. Moskovich R, Crockard HA. Atlantoaxial arthrodesis using interlaminar clamps: an improved technique. *Spine.* 1992;17:261–267.

61. Grob D, Jeanneret B, Aebi M, Markwalder T-M. Atlanto-axial fusion with transarticular screw fixation. *J Bone Joint Surg.* 1991;73B:972–976.

62. Jeanneret B, Magerl F. Primary posterior fusion C1/2 in odontoid fractures: indications, technique, and results of transarticular screw fixation. *J Spinal Disorders.* 1992;5:464–475.

63. Alexander E Jr, Forsyth HF, Davis CH Jr, Nashold BS Jr. Dislocation of the atlas on the axis: the value of early fusion of C1, C2, and C3. *J Neuro Surg.* 1958;15:353–371.

64. McDonnell DE. Intersegment tie bar cervical fusion: the Locksley procedure. *Joint Sectn Disord Spine Periph Nerves.* 4:97. Abstract.

10 Occipitocervical Instrumentation

Volker K. H. Sonntag, M.D., Curtis A. Dickman, M.D.

INTRODUCTION

Fusion techniques for occipitocervical stabilization have undergone continuous evolution. Subperiosteal dissection of the bone with onlay grafts was the initial technique used to promote fusion, but this technique had a high rate of failure, and pseudoarthrosis was common.[1-4]

Bone struts (ribs or iliac crest bone grafts), wired to the occiput and cervical vertebrae, subsequently became popular. Bone struts wired into position provided a method to obtain immediate internal fixation of unstable motion segments. These techniques have had reasonable success. However, failure rates have still ranged between 5% and 30%.[1,2,5-10]

Two components are critical for successful occipitocervical fusion: (1) immediate rigid vertebral fixation and (2) promotion of long-term bone union. These principles provided the foundation for technical developments. Metallic fixtures (eg, rods, pins, and screw plates) provide another method to obtain rigid internal fixation while bone healing occurs.[11-17] This chapter focuses on techniques using metallic implants and instrumentation for occipitocervical fusion.

THREADED STEINMAN PIN OCCIPITOCERVICAL FUSION

Optimum alignment of the craniovertebral junction and upper cervical spine must be restored before surgery for internal fixation and fusion. Reduction is achieved with positional adjustments, a halo ring, or Gardner-Wells tongs and traction. Alignment is then best maintained with rigid external immobilization using a halo brace. The adjunctive use of a halo brace maintains spinal alignment and protects the cervical spine from externally applied forces. Supplemental postoperative rigid external fixation also facilitates the formation of an osseous fusion. The halo brace is usually worn 12 to 16 weeks after surgery. The type of postoperative orthosis is individualized and depends on the type of fixation used, the pathology, and the quality and architecture of the patient's bone.

In surgery, patients are secured to the operating table in a prone position, and the alignment of the cervical spine is verified with radiographs. Stacked weights or a Mayfield headholder adaptor are used to support the patient and to secure the halo brace to the operating table (Fig. 10–1). Foam chest rolls are used to protect the chest and to allow adequate respiratory excursion. Patients are also fixed to the operating table with wide cloth tape to permit the table to be adjusted intraoperatively.

If the halo brace prohibits adequate access to the posterior occipitocervical region or iliac crest, the posterior bars or posterior vest of the brace can be removed and replaced at the completion of the operation. However, it is seldom necessary to disassemble the halo brace completely. The bars of the halo brace provide a support surface for the surgeon's hands and act as a handrest during the operative procedure. When a perioperative halo brace cannot be used, a Mayfield skull clamp is used to fixate the craniovertebral junction intraoperatively.

Access to the posterior occipitocervical region is achieved using a standard midline cervical exposure. A linear skin incision extends from the inion to the spinous process of C7. The nuchal fascia and posterior cervical muscles are divided in a midline sagittal plane, which offers a relatively avascular dissection. Subperiosteal dissection is used to expose the occiput and dorsal arches of the upper cervical vertebra. The suboccipital and cervical paraspinous muscles are swept laterally using lightweight, broad-surfaced periosteal elevators. Careful operative technique prevents dislocation of unstable vertebral segments. The laterally situated vertebral arteries should be avoided during the operative exposure.

Curettes are used to remove the soft tissue, interspinous ligaments, and ligamentum flavum from the vertebra to be fused and to remove the posterior occipitoatlantal membrane from the rim of the foramen magnum. Curettes are also used to decorticate the cervical facet joints to facilitate fusion.

Kerrison rongeurs are used to enlarge the posterior rim of the foramen magnum and to notch the laminae of the cervical vertebra. The ligamentum flavum must be removed completely. These maneuvers facilitate wire passage (Fig. 10–2).

Two burr holes are drilled into the occiput, 0.5 cm superior to the rim of the foramen magnum. The burr holes are waxed, and the dura is separated from the inner table of the skull toward the foramen magnum. Multistrand, flexible, braided cables; double-strand, twisted wires; or monofilament surgical wire is passed between each of the burr holes and the foramen magnum and sublaminar at the cervical levels to be fused. Multistrand steel cable is stronger and more resistant to fatigue than monofilament wire.[18]

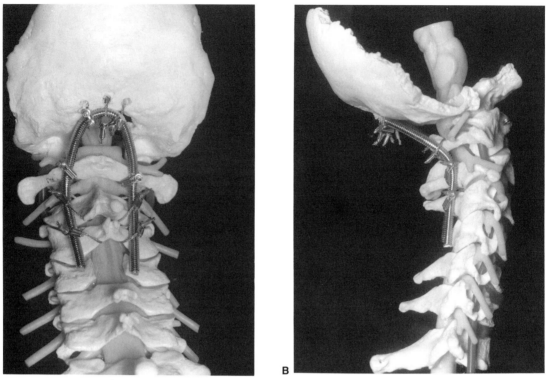

A   B

Figure 10–3.   (**A**). A $^5/_{32}$-inch threaded Steinman pin is bent into a U shape. (**B**). Secondary bends are place to fit the patient's lordotic contour. The pin is cut so the ends do not extend beyond the fused segments. Smooth contours, rather than sharp angles, are created. The pin is wired to the occiput and laminae or facets.

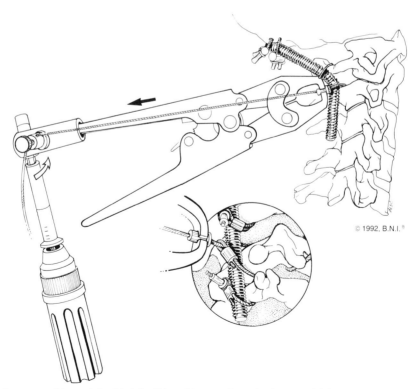

© 1992, B.N.I.®

Figure 10–4.   Songer, multistrand, braided flexible cables are fixated using special instruments. The cable tension is adjusted using a torque screwdriver and a tensiometer. The cable is secured with a metal crimp. (Reprinted with permission of Barrow Neurological Institute.)

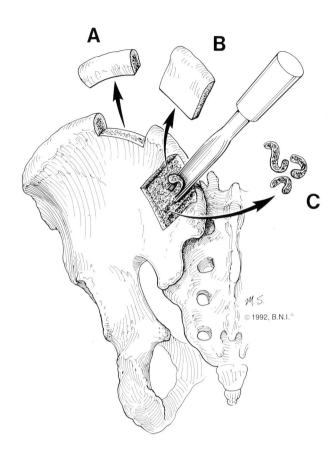

Figure 10–5. Autologous iliac crest bone grafts are usually obtained from the medial 6 or 8 cm of the ileum. Lateral incisions can cause buttock numbness from transection of the cluneal nerves. Grafts should be harvested with meticulous technique. The gluteal arteries are avoided by performing subperiosteal dissection. Retroperitoneal structures (eg, ureter), the sacroiliac joint, and the sciatic notch must be avoided. (**A**). Tricortical graft. (**B**). Unicortical graft. (**C**). Cancellous grafts. (Reprinted with permission of Barrow Neurological Institute.)

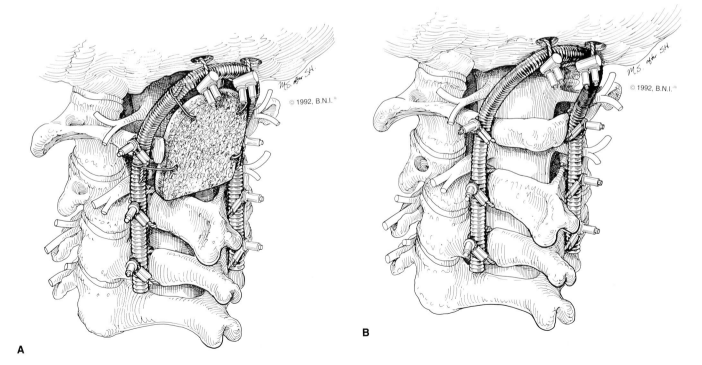

Figure 10–6. (**A**). The appearance of the fixation construct. Cancellous bone is added to promote fusion. (**B**). A plate of cortical bone from the iliac crest is wired to the construct after a posterior decompression has been performed. This re-creates the osseous contours, preserves the site of decompression, and provides a template for the fusion to form. (Reprinted with permission of Barrow Neurological Institute.)

Table 10–1. Type of Pathology Among 28 Patients Treated with Steinman Pin Occipitocervical Fusion.

PATHOLOGY	NO. OF PATIENTS
Rheumatoid arthritis	11
Congenital craniovertebral malformations	8
Occipitoatlantal dislocation	3
Unstable upper cervical fractures	4
Tumors	2

Follow-up ranged from 6 to 62 months (average follow-up, 25.6 months). Twenty-five patients achieved satisfactory long-term fixation. Osseous union was achieved in 23 cases (Fig. 10–7). Fibrous union occurred in two patients, both of whom had rheumatoid arthritis. Patients with fibrous unions had stable alignment of the instrumented segments without abnormal motion on flexion and extension radiographs. However, they had no evidence of new bone formation after long-term follow-up (26 and 41 months, respectively). These individuals are at risk for instrument breakage or delayed instability and are being followed on a long-term basis to monitor for late complications. One patient died 1 month after surgery from respiratory insufficiency. One patient has had progressive bony destruction due to tumor despite irradiation and chemotherapy. One patient was lost to long-term follow-up.

Instrument complications occurred in only two patients. Both patients had osseous unions. One woman with rheumatoid arthritis broke her Steinman pin 16 months after surgery (Fig. 10–8). Her postoperative radiographs demonstrated a

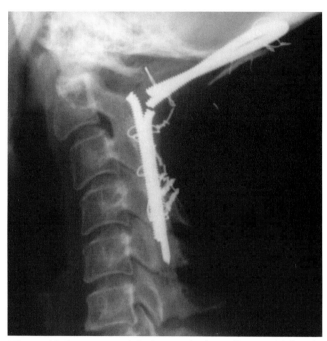

Figure 10–8. Fractured Steinman pin in a 62-year-old female with rheumatoid arthritis. The instrument breakage was asymptomatic and was associated with a solid fusion.

stable, well-aligned union despite the fractured pins. The broken Steinman pin caused no symptoms and was not removed. On follow-up 37 months postoperatively, she was without sequelae. In another patient, several facet wires broke after a solid fusion had formed. The cases of instrument failure emphasize that all metallic implants are susceptible to fatigue and may break or fail. A solid fusion must develop for long-term spinal stability. Rigid, precise instrumentation and meticulous preparation of the bone and autogenous grafts promote fusion.[19]

Other operative complications include one superficial wound infection that was treated with local care and oral antibiotics and resolved satisfactorily. Several patients complained of prolonged numbness or pain at the donor site. However, there were no major complications relating to the harvest of autogenous iliac bone.

LUQUE RECTANGLE OCCIPITOCERVICAL FUSION

The preoperative and operative techniques for occipitocervical fusion using the Luque rectangle or other metallic loops are identical to the techniques required for occipitocervical fusion using the threaded pin.[15–17] Steel rod constructs are available in a variety of sizes. The rectangles or loops must be contoured by the surgeon to fit the patient's cervical curvature. The closed configuration of the Luque rectangle requires that the inferior end of the rod be placed adjacent to the spinous processes or bent away from the spine. The constructs are wired to the occiput and laminae or to the facets of the cervical vertebra (Fig. 10–9). The rectangles and

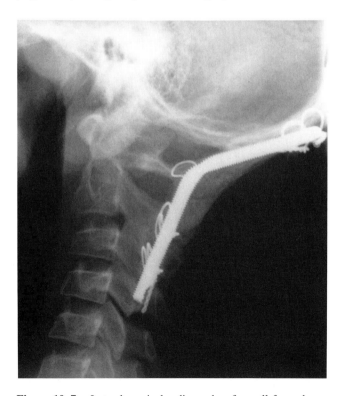

Figure 10–7. Lateral cervical radiographs of a well-formed osseous union in a 13-year-old male.

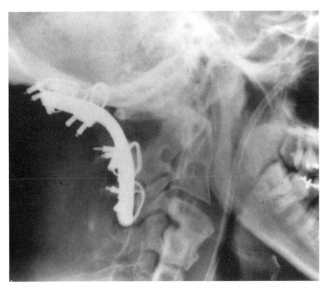

Figure 10–9. Lateral cervical radiograph of an occipitocervical fusion performed with a Luque rectangle and Songer cables. From Dickman CA, Locantro J, Fessler RG. The influence of transoral odontoid resection on stability of the craniovertebral junction. *J. Neurosurg.* 1992;77:525–530. (Reprinted with permission of *Journal of Neurosurgery*).

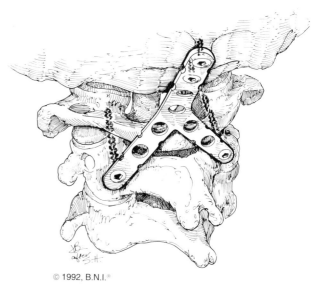

© 1992, B.N.I.®

Figure 10–10. Screw-plate fixation using an inverted Y plate. The plate is affixed to the spine with atlantoaxial facet screws. The occiput is fixated with short midline screws that are placed near the nuchal line. Bone grafts are added to ensure fusion. (Reprinted with permission of Barrow Neurological Institute.)

loops have smooth rod surfaces that can permit settling, telescoping, or vertical translocation of the instrumented segments. A wide diameter increases the resistance of the rods to fatigue and makes them less susceptible to breakage.

SCREW PLATE FIXATION FOR OCCIPITOCERVICAL FUSION

Steel or titanium screw plates have been used for occipitocervical fusion.[12,20,21] An inverted Y plate is affixed to the occiput and cervical spine with screws (Fig. 10–10). Occipital screws are placed into the midline crest of the occiput near the nuchal line. The thickness of the occipital bone must be assessed individually and measured precisely to avoid intradural penetration with the screws.[12,21] Grob found an average occipital thickness of 14 mm (range 10 to 18 mm) among 10 patients measured at the nuchal line.[12]

The plates can be fixated with several screw sites. The atlantoaxial articulations are immobilized using bilateral posterior transarticular facet screws. C1-C2 facet screws provide the most rigid mechanical fixation for the plate.[12] If C3 or lower cervical levels need to be fixated, lateral mass screws are also placed to affix the plate to these levels.

Atlantoaxial facet screws are placed in the following fashion.[20,22,23] A K wire is used to retract the C2 nerve root superiorly to visualize the C2 pedicle and C1-C2 facet during the drilling (Fig. 10–11). The posterior cortex of C2 is penetrated with a bone awl or drill beginning 2 to 3 mm medial and 2 to 3 mm above the C2-C3 facet joint. A pilot hole is drilled through the C2 pedicle, across the C1-C2 facet joint, into the C1 lateral mass. Lateral fluoroscopy is used to adjust and monitor the screw trajectory toward the dorsal cor-

tex of the C1 anterior arch. The screw is directed in the anteroposterior plane through the central axis of the C2 pedicle (0° to 10° medial) to avoid the dural sac medially and the vertebral artery laterally. A 2.5-mm-diameter drill and 3.5-mm-diameter screws are used.[20]

Lateral mass screws are placed into the C3 to C7 vertebrae with a similar technique.[13,20,24–26] Pilot holes are drilled in the bone, and self-tapping screws are inserted. Screws are inserted 1 mm medial to the center of the lateral mass. The drill and screws are directed 20° to 30° cephalad and 20° to 30° laterally. This trajectory avoids the vertebral artery and nerve roots and places screws bicortically within the lateral mass structure (Fig. 10–12).

This screw-plate technique for occipitocervical fusion provides immediate rigid fixation.[12,20,27] It avoids sublaminar wire passage and instrumentation within the spinal canal. Bone grafts are added to promote fusion. This technique is an excellent choice for patients who have several absent or fractured laminae that preclude wire fixation. Screw-plate techniques provide immediate rigid fixation if the bone quality is good. Adequate screw purchase sites must be achieved. Screws do not hold well in softened or diseased bone. Fusions can be restricted solely to the involved segments with this technique. This method of fixation is technically demanding, requires operative precision, and mandates expertise with cervical vertebral screw placement.

PREOPERATIVE CONSIDERATIONS

Occipitocervical fusion is indicated when the craniovertebral junction is unstable. The occipitoatlantal and atlantoaxial articulations are anatomically complex and permit a dy-

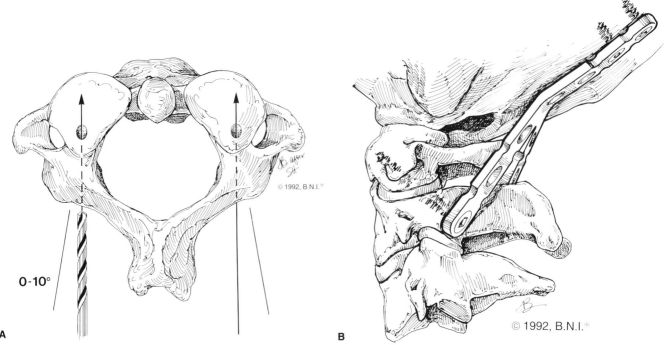

0-10°

A
B

Figure 10–11. (**A**). Posterior atlantoaxial facet screw placement. The screws enter C2 just above the C2 to C3 facet joint and pass through the center of the C2 pedicle, across the C1 to C2 facet, into the lateral mass of C1. A trajectory between 0° and 10° medially places the screw safely through the C2 pedicle. (**B**). Lateral fluoroscopic guidance is used to direct the screw toward the posterior cortex of the anterior arch of C1. (Reprinted with permission of Barrow Neurological Institute.)

namic, wide range of motion.[28] The broad range of normal mobility of the craniovertebral junction makes this region susceptible to injury, especially when secondarily affected by pathological processes. Degenerative diseases, rheumatoid arthritis, infections, tumors, congenital malformations, ligamentous injuries, fractures, or surgical procedures can precipitate permanent instability of the craniovertebral junction.

Instability of the occipitoatlantal joint and involvement of the occiput and multiple levels of the upper cervical spine are the principal indications for occipitocervical fusion. The occiput should not be routinely included into all upper cervical fusions.[1,2,7,19,28,29] The appropriate indications are mandatory. Occipitocervical fusion restricts additional movement and has a higher rate of nonunion compared to upper cervical fusions. Occipitocervical fusion is required when the occipitoatlantal joint is unstable or when widespread bone destruction or fractures preclude direct wiring and fixation of the atlas or axis.[1]

Compressive pathology of the craniovertebral junction may present with clinical signs of pain, myelopathy, brainstem dysfunction, occipital radicular pain, or vertebrobasilar insufficiency. The development of neurological deficits indicates that decompression and internal fixation are urgently needed.

When irreducible neural compression and spinal instability coexist, operative decompression must precede internal fixation. When compressive lesions are present, passing wire or placing instrumentation or tools into a stenotic canal can further compromise neural structures and exacerbate neurological deficits.

Surgical approaches must be directed specifically at the sites of neural compression. Anterior compression should be approached by an anterior route (ie, a transoral or anterolateral cervical approach). Posterior compressive lesions must be approached posteriorly. Posterior decompressive approaches can be followed immediately by a simultaneous arthrodesis in a single operative session. In comparison, no biomechanically satisfactory anterior fixations have been devised for occipitocervical fusion. When an anterior decompression is indicated, posterior arthrodesis is staged as a separate operative session.

SUMMARY

Occipitocervical fusion using instrumentation and grafts confers the advantage of providing immediate rigid fixation while bone fusion occurs. Threaded metallic pins and other implants have provided excellent results. Techniques should be simple and designed to avoid neurological injury and to maximize osseous stabilization and subsequent union. The threaded Steinman pin provides a versatile, adaptable means of restoring the occipitocervical contour. It is inexpensive, readily available, and provides excellent fixation. The threads of the pin provide a stable means of fixating the construct to avoid settling of the fusion. A wide-diameter, threaded, titanium Steinman pin facilitates rigid fixation and allows postoperative MRI. Screw plates provide an excellent

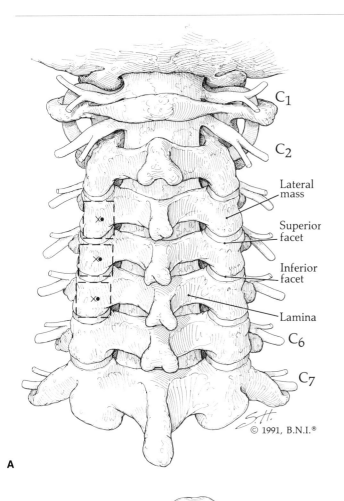

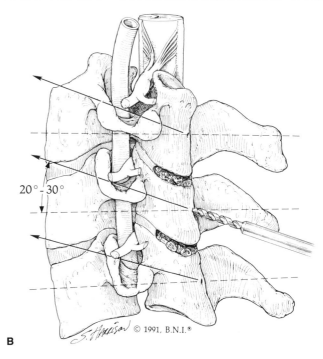

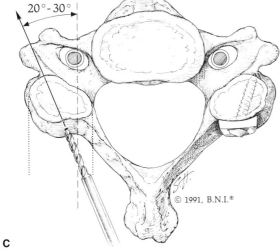

Figure 10–12. (**A**). Lateral mass screws are inserted into the lower cervical vertebrae (C3 to C7) by entering the bone 1 mm medial to the center of the lateral masses. (**B**). Bicortical screws are directed 20° to 30° cephalad. (**C**). The screws are directed 20° to 30° lateral. This trajectory avoids the nerve roots and vertebral arteries. (Reprinted with permission of Barrow Neurological Institute.)

alternative when the laminae cannot be wired or when a more rigid implant is required.

REFERENCES

1. Fielding JW, Hawkins RJ, Ratzan SA. Spine fusion for atlanto-axial instability. *J Bone Joint Surg.* 1976;58A:400–407.
2. Murphy MJ, Southwick WO. Posterior approaches and fusions. In: Cervical Spine Research Society, ed. *The Cervical Spine.* 2nd ed. Philadelphia, Pa: JB Lippincott; 1989:775–791.
3. Newman P, Sweetnam R. Occipito-cervical fusion. An operative technique and its indications. *J Bone Joint Surg.* 1969;51:423–431.
4. Pilcher LS. Atlo-axoid fracture-dislocation. *Ann Surg.* 1910;51:208–211.
5. Grantham SA, Dick HM, Thompson RC Jr, et al. Occipitocervical arthrodesis. Indications, technic and results. *Clin Orthop.* 1969;65:118–129.
6. Hamblen DL. Occipito-cervical fusion. Indications, technique and results. *J Bone Joint Surg.* 1967;49:33–45.

7. Menezes AH, VanGilder JC, Graf CJ, et al. Craniocervical abnormalities. A comprehensive surgical approach. *J Neurosurg.* 1980;53:444–455.

8. Wertheim SB, Bohlman HH. Occipitocervical fusion. Indications, technique, and long-term results in thirteen patients. *J Bone Joint Surg.* 1987;69:833–836.

9. Yashon D. Surgical management of trauma to the spine. In: Schmidek HH, Sweet WH, eds. *Operative Neurosurgical Techniques. Indications, Methods and Results.* 2nd ed, Vol 2. Orlando, Fla: Grune & Stratton; 1988:1449–1469.

10. Robinson RA, Southwick WO. Surgical approaches to the cervical spine. In: American Academy of Orthopedic Surgeons, ed. *Instructional Course Lectures.* Vol 17, St. Louis, Mo: CV Mosby; 1960:299–330.

11. Dickman CA, Douglas RA, Sonntag VKH. Occipitocervical fusion: posterior stabilization of the craniovertebral junction and upper cervical spine. *BNI Quarterly.* 1990;6:2–14.

12. Grob D, Dvorak J, Panjabi M, et al. Posterior occipitocervical fusion. A preliminary report of a new technique. *Spine.* 1991;16(suppl):S17–S24.

13. Roy-Camille R, Saillant G, Mazel C. Internal fixation of the unstable cervical spine by a posterior osteosynthesis with plates and screws. In: Cervical Spine Research Society, ed. *The Cervical Spine.* 2nd ed. Philadelphia, Pa: JB Lippincott; 1989:390–403.

14. Crockard HA, Pozo JL, Ransford AO, et al. Transoral decompression and posterior fusion for rheumatoid atlanto-axial subluxation. *J Bone Joint Surg.* 1986;68:350–356.

15. MacKenzie AI, Uttley D, Marsh HT, et al. Craniocervical stabilization using Luque/Hartshill rectangles. *Neurosurgery.* 1990;26:32–36.

16. Ransford AO, Crockard HA, Pozo JL, et al. Craniocervical instability treated by contoured loop fixation. *J Bone Joint Surg.* 1986;68:173–177.

17. Sakou T, Kawaida H, Morizono Y, et al. Occipitoatlantoaxial fusion utilizing a rectangular rod. *Clin Orthop.* 1989;239:136–144.

18. Songer MN, Spencer DL, Meyer PR Jr, et al. The use of sublaminar cables to replace Luque wires. *Spine.* 1991;16 (suppl):S418–S421.

19. Fielding JW. The status of arthrodesis of the cervical spine. *J Bone Joint Surg.* 1988;70:1571–1574.

20. Dickman CA, Sonntag VKH, Marcotte PJ. Techniques of screw fixation of the cervical spine. *BNI Quarterly.* 1992;8:9–26.

21. Heywood AWB, Learmonth ID, Thomas M. Internal fixation for occipitocervical fusion. *J Bone Joint Surg.* 1988;70: 708–711.

22. Magerl F, Seemann P-S. Stable posterior fusion of the atlas and axis by transarticular screw fixation. In: Weidner PA, ed. *Cervical Spine I.* New York, NY: Springer-Verlag; 1987: 322–327.

23. Weidner A. Internal fixation with metal plates and screws. In: Cervical Spine Research Society, ed. *The Cervical Spine.* 2nd ed. Philadelphia, Pa: JB Lippincott; 1989:404–421.

24. An HS, Gordin R, Renner K. Anatomic considerations for plate-screw fixation of the cervical spine. *Spine.* 1991;16(suppl):S548–S551.

25. Cherny WB, Sonntag VKH, Douglas RA. Lateral mass posterior plating and facet fusion for cervical spine instability. *BNI Quarterly.* 1991;7:2–11.

26. Heller JG, Carlson GD, Abitbol JJ, et al. Anatomic comparison of the Roy-Camille and Magerl techniques for screw placement in the lower cervical spine. *Spine.* 1991;16(suppl):S552–S557.

27. Hanson PB, Montesano PX, Sharkey NA, et al. Anatomic and biomechanical assessment of transarticular screw fixation for atlantoaxial instability. *Spine.* 1991;16:1141–1145.

28. White AA III, Panjabi MM. *Clinical Biomechanics of the Spine.* Philadelphia, Pa: JB Lippincott; 1978:1–199.

29. Dickman CA, Sonntag VKH, Papadopoulos SM, et al. The interspinous method of posterior atlantoaxial arthrodesis. *J Neurosurg.* 1991;74:190–198.

11   Posterior Atlantoaxial Screw Fixation

Noel I. Perin, M.D., F.R.C.S. (E.D.I.N.)

INTRODUCTION

Instability of the atlantoaxial complex can result from disruption of the bony or ligamentous elements, or both. Various methods have been described for the surgical stabilization of the unstable atlantoaxial complex. Historically, posterior wiring using the Gallie or Brooks technique, or a modification, was used to stabilize the unstable C1 to C2 complex.[1,2] Although these stabilization methods produced adequate results, patients had to be placed postoperatively in a halo vest to maintain alignment until bony fusion occurred. These techniques were also disadvantageous because they were dependent on the integrity of the posterior elements of the atlas and axis.

In 1979, Magerl developed a technique for placing screws in the C1 to C2 facet joint from a posterior approach.[3] These transarticular screws were independent of the posterior elements and were claimed to provide greater rotational stability. We have modified this technique so that we neither dissect the C2 nerve nor expose the C1 to C2 facet joint. We use C1 to C2 posterior Gallie wiring with an intervening H graft in selected patients. In the ensuing discussion, we will outline steps for the initial evaluation and management of patients with instability at the C1 to C2 complex, discuss the operative decision, and define the process and techniques for screw placement, including postoperative care and complications.

PATIENT MANAGEMENT

The initial management of patients with atlantoaxial instability treated with screw fixation is identical to that in patients treated with other techniques. Atlantoaxial instability can occur after traumatic injuries to the upper cervical spine. Type II odontoid fractures commonly produce instability and are associated with a high incidence of nonunion.[4–6] Jefferson's and Hangman's fractures only rarely produce instability. Rheumatoid arthritis is the other common cause of C1 to C2 instability. When these patients have both vertical and horizontal instability, they will need to undergo occipitocervical fusion.[7]

After the cervical spine alignment and general anatomy of the fracture are assessed with plain films, the patient is placed in cervical traction using Gardner-Wells tongs. We start with 5 lb of traction, which is usually sufficient to align the spine in most patients. The patient's head may need to be placed in neutral, extension, or flexion depending on the di-

rection of subluxation (anterolisthesis or retrolisthesis) to achieve adequate reduction. Lateral cervical spine films are obtained both after placing the initial weight and after making any adjustment of the weight or neck position. In acute traumatic cases of patients with neurological deficit, Methyl-Prednisolone is administered according to a previously published protocol.[8]

IMAGING EVALUATION

After the initial evaluation with plain films, all patients undergo computerized tomographic (CT) scans with bone windows to assess the fracture anatomy and canal dimensions. In odontoid fractures, CT scans with sagittal reformatting are necessary to delineate the fracture. Patients presenting with acute instability without neurological deficit and with a documented fracture do not undergo further studies. Patients with neck pain after acute trauma (with suspected or documented fracture in the C1 to C2 complex without subluxation) will have a flexion-extension lateral cervical x-ray. When there is uncertainty (eg, in the unconscious patient), the Gardner-Wells tongs, halo orthosis, or a firm cervical collar are maintained appropriately until the patient wakes up, at which time flexion-extension lateral cervical films are obtained.

Patients with chronic instability at the atlantoaxial joint should be evaluated with a magnetic resonance imaging (MRI) scan to document the presence of an inflammatory pannus or a pannuslike mass.[7] In cases of anterior compression, differentiation between bony and soft-tissue compression is essential to plan the operative approach. These patients should also have flexion-extension plain lateral cervical films to assess reducibility of the subluxation. Patients with chronic instability may need to be placed in cervical traction for several days to achieve reduction. In some cases MRI scans in flexion and extension may help to assess the varying degrees of compression.

INDICATIONS AND CONTRAINDICATIONS FOR PLACEMENT OF POSTERIOR TRANSFACETAL SCREWS

Indications

Posterior transfacetal C1 to C2 screw placement is an effective means to stabilize atlantoaxial instability and is suitable in both bony and ligamentous disruption. Posterior transfac-

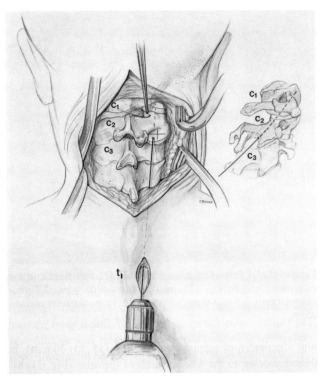

Figure 11–5. Drawing of the C1 to C2 complex shows the guide wire entering through a puncture wound in the skin at T1. The guide wire is passed under lateral fluoroscopic guidance into the pedicle of C2 toward the anterior tubercle of C1.

(2) entering the lower neck through a stab incision around C7 or T1; and (3) lifting the spinous process of C2 dorsally using a towel clip, again without compromising the reduction. The surgeon must exercise care when drilling so the drill bit does not bend excessively because it will break inside the pedicle, be difficult to retrieve, and hinder screw placement. When additional stability is required and the posterior elements of C1 to C2 are intact, a Gallie-type C1 to C2 wiring with an H graft may be performed.[3]

POSTOPERATIVE CARE

Patients get out of bed the day after surgery and wear a firm cervical collar for the next 6 weeks, and wear a soft collar for 6 weeks further. Lateral cervical spine films are obtained postoperatively once or twice during the first week and monthly until the collar is removed. If the patient shows any increase in neck pain or neurological deficit, repeat examination with a lateral x-ray of the cervical spine is indicated. After 3 months, the collar is removed and flexion and extension films of the cervical spine are taken.

COMPLICATIONS

Complications with posterior transarticular screw placement can occur during positioning of the patient, during exposure, or in the process of drilling.

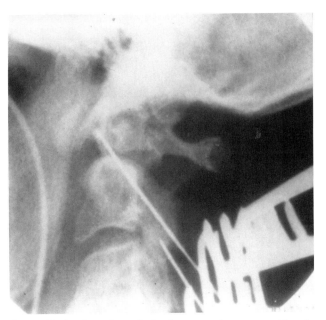

Figure 11–6. Lateral cervical spine x-ray shows one guide wire in place as a second is being placed on the opposite side.

Spinal Cord Injury

Fortunately, spinal cord injury is rare with posterior transarticular screw placement. All patients are monitored with somatosensory evoked-potential recordings, which warn of impending neurological problems from cord compression. Intubation and positioning the patient prone can be perilous for those with unstable spines. As described in the previous section, these maneuvers are performed with utmost care to avoid neurological injury.

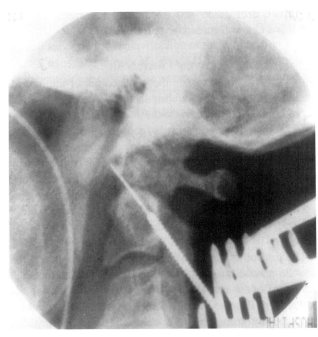

Figure 11–7. Lateral cervical spine x-ray shows the 2.7-mm cannulated drill being guided along the Kirschner wire under lateral fluoroscopic control toward the anterior tubercle of the atlas.

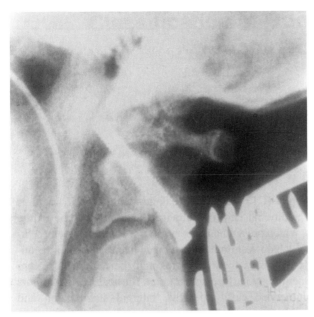

Figure 11–8. Lateral cervical spine radiograph shows the two 3.5-mm cannulated screws in place.

Spinal cord injury can also occur while placing the screw or during drilling. We expose the medial margin of the pedicle and keep a nerve hook on this medial wall to detect any breech of the medial wall before cord injury can occur.

Injury to the Nerve Roots or Vertebral Artery

In this approach, the surgeon can preserve the occipital nerve by not exposing the C1 to C2 facet joint. Therefore, the nerve with its venous plexus (just inferior to the joint) remains undisturbed. Injury to the vertebral artery is rare. By starting the drilling in the inferior medial quadrant and staying in the dorsal and medial aspects of the pedicle, we avoid injuring the artery, which is lateral to the pedicle. A preoperative CT scan should be obtained in every case to ascertain anomalous medial migration of the vertebral artery. These patients should not have a screw placed on that side.

Loss of Alignment, Screw Breakage, and Pullout

After initial reduction, loss of alignment will not occur unless a screw breaks or pulls out. Pullout occurs when the screws are overtightened, which can strip the threads. If the bone is soft as a result of osteoporosis or metabolic bone disease, screw pullout is likely and other means to stabilize the spine should be explored. A screw can break on one or both sides if external immobilization is not adequate until the bone graft is fused. In our series at 3-month follow-up, one patient presenting with bilateral screw breakage (Holfolo screw) showed neither change in clinical status on lateral

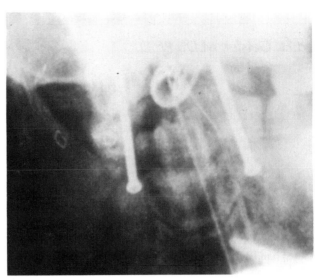

Figure 11–9. Anteroposterior radiographic study shows the screws traversing the C1 to C2 facet joint.

cervical spine x-ray nor movement on flexion and extension studies; thus intervention was not warranted.

CONCLUSION

Posterior transfacetal screw placement is a useful and safe technique in selected patients for stabilization of a reducible atlantoaxial subluxation, with or without additional posterior wiring with H graft. Because this method of stabilization does not require use postoperatively of a halo vest and does not depend on the integrity of the posterior elements of C1 to C2, posterior transfacetal screw placement is advantageous when compared with traditional wiring techniques.

REFERENCES

1. Brooks AL, Jenkins EB. Atlanto-axial arthrodesis by the wedge compression method. *J Bone Joint Surg.* 1978;60A:279–284.
2. Gallie WE. Fractures and dislocations of the cervical spine. *Am J Surg.* 1939;46:495–499.
3. Magerl F, Seeman PS. Stable posterior fusion of the atlas and axis by transarticular screw fixation. In: Kehr P, Weidner A, eds. *Cervical Spine I.* New York: Springer-Verlag; 1985:322–327.
4. Anderson LD, D'Alonzo RT. Fractures of the odontoid process of the axis. *J Bone Joint Surg.* 1971;56A:1663–1674.
5. Barbour JR. Screw fixation in fractures of the odontoid process. *S Austr Clin.* 1971;5:20–24.
6. Clark CR, White AA. Fractures of the dens, a multicenter study. *J Bone Joint Surg.* 1985;67A:1340–1348.
7. Thomson RC, Meyer TJ. Posterior surgical stabilization for atlantoaxial subluxation in rheumatid arthritis. *Spine.* 1985;10:597–601.
8. Bracken MB, Shepard MJ, Collins WF, et al. A randomized controlled trial of methyl prednisolone or naloxone in the treatment of acute spinal cord injury. *N Engl J Med.* 1990;322:1405–1411.

cal traction is utilized, the head is taped to prevent rotation of the neck and a pad is placed under the C6 to T1 area, to aid in placing the lower cervical spine into extension. Careful positioning is essential because anatomic alignment of the fracture fragments is required before screw insertions (minimal manipulation of the fragments is possible intraoperatively). The positioning is also necessary for maintaining fracture reduction during surgery, obtaining the surgical trajectory for the screw insertion, and for fluoroscopic evaluation of the drill, tap, and screw trajectory. Lower cervical extension is necessary to permit a direct line for drilling from the anterior inferior edge of C2 into the tip of the odontoid process. If this trajectory cannot be obtained intraoperatively, then the procedure must be abandoned.

Both anteroposterior (AP) and lateral fluoroscopy of the C1 to C2 area are necessary intraoperatively to perform this procedure. They can be obtained with two fluoroscope units draped in the field or one unit draped so that it is able to rotate between the two views. Before the start of surgery, the fluoroscopic beam angle, patient position, and operative height are adjusted for optimal visualization of the C2 body and the odontoid process. Minor adjustments of the head position are often required during positioning in most cases to obtain the best anatomic reduction of the odontoid fracture. The patient's jaw and teeth can obscure the anteroposterior view of the fracture when the mouth is closed. A gauze roll is placed in the patient's mouth to prevent these images from overlying that of the fracture site.

A horizontal skin incision is made from the midline to the anterior border of the sternocleidomastoid muscle on the right at the skin level, determined from where the drill trajectory line intersects the skin. Typically this occurs at the C5 level. The platysma muscle is transected in the line of the skin incision, and the fascial plane deep to the platysma and superficial to the medial strap muscles and lateral sternocleidomastoid is developed proximally to the level of C3. Blunt and sharp dissection are utilized to develop the plane between the strap muscles and the sternocleidomastoid muscle, allowing separation and lateral retraction of the carotid sheath from the medially retracted esophagus, larynx, and posterior pharynx. The anterior surfaces of the C3 or C4 vertebral bodies are exposed with this dissection. The dissection is then extended cephalad directly over the anterior longitudinal ligament until the inferior aspect of the anterior portion of C2 is exposed. The level and trajectory angle is verified with fluoroscopy. With sharp dissection, the anterior longitudinal ligament is cleared from a 1.0-cm-diameter area centered at the anterior inferior aspect of the body of C2. A small portion of the anterior center portion of the C2 to C3 disk and the superior anterior edge of the C3 body is removed to provide both the trajectory for the screw during insertion and act as a bed for the screw head.

Standard self-retaining cervical retractors with sharp blades are not used. The cephalad angulation of the surgical approach would cause the retractor teeth to be in contact with the pharynx or esophagus and possibly cause perfora-

tion. Hand-held Cloward blade retractors (Codman & Shurtleff, Inc., Randolph, Mass) and a Capsar self-retaining retractor with smooth blades (Aesculap, South San Francisco, Calif) are utilized during the deep dissection. Adjustments or removal of the wound retractors are commonly required during this procedure because the self-retaining blades obscure the fluoroscopic evaluation of the spine.

The starting point for drilling is the anterior inferior corner of the body of C2 slightly in the C2 to C3 disk space. A 2-mm drill (3M Minidriver, 3M Company, St. Paul, Minn) is drilled partially into the body of C2 and directed parallel to the midline in a trajectory that will penetrate the superior posterior portion of the tip of the odontoid. Often, this trajectory is obtained with the drill lying directly on the patient's chest. Under AP and lateral fluoroscopic control, the drill trajectory is adjusted as the drill is advanced in 2- to 3-mm intervals through the C2 body, across the odontoid fracture line, and finally penetrating the cortex near the top of the odontoid process. Typically, 8 to 12 fluoroscopy images with several trajectory corrections are necessary to obtain the desired drill trajectory (Figs. 12–5A and B). If a second screw is also inserted, a second 2-mm drill is drilled parallel and just lateral to the first in the same manner. Care is taken not to advance the first drill bit further while concentrating on the insertion of the second. The second drill bit also penetrates the superior cortex of the dens (Fig. 12–5C).

Once the position of the drill bit(s) is verified, the drill bit(s) is removed and screw length is determined with a depth gauge. The exact positioning of the depth gauge is verified with fluoroscopy. The drill hole is next tapped with a 3.5-mm tap (AO/ASIF Small Fragment Set, Synthes, Paoli, Pa), which facilitates screw insertion. A 4.0-mm cancellous screw long enough so that the threads of this screw penetrate the superior cortex of the odontoid process by 1 to 3 mm is used. Screw insertion is performed under biplanar fluoroscopic control also to assure that the screw is in the tapped drill hole (Fig. 12–5D). The second screw, if used, is inserted in a similar manner (Fig. 12–5E). The screws are tightened (Fig. 12–5F) snugly. The 4-mm cancellous screw has a smooth screw shank and hence obtains lag screw compression across the odontoid fracture when it is tightened. After the second screw crosses the fracture site, the fracture is internally fixated in the axis of rotation about the first screw (Figs. 12–6A and B). No bone grafting is performed.

Immediate stability of the odontoid screw fixation is tested intraoperatively with flexion and extension of the neck under fluoroscopic evaluation (Fig. 12–5G). The positions of the odontoid process C2 body and screw(s) should not change relative to one another. Motion will be present at the C1 to C2 joint. The surgical wound is irrigated and closed in layers over a suction drain. The patient is typically awakened in the operating room for a postoperative neurological examination.

Postoperatively, the patient has external orthosis for approximately 3 months. A cervicothoracic orthosis is used

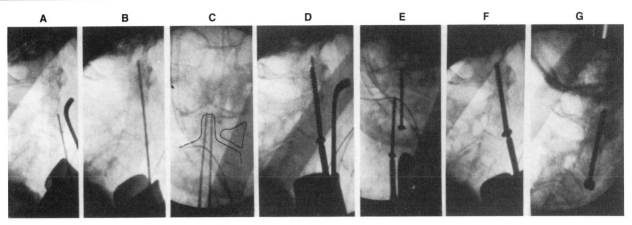

Figure 12–5. Intraoperative radiographs obtained during anterior screw placement for the internal stabilization of subtype II-P odontoid fractures. (**A**). Lateral fluorogram showing the start of the initial drill hole in the inferior anterior edge of the body of the dens with the drill 5 mm into the body. Note the image of the Cloward hand-held retractor elevating the posterior wall of the pharynx from the operative site. (**B**). The first drill tap hole completed with the drill bit extending through the superior posterior odontoid process cortex. (**C**). An antero-posterior intraoperative fluorogram of the two drill bits side by side through the cortex at the tip of the odontoid process. (**D**). Lateral cervical fluorogram with the first screw being advanced up the drill guide hole. The drill bit of the second screw hole is imaged as the parallel image that is best visualized as it extended superiorly beyond the tip of the screw. (**E**). Anteroposterior intraoperative fluoroscopy with one screw in place and the second screw being advanced up its guide hole. (**F**). Lateral cervical view while the two screws are being tightened with the matching screwdriver. (**G**). Patient moved manually in flexion to verify immediate mechanical stability of the screw fixation. See text for details of the surgical procedure. (Used with permission of Geisler FH, Cheng C, Poka A, Brumback RJ. Anterior screw fixation of posteriorly displaced type II odontoid fractures. *Neurosurgery.* 1989;25:30–38.)

unless other priorities required the use of a halo-vest device. These include the lack of patient compliance due to closed intracranial injury or personality disorder, or the presence of other cervical fractures requiring halo immobilization. The patient is permitted to assume the upright position and ambulate once the external orthosis is in place. Flexion/extension cervical lateral radiographs or lateral tomography are obtained to verify stability and union of the odontoid fracture (Figs. 12–6C and D) before the external orthosis is removed.

Of the eight patients who survived, we used a Philadelphia collar for postoperative cervical immobilization in three. One of these patients tolerated this orthosis poorly and a soft cervical collar was substituted. We initially used cervicothoracic orthosis braces (Yale)[81] for three patients. One of these patients developed an occipital pressure sore and was placed in a halo vest 1 month postoperatively. Two patients were definitively immobilized with a halo-vest device. One of them had additional anterior ring fractures of C1 accompanying his posterior ring fractures. The average length of postoperative external support was 3.1 months (range, 1.5 to 6.0 months).

A new set of surgical instruments has been developed recently by Dr Apfelbaum (Aesculap, South San Francisco, Calif) specifically for the anterior screw fixation of odontoid fractures.[55–57] This equipment offers several advantages over the equipment in the AO/ASIF small fragment set used in the first 9 of the 10 cases listed in Table 12–1 and described previously in the surgical technique section. The 10th case used this new instrumentation. Figure 12–7A shows this Type II-P fracture on initial presentation before

reduction, and Figure 12–7B shows the postoperative radiograph with a titanium lag screw internal fixation in the same patient.

The Apfelbaum instruments consist of three groupings according to their function: soft-tissue retractors, cannulated guide system, and a small angled handpiece drill. The soft-tissue retractors are a modification of the Caspar cervical retractor with an angled soft-tissue blade allowing retraction of the posterior wall of the pharynx (Fig. 12–8). Although this retractor combination provides good visualization of the screw entry site, the metal of the retractor can interfere with the fluoroscopic image (radiolucent blades are now available and should allow clear images). The author prefers hand-held retractors that are removed for imaging. The second component is a cannulated guide system that secures to the body of C3 with teeth at its base (Fig. 11–8). The drill guide provides both safety as it protects the soft tissue of the neck from injury with the tap or drill, and a steady base to perform drilling, taping, and screwing.

The measurement for screw length can be obtained from the drill bit because it has a scale etched on it and hence measuring the hole depth is not a separate step. The drill bit is powered by a small right-angle handpiece (Fig. 12–9). Figure 12–10 shows the use of the cannulated guide system in the surgical wound without the soft-tissue retractors during the drilling stage. Note that the soft-tissue retractors are not in the wound during the advancement of the drill bit. Optimal fluoroscopy images are obtained without the soft-tissue retractors. The cannulated system protects the soft tissues in the anterior neck from contacting the moving drill. The small right-angle handpiece is an advantage over standard in-line

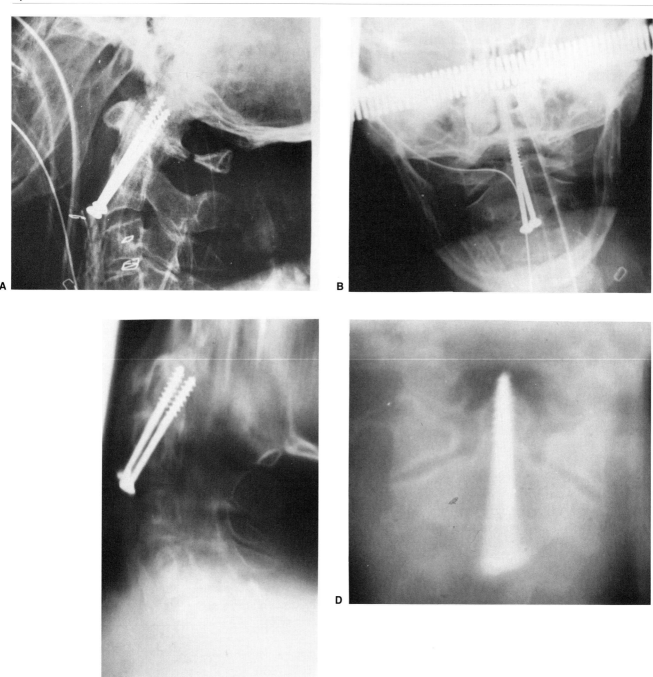

Figure 12–6. (**A**). Postoperative lateral cervical radiograph demonstrating good alignment between the odontoid process and the body of C2. The correct screw position is verified by the tip of the screws passing through the superior posterior cortex of the odontoid process. Note exact alignment of the bilateral posterior C1 arch fractures. (**B**). Postoperative anteroposterior cervical radiograph of the same patient. (**C**). Follow-up anteroposterior cervical tomogram of the same patient. (**D**). Follow-up anteroposterior cervical tomogram of the same patient. Both tomographic planes demonstrate continuity of the cortex at the previous fracture dislocation site, indicating a bony fusion on follow-up at 6 months. (Used with permission of Geisler FH, Cheng C, Poka A, Brumback RJ. Anterior screw fixation of posteriorly displaced type II odontoid fractures. *Neurosurgery.* 1989;25:30–38.)

drills in odontoid fixation, in which the drill bit's optimal trajectory is potentially compromised by contact between the bulk of the drill body and the patient's chest. Aesculap also provides titanium bone screws in a wide variety of lengths. The titanium screws have the advantage of reduced magnetic resonance imaging (MRI) scanning artifact compared to the stainless steel screws. Although the Apfelbaum instrumentation is not necessary to perform odontoid fixation, it is well customized for this application and appears to provide significant advantages in operative technique.

Other modifications and enhancements to anterior fixation of odontoid fractures have been reported. Meier et al[77]

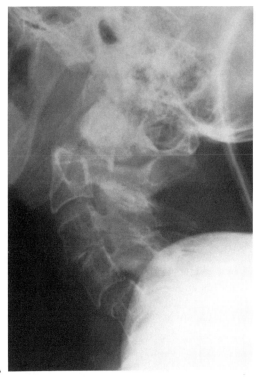
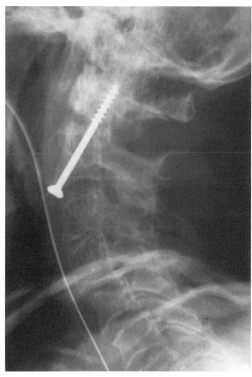

A   B

Figure 12–7. (A). Initial lateral radiograph of Type II-P odontoid fracture. This patient was realigned preoperatively and stabilized internally with a single titanium screw. (B). Postsurgical lateral radiographic of the same patient.

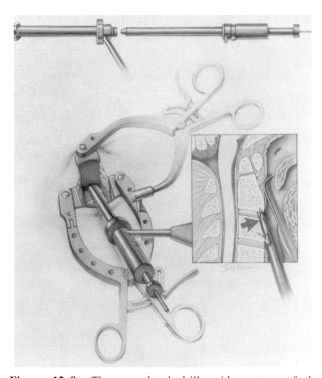

Figure 12–8. The cannulated drill guide system of the Apfelbaum instrumentation for anterior screw fixation of odontoid fractures. Also shown are the modified Caspar soft tissue retractors in the wound. Note the teeth in the cannulated guide system that secures it to C3. (Used with permission of Apfelbaum RI. *Anterior Screw Fixation for Odontoid fractures.* Tuttlingen, Germany: Aesculap; 1992.)

developed a cannulated screw system in which the fracture is first fixated with two Kirschner wires and then hollow screws are used over the wires to follow their trajectory. Neugebauer[82] has developed an endoscopic technique for placing the lag screw for anterior fixation of odontoid fractures. Lozes et al[64] described the use of a conical implant of biocompatible resorbable biopolymer instead of a metal screw. Thus, after healing of the fracture no metal remains to cause problems or interfere with future CT or MRI scans.

OPERATIVE AND POSTOPERATIVE COMPLICATIONS

There was one intraoperative complication: a broken drill bit that was retrieved from the body of C2. No postoperative infections or wound hematomas were recorded. No neurological deficits attributable to the operative procedure occurred. One patient developed an occipital decubitus from cervicothoracic postoperative bracing; it resolved with local wound care after the application of a halo vest. Two patients died in the postoperative period related to medical complications.

Intraoperative breakage of the drill bit in the body of C2 is potentially preventable with better patient positioning to allow a straight-line trajectory free of the anterior chest wall from the base of C2 to the tip of the odontoid process. The Apfelbaum instrumentation with the use of the right-angle drill would also have solved this technical problem. If the

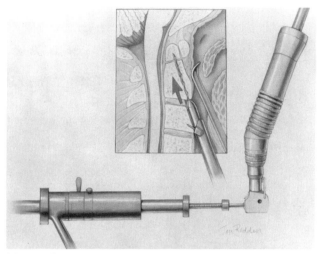

Figure 12–9. The cannulated drill guide and drill during the drilling of the trajectory hole. Note the smallness of the right-angle drill handpiece. The trajectory of the drill is perpendicular to the fracture line by having it start at the anterior inferior base of the C2 from within the C2 to C3 interspace. (Used with permission of Apfelbaum RI. *Anterior Screw Fixation for Odontoid Fractures.* Tuttlingen, Germany: Aesculap; 1992.)

drill trajectory is not aligned properly, the surgeon will tend to bend, and possibly break, the drill bit because the thoracic cage can interfere with correct drill placement.

The dissection for an anterior odontoid screw fixation can result in any of the reported complications associated with an anterior surgical approach to the cervical spine, including soft-tissue injury to the larynx, trachea, pharynx, and esophagus or damage to the nerve roots, spinal cord, and autonomic extraspinal nerves.[21,50] None of these complications occurred in our series.

No bone graft was used in this procedure because the surgery itself provides immediate reduction, compression, and stabilization of the fracture. The odontoid process healed to the body of C2 in all patients who survived. This high rate of fracture union was attributed to prompt surgical repair, the fracture compression inherent with this type of internal fixation, and the excellent contact of the anatomically aligned fracture surfaces. The use of this internal stabilization in the treatment of established nonunions of Type II odontoid fractures probably requires curretting the fibrous disunion so that cancellous bone contact is made at the fracture line.[55–57]

CONCLUSION

The results of this small clinical series and the literature review indicate that anterior odontoid screw fixation produced immediate stability and excellent long-term clinical results. The significant mechanical advantages, surgical safety, and low morbidity of this technique may result in it ultimately becoming the treatment of choice in Type II-P odontoid fractures displaced 4 mm or more with or without associated bilateral fractures of the posterior arch of C1. Excellent maintenance of fracture reduction and eventual fracture union occurred without the decrease in cervical motion inherent with alternative posterior arthrodesis treatment methods.

REFERENCES

1. Mixter SJ, Osgood RB. Traumatic lesions of the atlas and axis. *Ann Surg.* 1910;51:193–207.
2. Blockey NJ, Purser DW. Fractures of the odontoid process of the axis. *J Bone Joint Surg Br.* 1956;38:794–817.
3. Osgood RB, Lund CC. Fractures of the odontoid process. *N Engl J Med.* 1928;198:61–71.
4. Anderson LD, D'Alonzo RT. Fracture of the odontoid process of the axis. *J Bone Joint Surg Am.* 1974;56:1663–1674.
5. Donovan MM. Efficacy of rigid fixation of fractures of the odontoid process. Retrospective analysis of 54 cases. *Orthop Trans.* 1979;3:309.
6. Fielding JW, Hawkins RJ. Roentgenographic diagnosis of the injured neck. *American Association of Orthopaedic Surgeons:*

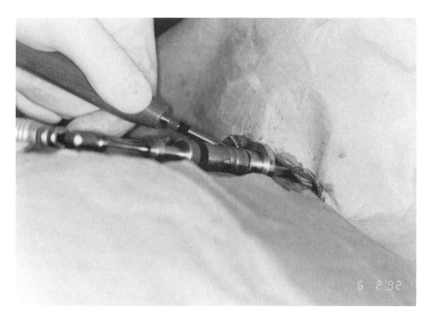

Figure 12–10. Operative use of the Apfelbaum cannulated guide system during the drilling operation. Note that the soft-tissue retractors are not in the wound during the advancement of the drill bit. Optimal fluoroscopy images are obtained without the soft-tissue retractors. The cannulated system protects the soft tissues in the anterior neck from contacting the moving drill.

Instructional Course Lectures. St. Louis, Mo: CV Mosby; 1976:149–170.

7. Pierce DS, Barr JS Jr. Fractures and dislocations at the base of the skull and upper cervical spine. In: Bailey RW, ed. *The Cervical Spine.* Philadelphia, Pa: JB Lippincott; 1983:196–206.

8. Southwick WO. Management of fractures of the dens (odontoid process). *J Bone Joint Surg Am.* 1980;62:482–486.

9. Dunn ME, Seljeskog EL. Experience in the management of odontoid process injuries: an analysis of 128 cases. *Neurosurgery.* 1986;18:306–310.

10. Ekong CEU, Schwartz ML, Tator CH, et al. Odontoid fracture: management with early mobilization using the halo device. *Neurosurgery.* 1981;9:631–637.

11. Hadley MN, Browner CM, Liu SS, et al. New subtype of acute odontoid fractures (type IIA). *Neurosurgery.* 1988;22:67–71.

12. Apuzzo MLJ, Heiden JS, Weiss MH, et al. Acute fractures of the odontoid process; an analysis of 45 cases. *J. Neurosurg.* 1978;48:85–91.

13. Bohler J. Anterior stabilization for acute fractures and nonunions of the dens. *J Bone Joint Surg Am.* 1982;64:18–27.

14. Brooks AL, Jenkins EB. Atlanto-axial arthrodesis by the wedge compression method. *J Bone Joint Surg Am.* 1978;60:279–284.

15. Clark CR, White AA III. Fractures of the dens. A multi-center study. *J Bone Joint Surg Am.* 1985;67:1340–1348.

16. Estridge MN, Smith RA. Transoral fusion of odontoid fracture. Case report. *J Neurosurg.* 1967;27:462–465.

17. Fang HSY, Ong GB. Direct anterior approach to the upper cervical spine. *J Bone Joint Surg Am.* 1962;44:1588–1604.

18. McLaurin RL, Vernal R, Salmon JH. Treatment of fractures of the atlas and axis by wiring with fusion. *J Neurosurg.* 1972;36:773–780.

19. Nakanishi T. Internal fixation of odontoid fracture (in Japanese). *Orthop Traum Surg.* 1980;23:399–406.

20. Salmon JH. Fracture of the second cervical vertebra: internal fixation by interlaminar wiring. *Neurosurgery.* 1977;1:125–127.

21. Verbiest H. Anterolateral operations for fractions or dislocations of the cervical spine due to injuries or previous surgical intervention. *Clin Neurosurg.* 1973;20:334–336.

22. Six E, Kelly DJ. Technique for C-1, C-2, and C-3 fixation in cases of odontoid fracture. *Neurosurgery.* 1981;8:374–377.

23. Waddell JP, Reardon GP. Atlantoaxial arthrodesis to treat odontoid fractures. *Canadian J Surg.* 1983;26:255–258.

24. Kelly DL, Alexander E, Courtland HD. Acrylic fixation of atlanto-axial dislocation. Technical note. *J Neurosurg.* 1972;36:366–371.

25. Bohler J. Fractures of the odontoid process. *J Trauma.* 1965;5:386–391.

26. Lind B, Nordwall A, Sihbom H. Odontoid fractures treated with halovest. *Spine.* 1987;12:173–177.

27. Dickson H, Engel S, Blum P. Odontoid fractures, systemic disease and conservative care. *Aust NZ J Surg.* 1984;54:243–247.

28. Cooper PR, Maravilla KR, Sklar FH. Halo immobilization of cervical spine fractures. *J Neurosurg.* 1979;50:603–610.

29. Chan RC, Schweigel JF, Thompson GB. Halo-thoracic brace immobilization in 188 patients with acute cervical spine injuries. *J Neurosurg.* 1983;58:508–515.

30. Fujii E, Kobayashi K, Hirabayashi K. Treatment in fractures of the odontoid process. *Spine.* 1988;13:604–609.

31. Sears W, Fazl M. Prediction of stability of cervical spine fracture managed in the halo vest and indications for surgical intervention. *J Neurosurg.* 1990;72:426–432.

32. Wang GJ, Mabie KN, Whitehill R. The nonsurgical management of odontoid fractures in adults. *Spine.* 1984;9:229–230.

33. Pepin JW, Bourne RB, Hawkins RJ. Odontoid fractures, with special reference to the elderly patient. *Clin Orthop.* 1985;193:178–183.

34. Hentzer L, Schalimtzek M. Fractures and subluxations of the atlas and axis. A follow-up study of 20 patients. *Acta Orthop Scand.* 1971;42:251–258.

35. Amyes EW, Anderson FM. Fracture of the odontoid process. *Arch Surg.* 1956;72:377–393.

36. Hadley MN, Browner CM, Sonntag VKH. Axis fractures: a comprehensive review of management and treatment in 107 cases. *Neurosurgery.* 1985;17:281–290.

37. Hadley MN, Sonntag VHK. Acute axis fractures. *Contemp Neurosurg.* 1987;9:1–6.

38. Maiman DJ, Larson SJ. Management of odontoid fractures. *Neurosurgery.* 1982;11:471–480.

39. Pierce DS, Barr JS. Use of the halo in cervical spine problems. *Orthop Trans.* 1979;3:125–126.

40. Schatzker J, Rorabeck CH, Waddell JP. Fractures of the dens (odontoid process). An analysis of 37 cases. *J Bone Joint Surg Br.* 1971;53B:392–405.

41. Griswold DM, Albright JA, Schiffman E, et al. Atlanto-axial fusion for instability. *J Bone Joint Surg Am.* 1978;60:285–292.

42. Levine AM, Edwards CC. Treatment of injuries in the C1-C2 complex. *Orthop Clin N Am.* 1986;17:31–44.

43. Ryan MD, Taylor TK. Odontoid fractures. A rational approach to treatment. *J Bone Joint Surg Br.* 1982;64:416–421.

44. White AM, Panjabi M. *Clinical Biomechanics of the Spine.* Philadelphia, Pa: JB Lippincott; 1978.

45. Dunham CM, Cowley RA. *Shock Trauma/Critical Care Handbook.* Rockville, Md: Aspen Publishers; 1986.

46. Lewallen RP, Morrey BF, Cabanela ME. Respiratory arrest following posteriorly displaced odontoid fractures. Case reports and review of literature. *Clin Orthop.* 1984;188:187–190.

47. Fried LC. Atlanto-axial fracture-dislocations. Failure of posterior C1 to C2 fusion. *J Bone Joint Surg Br.* 1973;55B:490–496.

48. Autricque A, Lesoin F, Francke JP, et al. Choice of a technique of stabilization in surgical treatment of recent fractures of the odontoid process. 90 cases. *Neurochirurgie.* 1988;34:410–419.

49. Jeanneret B, Magerl F. Primary posterior fusion C1/2 in odontoid fractures: indications, technique, and results of transarticular screw fixation. *J Spinal Disord.* 1992;5:464–475.

50. Horowitz NH, Rizzoli HV. *Postoperative Complications of Extracranial Neurological Surgery.* Baltimore, Md: Williams & Wilkins; 1987.

51. Jeanneret B, Vernet O, Frei S, et al. Atlantoaxial mobility after screw fixation of the odontoid: a computed tomographic study. *J Spinal Disord.* 1991;4:203–211.

52. Borne GM, Bedou GL, Pinaudeau M, et al. Odontoid process fracture osteosynthesis with a direct screw fixation technique in nine consecutive cases. *J Neurosurg.* 1988;68:223–226.

53. Lesoin F, Autricque A, Franz K, et al. Transcervical approach and screw fixation for upper cervical spine pathology. *Surg Neurol.* 1987;27:459–465.

54. Geisler FH, Cheng C, Poka A, et al. Anterior screw fixation of posteriorly displaced type II odontoid fractures. *Neurosurgery.* 1989;25:30–37.

55. Apfelbaum RI. Anterior screw fixation of odontoid fractures. In: Camins MS, O'Leary PF, eds. *Diseases of the Cervical Spine.* Baltimore, Md: Williams & Wilkins; 1992:603–613.

56. Apfelbaum RI. Anterior screw fixation of odontoid fractures. In: Rengachary SS, Wilkins RH, eds. *Neurosurgical Operative Atlas.* Vol 2. Baltimore, Md: Williams & Wilkins; 1992:189–199.

57. Apfelbaum RI. *Anterior Screw Fixation for Odontoid Fractures.* Tuttlingen, Germany: Aesculap; 1992.

58. Pentelenyi T, Szarvas I, Bodrogi L. Up-to-date method of treatment of most frequent axis-injuries: screw-fixation of the odontoid fractures. *Acta Chir Hung.* 1988;29:349–357.

59. Hasegawa T, Yamano K, Hamada Y, et al. Intra-operative screw trimming in direct screw fixation of the odontoid process fracture—technical note. *Acta Neurochir (Wien).* 1992;115:60–61.

ture—technical note. *Acta Neurochir (Wien).* 1992;115:60–61.

60. Pentelenyi T, Szarvas I, Bodrogi L. Screw fixation of odontoid fractures: preliminary report. *Injury.* 1988;19:139–142.

61. Hacker R, Golden PF. Internal fixation of the odontoid: a newer approach to an old problem. *Nebr Med J.* 1991;76:325–329.

62. Knoringer P. Treatment of fresh fractures of the dens axis by compression screw osteosynthesis. *Neurochirurgia Stuttg.* 1984;27:68–72.

63. Gilsbach J. Screw fixation of the odontoid process. A functional procedure (letter). *Neurochirurgie.* 1992;38:54–55.

64. Lozes G, Fawaz A, Jomin M, et al. Direct osteosynthesis of fractures of the odontoid process using a biodegradable implant (B.O.P.). *Neurochirurgie.* 1988;34:355–358.

65. Autricque A, Lesoin F, Villette L, et al. Screwing of the odontoid process via the anterior intermaxillo-hyoid retropharyngeal approach. *Neurochirurgie.* 1987;33:156–160.

66. Borne G, Bedou G, Omeiri SE, et al. Osteosynthesis of fractures of the odontoid process by direct screwing. Preliminary reflections on 2 surgically treated cases. *Neurochirurgie.* 1987;33:152–155.

67. Moossy JJ, Hanley EN. Anterior screw fixation of odontoid fractures (letter). *Neurosurgery.* 1989;25:847.

68. Aebi M, Etter C. Ventral direct screw fixation in dens fractures. *Orthopade.* 1991;20:147–153.

69. Grob D, Magerl F. Surgical stabilization of C1 and C2 fractures. *Orthopade.* 1987;16:46–54.

70. Autricque A, Lesoin F, Jomin M. Screw fixation of the odontoid process. *Presse Med.* 1988;17:1647–1648.

71. Asfora WT, Free TW, Johnson JH. Odontoid fracture in the elderly: a case report of the screw fixation technique. *S D J Med.* 1992;45:175–177.

72. Grosse A, Bohly J, Taglang G, et al. Screw fixation of fractures of the odontoid process. *Rev Chir Orthop Reparatrice Appar Mot.* 1991;77:425–431.

73. Etter C, Coscia M, Jaberg H, et al. Direct anterior fixation of dens fractures with a cannulated screw system. *Spine.* 1991;16:S25–S32.

74. Montesano PX, Anderson PA, Schlehr F, et al. Odontoid fractures treated by anterior odontoid screw fixation. *Spine.* 1991;16:S33–S37.

75. Etter C, Coscia M, Ganz R, et al. Bone screw osteosynthesis of dens fractures. Technical surgical aspects and results. *Unfallchirurg.* 1989;92:220–226.

76. Bohler J. Screw-osteosynthesis of fractures of the dens axis (author's transl). *Unfallheilkunde.* 1981;84:221–223.

77. Meier U, Knopf W, Klages G, et al. Instrumentation for hollow screw osteosynthesis of basal dens axis fractures. *Zentralbl Neurochir.* 1987;48:303–307.

78. Barth H, Lang G. Double compression screw osteosynthesis in the treatment of fresh fractures and pseudarthroses of the dens axis. *Zentralbl Chir.* 1989;114:263–270.

79. Heller JG, Alson MD, Schaffler MB, et al. Quantitative internal dens morphology. *Spine.* 1992;17:861–866.

80. Schaffler MB, Alson MD, Heller JG, et al. Morphology of the dens. A quantitative study. *Spine.* 1992;17:738–743.

81. Sypert GW. External spinal orthotics. *Neurosurgery.* 1987;20:642–649.

82. Neugebauer R. Tissue-preserving ventral compression osteosynthesis of dens axis fractures using endoscopy and special instruments. *Unfallchirurg.* 1991;94:313–316.

13 Interspinous, Laminar, and Facet Posterior Cervical Bone Fusions

John C. VanGilder, M.D.

INTRODUCTION

The object of a cervical fusion is to establish a bony union between vertebrae. Subsequent to the initial report by Albee in 1911, fusions have been used to treat a variety of spinal disorders.[1] The ultimate goal of these surgical procedures is to decrease pain and to preserve or improve any neurological deficit associated with spinal pathology. Paralleling significant advances in diagnostic techniques, a variety of operative procedures have been developed for spinal stabilization using both metal devices and acrylic material. Despite these alternative procedures, bony fusion remains the most effective of these difficult procedures.

There are three anatomic bone areas that are utilized for posterior fusion of the cervical spine: the spinous processes, laminae, and facets. Which fusion technique selected is dependent on an understanding of the biomechanics of the cervical spinal column, underlying pathology, and principles of fusion.

Biomechanics

The basic function of the cervical spinal column is to allow neck motion, transmit load, and protect the spinal cord and nerve roots. The cervical spine can be divided into upper (C1 to C2), middle (C3 to C5), and lower (C5 to C7) segments. The subsequent contents of this chapter are concerned only with the middle and lower cervical spine.

The annulus fibrosis is a major stabilizing structure between the vertebral bodies.[2] It is subject to compressive loading stress, tensile stress secondary to flexion, extension and lateral bending, and shear stress from axial rotation. Rotation and bending are interdependent, and these stress forces are considered to be coupled.

The C3 to C7 interarticular facets are oriented at a 45° angle to the vertical in the sagittal plane. Accordingly, with lateral bending there is simultaneous rotation. This coupling motion is maximal at C2 to C3 and decreases slightly in the more caudal vertebra because of an increase in the facet angle. Because of this coupling, the spinous processes form a convex curve to the opposite side with lateral bending.[2] In contrast, the majority of flexion-extension motion is at the midcervical area, or C5 to C6.

The intervertebral disks in combination with the anterior and posterior ligaments are the major structures responsible for cervical spine stability.[3] Panjabi and White have divided the cervical spine into anterior and posterior functional units.[4] The anterior elements consist of the posterior longitudinal ligament and all structures anterior to it. The posterior elements are all structures dorsal to the posterior longitudinal ligament. If either of the functional spinal units is destroyed or unable to function, the spine should be considered unstable.[5] Conversely, if one of these units is only subtotally damaged, with one or more of its elements intact, the spinal column is probably stable. In general, if the anterior elements are destroyed, the spine is more unstable in extension, and if the posterior elements are destroyed, it is more unstable in flexion.

Assessment of Instability

Controlled, monitored axial traction for stretch test may be helpful to evaluate ligamentous integrity.[6] Axial traction loads are applied up to a maximum of one third of the patient's body weight or to a maximum of 65 pounds. The test is abnormal if differences greater than 1.7 mm of interspace separation or greater than 7.5° of angle change occurs between the vertebrae.

Lateral cervical spine roentgenographs should be obtained with 72 inches of tube-to-film distance to standardize magnification error. Under these conditions, sagittal plane translation should not exceed 3.5 mm on either static or flexion/extension views in a patient over 7 years of age.[6] More than 20% sagittal plane angulation on dynamic views should be considered potentially unstable. On static roentgenographs, more than 11° relative (pathologic minus normal angle) sagittal angulation should be considered unstable.

The degree of neurological deficit following a spinal injury influences assessment of instability in a more subjective fashion. Although spinal cord damage may occur with intact supporting spinal column structures, in general, when neurological deficit is present, these supporting structures have been significantly altered and may be clinically unstable.[7] Similarly, clinical judgment must be used to assess the magnitude of loads anticipated on the patient's spine following injury where criteria of instability are inconclusive.

Principles of Bone Fusion

In a successful posterior spinal fusion, there is an adequate summation of osteogenic, osteoinductive, and osteoconductive forces. Bone growth is a cellular process and the fusion site is the principal source for viable cells. The fusion site

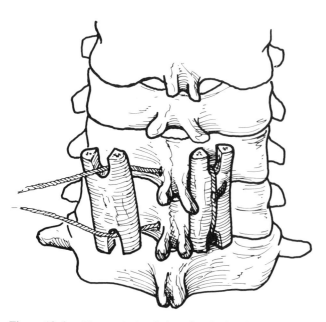

Figure 13–2. The surgical technique for placing the wire through the spinous process, preparing the bone graft, and securing the bone graft.

in layers with interrupted sutures. The patient is maintained in 3 to 5 pounds of skeletal traction for 1 to 3 days subsequent to surgery. Prior to ambulation, the patient is immobilized in a halo brace or cervical orthosis until the fusion is solid. The immobilization period is usually 3 months.

Results

Seventy-four interspinous fusions have been done in our neurosurgical clinic over 16 years. The most common etiology of instability was trauma. There have been no cases of increased neurological deficit following surgery, and there was one case of fusion failure, a 1.3% incidence.

POSTERIOR INTERLAMINAR FUSION

Those patients with extensive disruption of the anterior stabilizing ligaments and with rotational instability not requiring laminectomy are best treated with an interlaminar fusion. This technique differs from the spinous process fusion in that there is two-point stabilization of the posterior elements. The fusion usually incorporates two vertebrae above and one vertebra below the site of instability for optimal stabilization.

The exposure of the posterior elements and preparation of the donor and receptor sites for the bone grafts are similar to

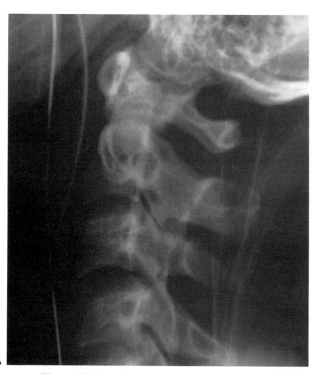

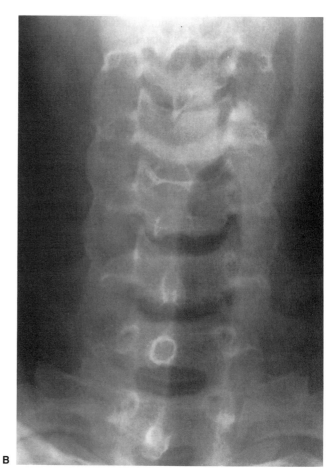

A   B

Figure 13–3. (**A**). Preoperative C3 to C4 unstable subluxation lateral. (**B**). Anterior-posterior roentgenograph.

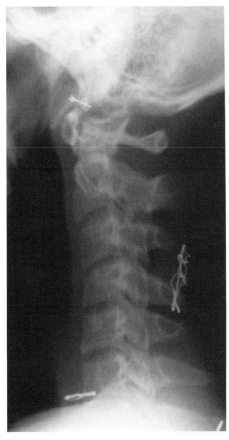 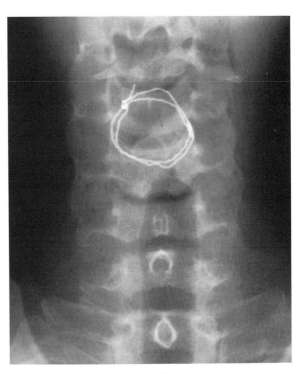

Figure 13–4.   Lateral (**A**) and anterior-posterior (**B**) roentgenograph of C3 to C4 subluxation 6 months postoperation.

that described for posterior spinous process fusion. The laminae are notched superiorly and inferiorly using a small Kerrison rongeur. The superior indentation is placed laterally in relation to the inferior notch. This notching will assist in the establishment of a plane to separate the ligamentum flavum and dura from the ventral lamina. The separation is completed with a Mixter clamp or Woodson dissector, and a single twisted wire is passed bilaterally under each lamina. Extreme care must be made in this maneuver to avoid damage to the spinal cord (Fig. 13–5).

The donor graft is then notched medially and laterally at the level of each lamina. After placing the donor graft into position dorsal to the lamina, the caudal portion of the wire is placed medially around the graft and the superior portion of the wire laterally. The individual wires are twisted in a clockwise direction until the donor graft fits snugly against the lamina (Fig. 13–6). This process is best initiated in the center of the fusion. The remaining wires are tightened in an alternating fashion around the rostral and caudal vertebra lamina.

A lateral roentgenogram is obtained to ensure that the cervical spine is aligned satisfactorily and the surgical incision is closed in layers (Fig. 13–7). Postoperatively, the patient is maintained in skeletal traction of 3 to 5 pounds for 2 to 4 days until application of an external stabilizing orthosis.

Similar to the interspinous fusion, the halo brace is preferred for external fixation compared to a cervicothoracic brace. The orthosis should remain in place for 3 to 4 months minimum or until the fusion demonstrates radiographic evidence of stability.

Results

Our experience is represented by 83 laminar fusions, the majority for instability secondary to trauma and seven cases from tumor. There were no cases of increased neurological deficit secondary to surgery. There was a fusion failure incidence of 2.4% (two cases) and 1% infection rate (one case).

LAMINECTOMY AND FACET FUSION

Laminectomy is indicated in those patients with spinal cord posterior compression from bone elements or when it is necessary to decompress the cervical cord for infection, tumors, or soft-tissue hypertrophy. In those pathologic states where the spinal cord is compromised from ventral pathology, anterior decompression is the procedure of choice.

Laminectomy alone does not result in instability. Interfacet fusion is indicated following laminectomy in those patients who have an unstable spinal column from damage to capsular ligaments, anterior and posterior longi-

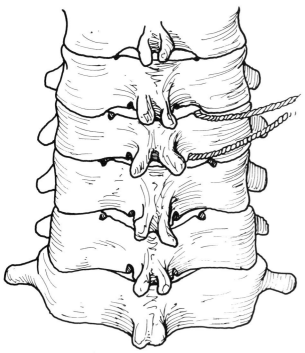

Figure 13–5. Placement of wire under the laminae.

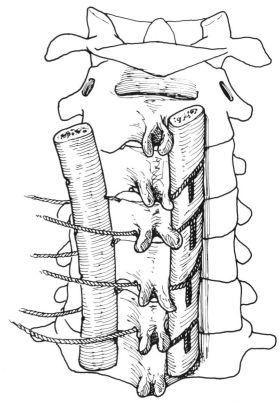

Figure 13–6. Technique of placement and securing the graft to the laminae.

tudinal ligaments, and–or supporting vertebral bone structure. Facet fusion is done immediately following laminectomy by passing wires through the facets and binding two longitudinal donor grafts to each vertebra to be fused. In most cases, this fusion technique adds immediate strength to an unstable spine to convert it to a stable one.[18]

Operative Technique

Precautions with patient transfer, intubation, and positioning on the operating table are similar to those described previously for interspinous and interlaminar fusions. The patient is maintained in 5 to 10 pounds of cervical traction throughout the operative procedure until the graft is secured in place and satisfactory spinal alignment is confirmed by lateral roentgenograms.

A midline cervical incision is made posterior to the spinous processes of the vertebra to be fused through the skin, subcutaneous tissue, and ligamentum nuchae to the spinous process. The muscles are dissected off of the spinous processes and lamina in a subperiosteal plane using cutting current and the two-periosteal technique as described previously. The tissues are dissected laterally to expose the bony facets to their lateral border. The ligamentous structures are densely adherent to the facets, and dissection is best accomplished using both sharp instrumentation and low-voltage cutting current. This must be done meticulously because venous bleeding may be troublesome, especially at the C2 to C3 level.

The spinous processes and laminae are removed in a rostral-to-caudal direction. The removal of the lamina should extend laterally to the medial border but not into the facets. The ligamentum flavum is resected to identify the dura mater. If it is necessary to expose the spinal cord, the dura is opened longitudinally in the midline. Following the surgical procedure in or around the spinal cord, the dura is closed with interrupted sutures with or without a dural graft to ensure that no constriction of the spinal cord is present.

The recipient site for the graft is prepared by ensuring that all soft and ligamentous tissue has been removed from the posterior facets. The articulation between the superior and inferior facets is exposed by inserting and rotating a Freer elevator between the joints. The articular cartilage of the superior and inferior facets is then removed with a small angled curet. A 2- to 3-m-diameter hole is drilled through the midportion of the inferior facet at a right angle to the articular joint. During this maneuver, a Freer elevator is placed between the inferior and superior facets to prevent damage to the nerve root, vertebral artery, and superior facet from the burr. The proper 90° angle is facilitated using an angled handpiece attached to the drill (Fig. 13–8).

Twisted number 25 wire (prepared as described previously) is inserted into each hole. The wire emerging between the facet is grasped by an Allis clamp, and a similar instrument is applied proximally to the wire. This enables the twisted wire to be passed through the facet without a "sawing" effect and damage to the bone (Fig. 13–9).

The donor bone graft, either from a rib or posterior iliac crest, is obtained and cut to the desired length depending on the area to be fused. The donor graft from these sites will have a concave/convex surface, enabling it to fit snugly on the recipient site conforming to the lordotic curve of the cervical spine. Two 3-mm-diameter holes are made in the cen-

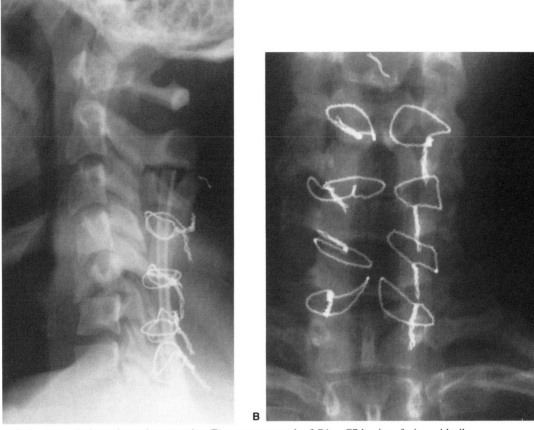

Figure 13–7. Lateral (**A**) and anterior-posterior (**B**) roentgenograph of C4 to C7 laminar fusion with rib.

ter of the graft, and the wire entering the facet is passed through this hole. The portion of the wire that emerges from the facet encircles the medial border of the graft. The two ends are then approximated by twisting the wires together (Fig. 13–10). This technique secures the graft firmly over the facets and prevents its migration medially to avoid any compression of the spinal cord.

Similar to the interlaminar fusion, when securing the donor graft to the facets, the surgeon should begin the process in the midportion of the fusion; the wires are then tightened by alternating the procedure in the rostral and caudal vertebrae throughout the fusion. If there is concern about the stability of the spine, the fusion can extend one segment beyond the laminectomy site and incorporate it into the spinous process or the lamina of the adjacent vertebra. The incision is then closed in layers approximating the muscle, fascia, subcutaneous tissue, and skin with interrupted sutures.

The patient postoperatively is usually maintained in the supine position for 2 to 3 days until the operative pain subsides. A cervicothoracic orthosis or halo brace is used to maintain cervical spinal immobilization and the patient ambulated. The fusion is followed by serial radiographs until fusion is well established and there is no motion on forced

flexion-extension radiographs (Fig. 13–11). The fusion is usually stable 5 to 10 months after the operative procedure.

Results

One hundred seven laminectomies with facet fusion have been done in our clinic. The etiology of cervical instability in these cases is as follows:

• Trauma: 63 cases

• Rheumatoid arthritis: 21 cases

• Tumors: 15 cases

• Osteoarthritis: 7 cases

• Osteoporosis imperfecta: 1 case.

There was one patient with transient increased neurological deficit subsequent to surgery, three cases of fusion failure (3%), and one infection.

SUMMARY

Three different operative techniques have been described in this chapter. Several modifications of these posterior stabilization and fusion operations are often employed dependent on the etiology and mechanics of the spine instability. Two examples of these modifications are illustrated in Figures 13–12 and 13–13.

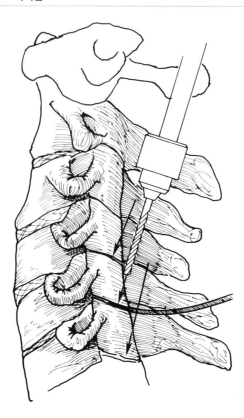

Figure 13–8.   Cervical spine (lateral view) to illustrate the angle for placing a hole in the inferior facet. A Freer elevator is between the facets to prevent damage to the soft tissue.

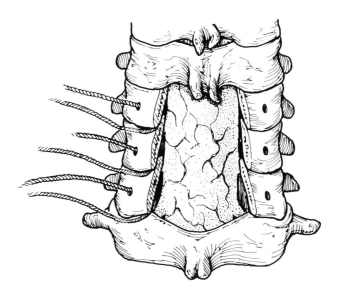

Figure 13–9.   Wire placement through the inferior facets.

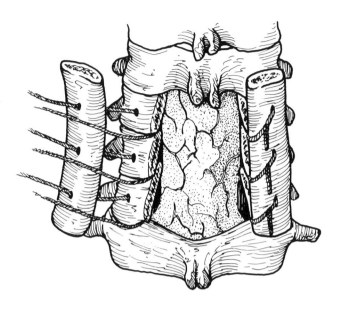

Figure 13–10.   The technique of placing wires in the graft and securing the graft over the facets.

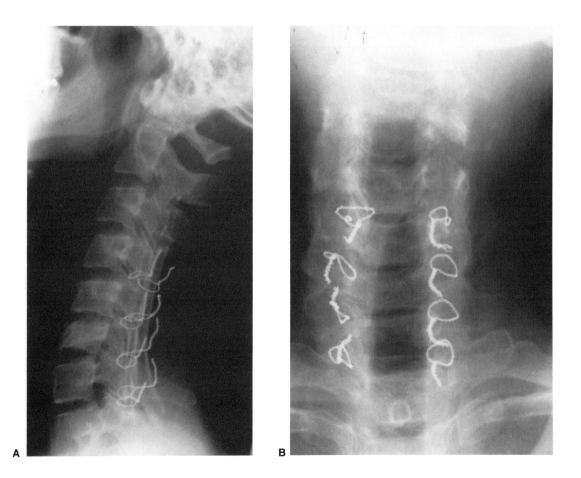

Figure 13–11.   Lateral (**A**) and anterior-posterior (**B**) roentgenograph of C4 to C7 laminectomy and interfacet fusion.

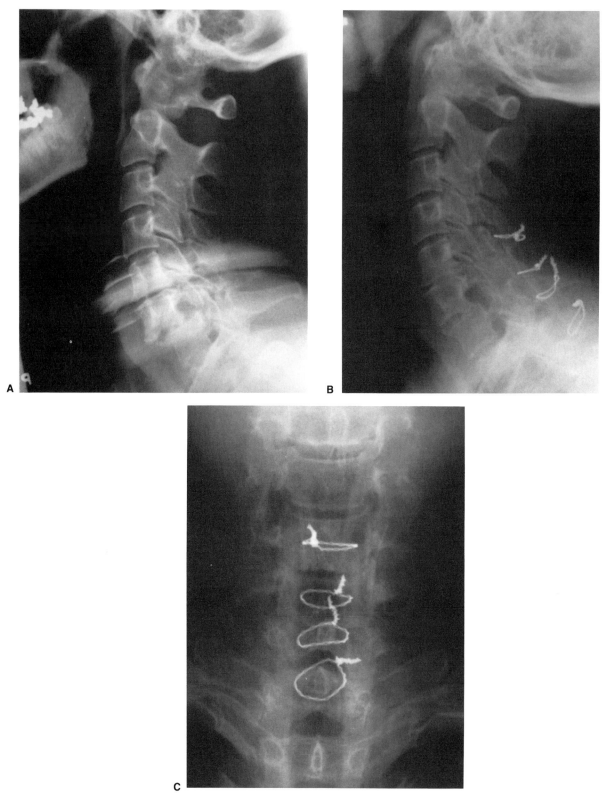

Figure 13–12.   Preoperative lateral roentgenograph of C6 to C7 subluxation (**A**), postoperative lateral (**B**), and anterior-posterior (**C**) roentgenograph of C6 to T1 spinous process fusion.

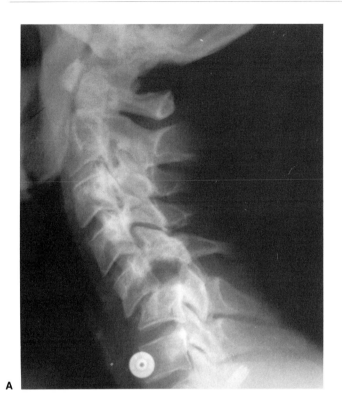

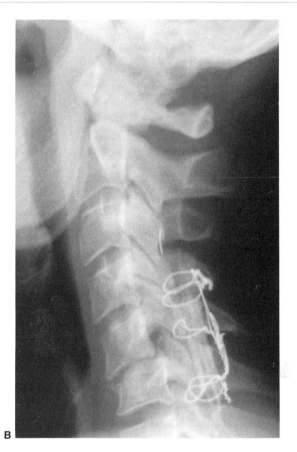

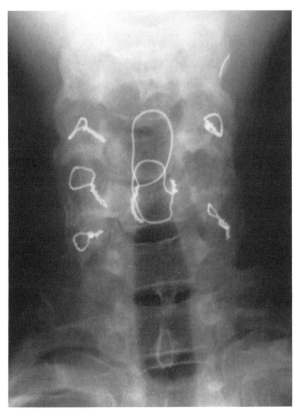

Figure 13–13.   Preoperative lateral roentgenograph (**A**) of C5 to C6 subluxation, postoperative lateral (**B**), and anterior-posterior (**C**) roentgenograph of facet fusion combined with interspinous stabilization.

REFERENCES

1. Albee FH. Transplantation of a portion of the tibia into the spine for Potts disease. *JAMA*. 1911;57:885–886.
2. White AA III, Panjabi MM. *Clinical Biomechanics of the Spine*. 2nd ed. Philadelphia, Pa: JB Lippincott; 1990.
3. Munro P. Treatment of fractures and dislocations of the cervical spine complicated by cervical cord and root injuries: a comparative study of fusion vs. nonfusion therapy. *N Engl J Med*. 1961;264:573–582.
4. Panjabi MM, White AA III, Johnson RM. Cervical spine mechanics as a function of transection of components. *J Biomech*. 1975;8:327–336.
5. White AA III, Johnson RM, Panjabi MM, Southwick WO. Biomechanical analysis of clinical stability in the cervical spine. *Clin Orthop*. 1975;109:85–96.
6. White AA III, Panjabi MM. *Clinical Biomechanics of the Spine*. 1st ed. Philadelphia, Pa: JB Lippincott; 1978.
7. Gosch HH, Gooding E, Schneider RC. An experimental study of cervical spine and cord injuries. *J Trauma*. 1972;12:570–575.
8. Nilsson OS, Bauer NCF, Brovjo O, Tornkvist H. Influence of indomethacin on heterotopic bone formation in rats: importance of length of treatment and age. *Clin Orthop*. 1986;207:231–245.
9. Simmons JW. Treatment of failed posterior lumbar interbody fusion (PLIF) of the spine with pulsing electromagnetic field. *Clin Orthop*. 1985;193:127–132.
10. Hartman JJ, McCurran RF, Robertson WW. A pedicle bone grafting procedure for failed lumbosacral spine fusion. *Clin Orthop*. 1983;178:223–227.
11. Stabler CL, Eismont FJ, Brown MD, et al. Failure of posterior cervical fusions using cadaveric bone graft in children. *J Bone Joint Surg*. 1985;67A:371–375.
12. Gepstein R, Nakamure K, Latta M, et al. Posterior spinal fusions with various types of bone grafts. *Trans Orthop Res Soc*. 1986;11:203.
13. Brown MD, Madinin TJ, Davis PB. A roentgenographic evaluation of frozen allografts in anterior cervical spine fusion. *Clin Orthop*. 1976;119:231–236.
14. Sypert GW. Anterior decompression and fusion for cervical myelopathy. Disorders of the Cervical Spine—Chapt. 36. Camins ME, O'Leary PE, eds. Baltimore, Md: Williams & Wilkins; 1992.
15. Crutchfield WG. Skeletal traction in the treatment of injuries to the cervical spine. *JAMA*. 1954;155:21–22.
16. VanGilder JC, Menezes AH, Dolan KD. *The Craniovertebral Junction and Its Abnormalities*. Mt. Kisco, NY: Futura; 1987:chap 9.
17. Johnson RM, Owen JR, Panjabi MM, et al. Immediate strength in anterior cervical fusion techniques. *Orthop Trans*. 1980;4:42.
18. Callahan RA, Johnson RM, Margois RN, et al. Cervical facet fusion for control of instability following laminectomy. *J Bone Joint Surg*. 1977;594:991–1002.

14 Methyl Methacrylate in Spinal Stabilization

Thomas A. Duff, M.D.

INTRODUCTION

It has been over 30 years since methyl methacrylate was first employed in spinal surgery. Knight initially used acrylic in place of a posterior bone inlay for treatment of patients suffering chronic pain due to spondylosis, osteoarthritis, or unhealed fractures.[1] Since then acrylic has been utilized in a variety of surgical techniques for a spectrum of spinal disorders causing instability.[2-11] Perceptions that acrylic alone could not reliably provide long-term stabilization led some to caution against its use without bone grafts under any circumstances. Other surgeons sanctioned employment of acrylic only in patients with spinal instability secondary to metastatic disease that portended a limited remaining lifetime.[7,9]

To some extent the concerns about acrylic were understandable, for previous experience with a wide spectrum of stabilizing devices, particularly those used in orthopedic surgery, had shown that many of these would loosen over time. Indeed, some of the skeptics' worst fears were reinforced by reports of recurrent subluxation in patients who had undergone acrylic stabilization. As with virtually any new technique or material, however, acrylic had sometimes been employed in inappropriate situations and at other times in an inappropriate manner. The following section reviews the indications for acrylic stabilization, and the subsequent section describes technical aspects that contribute to successful stabilization.

INDICATIONS

The use of acrylic without bone grafts for spinal stabilization should be limited to fracture/dislocations of the cervical spine. Despite the favorable experience reported by Knight,[1] chronic disorders associated with spinal instability, such as os odontoidium or rheumatoid arthritis, cannot be stabilized reliably by any technique that relies solely on instrumentation because there is always a risk that the device will loosen over time. In addition, acrylic in the absence of other reinforcing material has no demonstrated ability to cope with the stresses that occur in the lower thoracic or lumbar spine. Instability in these regions should be treated with metal plates or rods, generally in conjunction with bone grafting.

With regard to fractures of the cervical spine, there are two basic criteria governing the appropriateness of stabiliza-

tion with acrylic. The first is whether with reduction, either preoperatively or intraoperatively, the fractured bone elements essential for stability can be brought together to allow fusion. The second issue is whether the spinal cord or nerve roots in patients with neurological deficit are free from anterior impingement by bone, ruptured disk, or hematoma. If both of these conditions are met, posterior stabilization with acrylic without an inlay bone graft may be a surgical option.

Over the years there has been considerable debate about the type of surgical stabilization required for patients in whom there is extensive ligamentous damage. From the vigor of this debate it would be difficult for an outside observer to realize that there are no reliable indicators for assessing the likelihood that ligamentous damage is so severe that healing cannot take place. In my own series of patients with cervical spine fracture/dislocations, no one has been excluded from acrylic stabilization simply on the basis of an associated ligamentous injury that might be presumed to be severe. Perhaps the most succinct statement for the indication of acrylic stabilization is this: If the patient is a candidate for a halo-type brace and can safely tolerate general anesthesia, he or she is a potential candidate for acrylic stabilization. A reasonable approach is to discuss the pros and cons of each method of treatment and to do whichever the patient prefers.

The use of acrylic and bone together in posterior stabilization of the cervical spine entails difficulties because the acrylic leaves little space for a bone inlay and restricts the availability of the necessary vascular supply to the graft. One method for avoiding this problem is to place acrylic on one side and bone on the other.[11] If bone grafting is deemed necessary, anterior cervical spine procedures can also be considered.

TECHNIQUE

Several methods for posterior stabilization of cervical spine fracture/dislocations with acrylic have been shown to be effective in large series of patients. Perhaps the most widely used technique involves placement of interspinous wires and spinous process pins, which are then encased in acrylic.[3,10] The method described in this section has likewise been demonstrated to achieve reliable stabilization of acute cervical spine fracture/dislocation in a large series of patients.[5,6] There is no assumption, however, that it is the preferred

147

method, and surgeons must judge the various techniques on their intrinsic merits and on their track record.

The procedure is designed to meet at least four criteria important for successful stabilization with methyl methacrylate. The first is that the acrylic needs to be anchored to something other than to the posterior vertebral elements themselves because these do not possess sufficient contours to become locked within an acrylic mold. The second is that the anchoring material should not be prone to erode through bone. The third is that the anchors should be such that they can be encased entirely in the methyl methacrylate. The fourth is that the amount of acrylic must be sufficient to meet the stresses imposed on it.

The basic features of the technique are the placement of ¾-inch stainless steel screws into stable bone elements immediately above and below the level of the fracture, tightening a loop of 18-gauge stainless steel wire around the exposed shaft of screws on each side, and completely encasing the screws and wires with methyl methacrylate. The basic technique is applicable to fracture/dislocations at all levels of the cervical spine.

In the case of fractures involving the lower cervical spine (C3 to C7), the screws are inserted into the lateral masses of the vertebrae above and below the one(s) that is fractured (Fig. 14–1). For odontoid and Hangman's fractures, the upper set of screws is inserted obliquely into the marrow shaft of the posterior arch of C1 (Fig. 14–2). For fractures of C1, the upper set of screws is inserted in the occipital bone (Fig. 14–3).

There are two helpful hints for drilling the screw holes. First, because the posterior surface of the lateral masses and of the arch of C1 are somewhat irregular and sloping, the tendency of the drill tip to precess can be prevented by initiating the hole with a small curette. Second, drilling the screw holes with the power drill requires an appropriate level of caution to avoid excessive penetration and potential injury to the vertebral arteries or cerebellum. A small piece of bone wax on the drill bit approximately ½ inch from the tip can serve as an indicator of drill depth; the last few millimeters of drilling through the anterior cortex of the lateral mass is best done using gentle, intermittent pressure. The risk of excessive penetration could, if desired, be further decreased by use of an adjustable guard on the drill bit. The screws are then inserted to leave the upper third of the shaft exposed. For the sake of additional strength to the construct, 18-gauge wires can be looped around the heads of screw on each side and tightened. These loops should not be in contact with bone or soft tissues so that they can then be encased completely with acrylic. Each acrylic side strut should measure at least 1.5 cm in width and in depth.

Posterior stabilization with acrylic overcomes a number of disadvantages known to occur with certain other methods of stabilization. First, procedures that rely on interspinous or interlaminar wires to provide even temporary stability carry a potential for failure. The reasons for failure include unequal tension on the wires leading to sequential breakage, loosen-ing due to bending and/or to erosion of bone, slippage of interspinous wires as illustrated in Figure 14–1B, and the risk of spinal cord injury from interlaminar wiring. Second, other devices, such as metal hooks designed to grasp the lamina, require removal of the ligamentum flavum and again provide resistance primarily to anterior subluxation.

One could question whether any surgical procedure should be carried out in cases where a halo-type brace might suffice. The answer to this question is derived in part from the published results of treatment with halo-type fixation, which indicate that failure rates, as defined by the need for subsequent surgical stabilization, range between 20% and 30%.[12] Any surgical technique that carried this rate of failure would be subject to severe criticism. What justifies the halo brace is not so much the avoidance of general anesthesia and surgery but rather the avoidance of fusion across vertebrae and the potential decrease in range of neck motion.

It is interesting to note that despite continued claims for the necessity of bone inlays in the treatment of cervical spine fracture/dislocations, there are very few reports on the long-term outcome of a large, consecutive series of patients treated by this method. In other words, the information on outcome from posterior stabilization with methyl methacrylate has been more clearly defined than that of bone inlays. Correction of this discrepancy would shed light on the relative merits of the various techniques used to stabilize cervical spine fracture/dislocations.

REFERENCES

1. Knight G. Paraspinal acrylic inlays in the treatment of cervical and lumbar spondylosis and other conditions. *Lancet.* 1959;2:147–149.
2. Alexander E Jr. Posterior fusions of the cervical spine. *Clin Neurosurg.* 1981;28:273–296.
3. Branch CL Jr, Kelly DL Jr, Davis CH Jr, McWhorter JM. Fixation of fractures of the lower cervical spine using methylmethacrylate and wire; technique and results in 99 patients. *Neurosurgery.* 1989;25:503–513.
4. Clark CR, Keggi KJ, Panjabi MM. Methylmethacrylate stabilization of the cervical spine. *J Bone Joint Surg Am.* 1984;66:40–46.
5. Duff TA. Surgical stabilization of traumatic cervical spine fracture dislocation using methyl methacrylate. Long-term results in 26 patients. *J Neurosurg.* 1986;64:39–44.
6. Duff TA, Khan A, Corbett JE. Surgical stabilization of cervical spinal fractures with methyl methacrylate. Technical considerations and long-term results in 52 patients. *J Neurosurg.* 1992;76:440–443.
7. Hansebout RR, Blomquist GA Jr. Acrylic spinal fusion. A 20-year clinical series and technical note. *J Neurosurg.* 1980;53:606–612.
8. Kelly DL Jr, Alexander E Jr, Davis CH Jr, Smith JM. Acrylic fixation of atlanto-axial dislocations. Technical note. *J Neurosurg.* 1972;36:366–371.
9. McAfee PC, Bohlman HH, Ducker T, Eismont FJ. Failure of stabilization of the spine with methylmethacrylate. A retrospective analysis of twenty-four cases. *J Bone Joint Surg Am.* 1986;68:1145–1157.

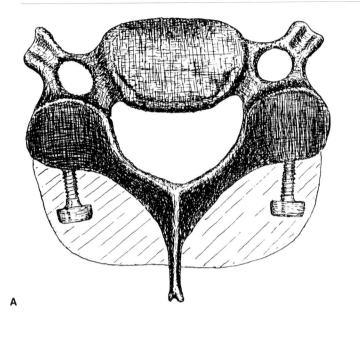

A

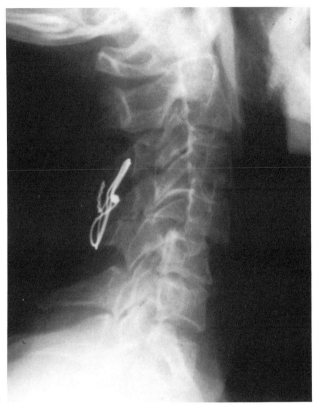

B

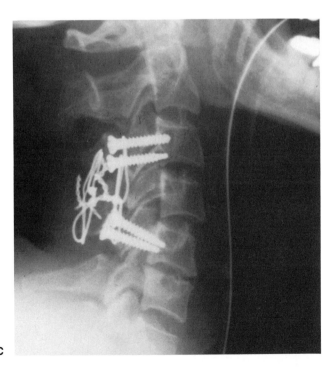

C

Figure 14–1. (**A**). Diagram of axial view of a cervical vertebra showing placement of screws, wire, and acrylic for stabilization of fractures of lower cervical spine. (**B**). Lateral cervical spine radiograph of patient referred for recurrent arm pain following attempted stabilization of C4 fracture with wire and bone. (**C**). Lateral cervical spine radiograph of same patient following stabilization with screws, wire, and acrylic.

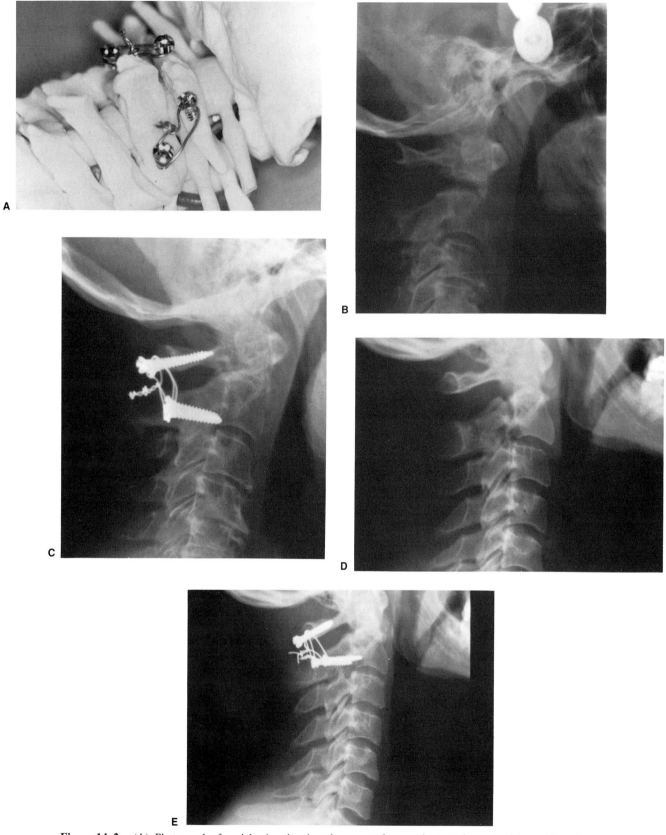

Figure 14–2. (**A**). Photograph of model spine showing placement of screws in posterior arch of C1 and lateral masses of C2 for stabilization of odontoid and Hangman's fractures. (**B**). Lateral cervical spine radiograph demonstrating odontoid fracture. (**C**). Lateral radiograph following stabilization with screws, wire, and acrylic. (**D**). Lateral cervical spine radiograph showing Hangman's fracture. (**E**). Lateral radiograph following stabilization with screws, wire, and acrylic.

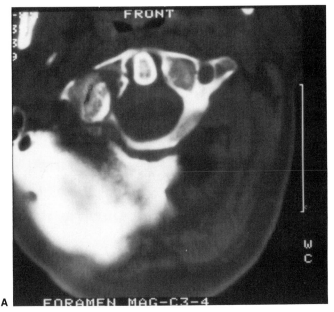

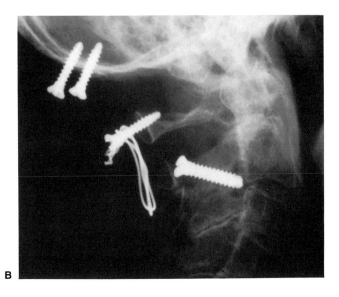

Figure 14–3. (**A**). Axial CT scan showing an atlas fracture. (**B**). Lateral cervical spine radiograph after stabilization with screws, wire, and acrylic.

10. Six E, Kelly DL Jr. Technique for C-1, C-2, and C-3 fixation in cases of odontoid fracture. *Neurosurgery.* 1981;8:374–377.
11. Whitehill R, Cicoria AD, Hooper WE, Maggio WW, Jane JA. Posterior cervical reconstruction with methyl methacrylate cement and wire: a clinical review. *J Neurosurg.* 1988;68:576–584.
12. Sears W, Fazl M. Prediction of stability of cervical spine fracture managed in the halo vest and indications for surgical intervention. *J Neurosurg.* 1990;72:426–432.

15 Posterior Cervical Plate Stabilization with the AME Haid Universal Bone Plate System

Vincent C. Traynelis, M.D., Regis W. Haid, M.D.

INTRODUCTION

Posterior cervical fusions have been performed for years using many different wiring techniques. Following such procedures, external immobilization is usually necessary until bony fusion occurs. Cervical articular mass plates, compared to wire/bone constructs, provide superior internal stability. Advantages of lateral mass plates include ease of application, lack of dependence on intact posterior spinal elements, and immediate rigid fixation. Because of these qualities, articular mass plates have gained widespread popularity. Roy-Camille, using plates constructed with vitallium (Roy-Camille plates, Benoist-Girard et Compagnie, Bagneux, France) was the first surgeon to publish a great deal of experience with these devices.[1,2] In 1989 Haid developed a titanium alloy implant (AME Haid Universal Bone Plate System, American Medical Electronics, Inc., Richardson, Tex) that represented a major design improvement because titanium causes less distortion of x-ray and magnetic resonance (MR) images than stainless steel (Fig. 15–1).[3] Both stainless steel and titanium are fully biocompatible; therefore, posterior articular mass plates do not need to be removed after implantation. The biomechanics, indications for placement, complications, and outcome for both the Roy-Camille and Haid plates are similar.

BIOMECHANICS

The biomechanical properties of posterior articular mass plates have been studied in several laboratories.[2,4–6] Roy-Camille et al compared lateral mass plating to posterior wiring in a cadaveric model of posterior ligamentous instability.[2] They reported that lateral mass plates increased stability in flexion and extension by 92% and 60%, respectively.[2] Posterior wiring did not produce any resistance to extension and increased flexural stability by only 33%. Coe et al concluded that the Roy-Camille plate effectively restored stiffness in flexion, extension, and torsion in a cadaveric model of posterior ligamentous instability.[4] The stability of cervical lateral mass plates has been documented by other investigators as well.[5,6] Overall, biomechanical testing indicates that posterior articular mass plates probably provide the same or superior biomechanical support as standard posterior wiring techniques.

INDICATIONS

Lateral mass plates have been used to stabilize the spine from C2 to T1. These devices are most frequently employed in the treatment of posttraumatic instability when conservative management is inappropriate or has failed.[1,7–14] They have also been used to stabilize patients with neoplasms and degenerative instability.

Persistent or extensive posterior ligamentous instability is stabilized effectively with lateral mass plates. Patients requiring surgical reduction of facet dislocations are excellent candidates for lateral mass stabilization. Although fixation across the involved segment is usually adequate to achieve stabilization in patients with either ligamentous injury and–or facet dislocation, one may wish to plate additional levels in cases of severe instability.[1,2,7–9,12,14] Certainly if multilevel instability is present preoperatively, longer plates are indicated.

Ligamentous extension injuries of the cervical spine are difficult to stabilize with a posterior construct, and alternative treatments should be considered. If one chooses to treat anterior ligamentous instability with lateral mass plates, fixation should extend a segment above and below the region of injury.[2,7]

Instability secondary to fractures can be managed with articular mass plates. These devices are particularly useful when laminar and spinous process fractures preclude sublaminar or spinous process wiring. Stabilization of cervical fractures usually requires multilevel fixation. Fractures that involve the facet and–or pedicle may be managed by plating to the lateral masses above and below the fracture using a three-hole plate. No screw is placed into the middle hole on the injured side so that the plate bridges the actual fracture site. The noninjured side should be secured with a three-hole

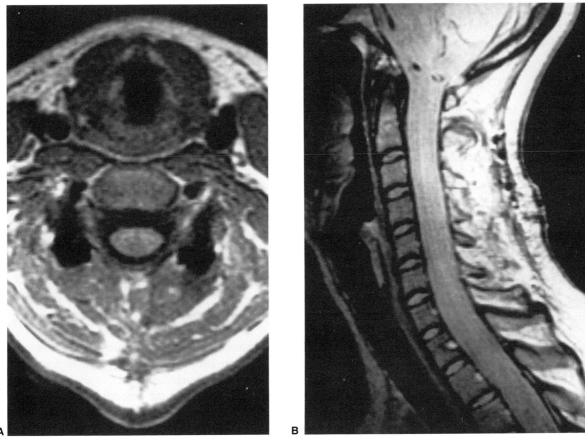

Figure 15–1.   Axial (**A**) and sagittal (**B**) MR images of a patient stabilized with titanium articular mass plates demonstrate minimal signal distortion and excellent visualization of the neural structures.

plate with screws placed in each hole.[8,15] Ideally, plates should be bilateral and symmetrical.

Vertebral body and–or disk injuries are likely to produce anterior compression of the cervical roots or cord. Patients with significant ventral canal compromise (from either disk or bone) and an incomplete neurological deficit almost invariably require an anterior approach for adequate decompression; therefore, posterior decompression is contraindicated. Some surgeons recommend posterior fusion in patients with complete neurological injuries and anterior compression; however, it is our opinion that ventral lesions are best treated via a ventral approach. Persistent instability following ventral decompression is often associated with injury to the posterior ligaments and may be managed with articular mass plates. This 360-degree operation may be performed under a single anesthetic or may be staged. Cervical instability associated with a vertebral body fracture without anterior canal compromise may be treated by lateral mass plate fixation. In these cases, a multilevel fixation will minimize the risk of developing a postoperative kyphotic deformity.[1,7–9,11] If, however, there is a greater than 25% loss of vertebral body height, an anterior approach may be more effective at preventing progressive kyphosis.

Instability following bony metastatic tumor resection has been managed with lateral mass plates.[11,15] It is important in these cases to achieve fixation in disease-free bone, and the spine should be stabilized well above and below the affected level(s).[2] Lateral mass plates are useful in the treatment of some benign tumors such as neurofibromas. When these neoplasms cause bony erosion or an extensive laminectomy is necessary for excision, posterior plate stabilization may be considered at the time of the primary operation.

Lateral mass plates have been used successfully in patients with spondylosis who require fusion.[2,11] These plates may be placed to prevent or treat postlaminectomy kyphosis. Although kyphosis following laminectomy can be stabilized posteriorly (following realignment), in this situation, posterior constructs, including articular mass plates, are at a mechanical disadvantage, and rigid external immobilization and–or anterior fusion may also be necessary.[15–17] We advocate that such kyphotic deformities initially be approached anteriorly with strut graft placement and that anterior plating be considered. Following strut grafting, posterior stabilization with plates may be utilized additionally.

Patients with poor bone quality are often difficult to stabilize by any method. Significant osteoporosis is a major

injury is unilateral, all three levels are stabilized with screws on the noninjured side.

Bicortical screw fixation is desirable, and frequently the drill can be felt to penetrate the inner cortex.[5] If penetration of the inner cortex is not appreciated, bicortical purchase is often accomplished because the screws are 4.5 mm longer than the drill bit.

The Haid UBP is secured with 3.5-mm-diameter self-tapping screws that are 15.5 mm long. It is essential that the implanted components are compatible; therefore, these screws are constructed of the same material as the plate. The screws are inserted in the same trajectory used for drilling, and complete tightening is performed in a sequential fashion once all screws are in place (Fig. 15–4).[21] The plates should be positioned so that one may read the imprinted serial numbers. The screws will seat into the plate and become snug with two-finger tightening.

Infrequently, a screw will strip or not tighten satisfactorily for other reasons. This problem may be rectified by replacing the original screw with a recovery screw. These screws have a 4.5 mm diameter (as opposed to the 3.5 mm diameter of the standard Haid UBP screw). It may not be wise to use recovery screws in extremely small articular masses because they may split the mass into two pieces. Alternatively, an inadequate purchase may be salvaged by removing the screw, placing a small amount of methyl methacrylate in the hole, and then replacing the screw.[15]

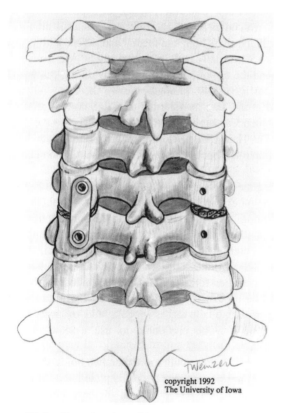

copyright 1992
The University of Iowa

Figure 15–4. Posterior view of the cervical spine with a two-hole plate in place. A second plate will be positioned before final screw tightening.

After the plate is secured, the posterior elements may be grafted as described previously. The spinous processes may also be wired together at the plated levels in cases of severe instability.[7,9] Spinous process wiring only increases stability in flexion loading; however, it is stress in this direction that is usually the primary concern.

At this point, the traction is discontinued. The neck may be flexed gently and extended under direct vision to ensure that stability has been achieved. This maneuver is important in the trauma patient who may have previously unrecognized instability at other levels. The wound is closed in the standard fashion.

A postoperative neurological examination is performed and anteroposterior and lateral cervical spine roentgenograms are obtained immediately after reversal of the effects of anesthesia. New neurological deficits and–or significant radiographic abnormalities must be addressed promptly. The rapidity with which the patient may be mobilized is variable. Patients with no or minimal neurological deficits may be allowed to be out of bed the evening after surgery. On the other hand, severely ill patients (eg, those with quadriplegia, multiple trauma, etc) must often be mobilized more gradually.

Generally, the cervical spine is immobilized in a collar for 3 months. Patients with associated vertebral body fractures, ankylosing spondylitis, total ligamentous disruption, and so on may require a cervicothoracic brace, minerva jacket, or halo vest until fusion occurs.[1,2,7–9,11,13–15,18,20,21]

RESULTS

Traynelis has reviewed the literature concerning lateral mass plating in an attempt to assess the outcome of these procedures.[26] Perioperative mortalities have occurred with posterior cervical plating procedures; however, with one exception, mortality has not been directly related to the plating procedure.[1,12] Honnart et al described a patient who suffered a cardiac arrest secondary to severe intraoperative hemorrhage.[12] The authors stated that a "vertebral artery injury was recognized at the time of reduction of dislocation"; no other details are provided.[12]

The spinal cord and the vertebral artery are theoretically at risk for injury during drilling and screw placement. A review of 490 published cases revealed only the aforementioned case of vertebral artery injury (which does not appear to be secondary to either drilling or screw placement) and no cases of spinal cord injury.[26] The low risk of injury to these structures was confirmed in an anatomic investigation of the Roy-Camille and Magerl techniques for screw placement. This study, by Heller et al, failed to demonstrate any screw in close proximity to the spinal cord or the vertebral artery.[23] Although one must consider and respect these structures when placing articular mass plates, the risk of injury to them is low.

In contrast to the spinal cord and vertebral artery, cadaveric studies suggest that drilling and screw placement can injure the cervical roots.[23] Clinically, however, root dysfunction following posterior articular mass plating is rare. Root deficits secondary to drilling or screw placement were not reported in a combined review of almost 500 patients.[26]

Inadvertent violation of a facet joint may lead to either ankylosis of an additional segment or screw loosening.[7] This problem is best prevented by carefully planned drill trajectories, and the risk of its occurrence probably decreases with experience.[23] Screw loosening is infrequent and usually occurs in the setting of osteoporosis or incorrect screw placement. Properly positioned screws, however, will occasionally loosen, sometimes months after surgery. If the spine is stable, minor screw backout is usually of no consequence.[1,7,9]

Infection is an inherent risk of all surgical procedures. Wound infections have been managed successfully without removing the plates; in fact, instability secondary to infection has been treated with application of posterior articular mass plates.[1,7,9] Persistent osteomyelitis or serious soft-tissue infections may require plate removal.

The overall fusion rate for posterior articular mass plates is 98%.[26] A few patients may develop kyphosis that, when it occurs, is usually minor and requires only observation.[7,9] Significant or increasing kyphosis requires a more aggressive approach.

Finally, it must always be remembered that osteoporosis is a relative contraindication to spinal plating.[2,18] This condition is associated with screw pullout, which may lead to a loss of reduction; therefore, if osteoporotic patients must be treated with lateral mass plates, they should be immobilized rigidly in the postoperative period.[1,9,11]

CONCLUSION

Lateral mass plate fixation is simple, safe, and effective. The advantages of this system include fixation independent of posterior element integrity, maintenance of normal cervical lordosis, multisegmental capability, and MRI compatibility. Although the risk of injury to the neural elements and vertebral artery is small, this must be considered the major disadvantage of posterior lateral mass plating. Poor bone quality is a contraindication for lateral mass plating. Overall, lateral mass plates are an excellent means of achieving posterior internal fixation of the cervical spine.

REFERENCES

1. Cooper PR, Cohen A, Rosiello A, Koslow M. Posterior stabilization of cervical spine fractures and subluxations using plates and screws. *Neurosurgery*. 1988;23:300–306.
2. Roy-Camille R, Saillanr G, Mazel C. Internal fixation of the unstable cervical spine by posterior osteosynthesis with plates and screws. In: The Cervical Spine Research Society Editorial Committee, ed. *The Cervical Spine*. 2nd ed. Philadelphia, Pa: JB Lippincott; 1989:390–404.
3. Savolaine ER, Ebraheim NA, Andreshak TG, Jackson WT. Anterior and posterior cervical spine fixation using titanium implants to facilitate magnetic resonance imaging evaluation. *J Orthop Trauma*. 1989;3:295–299.
4. Coe JD, Warden KE, Sutterlin CE III, McAfee PC. Biomechanical evaluation of cervical spinal stabilization methods in a human cadaveric model. *Spine*. 1989;14:1122–1131.
5. Gill K, Paschal S, Corin J, Ashman R, Bucholz RW. Posterior plating of the cervical spine. A biomechanical comparison of different posterior fusion techniques. *Spine*. 1988;13:813–816.
6. Montesano PX, Juach EC, Anderson PA, Benson DR, Hanson PB. Biomechanics of cervical spine internal fixation. *Spine*. 1991;16:S10–S16.
7. Anderson PA, Henley MB, Grady MS, Montesano PX, Winn HR. Posterior cervical arthrodesis with AO reconstruction plates and bone graft. *Spine*. 1991;16:S72–S79.
8. Borne G, Bedou G, Pinaudeau M, El Omeiri S, Cristino G. Treatment of severe lesions of the lower cervical spine (C3-C7). A clinical study and technical considerations in 102 cases. *Neurochirurgia Stuttg*. 1988;31:1–13.
9. Cherny WB, Sonntag VKH, Douglas RA. Lateral mass posterior plating and facet fusion for cervical spine instability. *BNI Quarterly*. 1991;7:2–11.
10. Domenella G, Berlanda P, Bassi G. Posterior-approach osteosynthesis of the lower cervical spine by the R. Roy-Camille technique. (Indications and first results). *Ital J Orthop Traumatol*. 1982;8:235–244.
11. Ebraheim NA, An HS, Jackson WT, Brown JA. Internal fixation of the unstable cervical spine using posterior Roy-Camille plates: preliminary report. *J Orthop Trauma*. 1989;3:23–28.
12. Honnart F, Patel A, Furno P. Fractures of cervical spine with neurological lesion treated by reduction and fixation with plates. *Ann Acad Med Singapore*. 1982;11:186–193.
13. Nazarian SM, Louis RP. Posterior internal fixation with screw plates in traumatic lesions of the cervical spine. *Spine*. 1991;16:S64–S71.
14. Savini R, Parisini P, Cervellati S. The surgical treatment of late instability of flexion-rotation injuries in the lower cervical spine. *Spine*. 1987;12:178–182.
15. Haid RW Jr, Papadopoulos SM, Sonntag VKH, Cooper PR. Posterior cervical stabilization with lateral mass osteosynthetic plate technique. *Levtech Technical Bulletin*. Jacksonville, Fla: Levtech Inc.; 1991.
16. Callahan RA, Johnson RM, Margolis RN, Keggi KJ, Albright JA, Southwick WO. Cervical facet fusion for control of instability following laminectomy. *J Bone Joint Surg Am*. 1977; 59A:991–1002.
17. Heller JG, Whitecloud TS III. Post-laminectomy instability of the cervical spine. In: Frymoyer JW, Ducker TB, Hadler NM, Kostuik JP, Weinstein JN, Whitecloud TS III, eds. *The Adult Spine*. Vol 2. New York: Raven Press; 1991:1219–1240.
18. Weidner A. Internal fixation with metal plates and screws. In: The Cervical Spine Research Society Editorial Committee, ed. *The Cervical Spine*. 2nd ed. Philadelphia, Pa: JB Lippincott; 1989:404–421.
19. Horwitz NH, Rizzoli HV. Laminectomy: general complications. In: Horwitz NH, Rizzoli HV, eds. *Postoperative Complications of Extracranial Neurological Surgery*. Baltimore, Md: Williams & Wilkins; 1987:3–29.
20. Murphy MJ, Daniaux H, Southwick WO. Posterior cervical fusion with rigid internal fixation. *Orthop Clin North Am*. 1986;17:55–65.
21. Aebi M. Surgical treatment of cervical spine fractures by AO spine techniques. In: Bridwell KH, DeWald RL, eds. *The Textbook of Spinal Surgery*. Philadelphia, Pa: JB Lippincott; 1991:1081–1105.
22. Ebraheim NA, Hoeflinger MJ, Salpietro B, Chung SYM, Jackson WT. Anatomic considerations in posterior plating of the cervical spine. *J Orthop Trauma*. 1991;5:196–199.

23. Heller JG, Carlson GD, Abitbol J-J, Garfin SR. Anatomic comparison of the Roy-Camille and Magerl techniques for screw placement in the lower cervical spine. *Spine.* 1991;16:S552–S557.

24. An HS, Gordin R, Renner K. Anatomic considerations for plate-screw fixation of the cervical spine. *Spine.* 1991;16:S548–S551.

25. Montesano PX, Jauch E, Jonsson H Jr. Anatomic and biomechanical study of posterior cervical spine plate arthrodesis: an evaluation of two different techniques of screw placement. *J Spinal Disord.* 1992;5:301–305.

26. Traynelis VC. Anterior and posterior plate stabilization of the cervical spine. *Neurosurg Quarterly.* 1992;2:59–76.

16 Axis Fixation System for Posterior Cervical Reconstruction

Chester E. Sutterlin III, M.D.

INTRODUCTION

The Axis Fixation System was developed as a long bone and pelvis plate and screw implant. The perceived need for use of Axis to provide a better method for posterior fixation of the cervical spine was based on analysis of other implants. The attributes and deficiencies of the previously available devices were recognized by clinical utilization of them for a variety of spinal disorders, as well as by biomechanical testing in animal and human cadaveric models.[1–3] A direct design effort of 2 years' duration began in early 1991 and included: (1) characterization of the advantages and deficiencies of currently available methods and devices for posterior cervical fixation; (2) development of a list of desirable features and functions of a new bone fixation system; (3) design of such a system along with instrumentation specific for posterior cervical application; (4) mechanical testing of the system's components to assure adequate strength and durability; (5) clinical utilization of the system to evaluate efficacy and safety; and (6) application of the system by other investigators to assure a nonbiased critical review of the unique features of the implant and instruments and to encourage further mechanical and biomechanical testing of the device.

Characterization of Current Devices

Although wiring techniques vary, they are the standard by which all posterior cervical fixation systems should be measured. In general, they are relatively simple in concept, easy to perform, and utilize readily available and inexpensive materials. Wire fixation represents an eloquent and efficient use of material when instability is not great and complex or large-magnitude loading forces are not expected. Wiring techniques have a proven track record with long-term documentation of performance. To encourage a surgeon to supplement and–or replace his or her wiring armamentarium with a new technique requires that the surgeon agree that wiring performs poorly in certain situations and that a newer method, although not yet documented with long-term study, has conceptually recognizable advantages.

Wires perform best when attached to nonosteoporotic bone to resist flexion, with an intact anterior column for axial compressive load bearing. Wires perform poorly when bone is osteoporotic, the laminae are fractured or have been removed, forces other than flexion are involved (rotational forces may be resisted partially by wires, although facet wirings are prone to pullout), and when anterior column axial load-bearing capabilities are compromised. Finally, most wires and cables are constructed with stainless steel, which interferes with postoperative magnetic resonance imaging (MRI) and computed tomography (CT) scan quality.[4] Titanium does not distort scan images; however, titanium wire is brittle and difficult to use. Titanium cable is less readily available at present.

Posterior interlaminar clamps are stronger than wire and resist flexion efficiently. When used properly with the appropriate bone-grafting technique, some effect can be gained at resisting rotation; however, translational, bending, and extension forces are counteracted less effectively, and dislogment of the implant can occur by rotation of the motion segment or by spinal extension. Posterior interlaminar clamps require intact laminae for proper placement. Sublaminar hook position is often precariously close to the spinal cord, and cord compression has been documented following use of this device.

Options for lateral mass plating, using both stainless steel and titanium, are numerous. Most often, generic long-bone plates, in which minimal specific adaptive changes have been made, are utilized for posterior cervical fixation. The instrumentation necessary to apply these plates was not developed for ease of use within cervical wound dimensions given the requisite angles of approach and depths of penetration. There are numerous advantages of posterior cervical plating, including superb attachment to bone, which may even be achieved in the face of mild to moderate osteoporosis. Lateral mass plates effectively resist flexion forces as well as translation, lateral bending, and rotation. Improved resistance to extension can be achieved as compared to posterior wiring techniques, although an anterior tension band is most effective in this regard. Resistance to flexion can be realized even in the face of impaired anterior axial compressive load-bearing capabilities if posterior lateral mass plating is supplemented with posterior interspinous wire or cable use. Plate use is not precluded by laminar fractures or removal (except for those plates that hook beneath a lamina) and can be used following keyhole foraminotomy or to span fractured facets. Some types can be stacked to achieve long occipitocervical constructs, but most are used for short segment fixation only.

Variations in patient size and age, the anatomic configuration of the lateral masses, and the spatial relation of the cervical segments (ie, deformity) contribute to the frequent inability of the hole spacing of most lateral mass plates to match the bony lateral mass itself. Often they "just don't line up," particularly in multilevel constructs. Some plates are not bendable to match normal cervical contours, especially lordosis, and when bending is possible, it occurs at the plate holes, which weakens both the static and fatigue strengths of the plate. Some plates cannot be twisted to match contours, and most cannot be bent to match medial-lateral alignments. The dimensions of the plate holes in relation to screw diameter determines the achievable screw angulation. The ability to insert a screw through a plate at any angle allows the surgeon to obtain fixation within anatomic restraints while avoiding neural or vascular injury. Most available systems are restrictive in this regard, and some screws themselves are poorly designed to resist pullout, which is critical in achieving a proper tension band effect.

AXIS SYSTEM DESIGN

Based on the characterization of available posterior cervical fixation methods, the goals for the Axis System (Danek Group, Inc., Memphis, Tenn) can be outlined clearly. Succinctly stated, the objective was to include all desirable features of the existing implants and to address all deficiencies by altering design. The system consists of plates and screws made of titanium for MRI and CT compatibility. The plates are segmental with variation in intersegmental spacing of 11 mm, 13 mm, and 15 mm to accommodate small and large individuals. Easily bendable trial templates are included to match each hole spacing (Fig. 16–1). The plates are available in two-, four-, six-, and eight-hole lengths and may be cut with a standard bolt or rod cutter. Bending of the plates to match or create cervical lordosis is possible, as is plate twisting and medial-lateral bending. When the plate is bent into lordosis, it bends at the predetermined scored sections in a predictable manner and not through the holes. In addition, the cross-sectional area of the plate at the holes is greater than that at the scored sections; therefore, should the plate break, it will fail at a predictable location within determined strength parameters.

At each segment a figure-eight slot allows for variability in screw placement. In addition, screws may be angled medially or laterally up to approximately 30° (Fig. 16–2) to allow for alternative lateral mass techniques. The screws can achieve even greater cephalad and caudad angulation (Fig. 16–3). The plate has an arch on its ventral surface for increased strength and to allow for bone grafting beneath the plate. Future modifications will allow for occipitocervical fixation and for attachment to the TSRH system (Texas Scottish Right Hospital System, Danek Group, Inc., Memphis, Tenn) for cervicothoracic constructs. The possi-

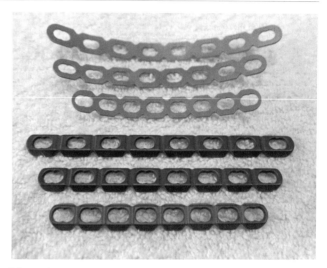

Figure 16–1. Axis templates and plates. Above: From top to bottom are shown 15-mm, 13-mm, and 11-mm trial templates that are easily bendable into a lordotic curvature. Below: Corresponding eight-hole, segmented axis plates with 15-mm, 13-mm, and 11-mm intersegmental spacings. Note that two options exist for screw placement at each segment.

bility, therefore, will exist for continuous posterior fixation from the occiput through the cervical, thoracic, and lumbar areas of the spine to the sacrum and ilium of the pelvis. Modifications will allow for rod usage with screws as well as plates. In addition, supplemental points of fixation can be made using titanium cable.

The screws are made of titanium. The basic lateral mass screws are 3.5-mm cancellous screws available in 2-mm increments from 10 to 24 mm. A 4.0-mm cancellous screw is

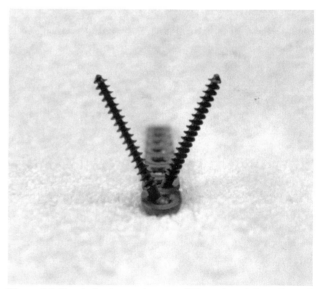

Figure 16–2. Axis plate and screws. When viewed from the end, with the plate turned over (ie, dorsal surface of plate is down), it can be appreciated that the 4.0-mm screws can achieve nearly 30° of angulation medially or laterally. Also note the concave contour of the plate's ventral surface (side facing up in this illustration). This contour increases bending strength and allows for bone graft placement beneath the plate.

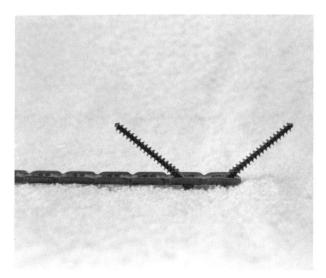

Figure 16–3. Axis plate and screws viewed from the side. Note the extreme angulation that can be achieved in a cephalad and/or caudal direction.

available for use as the primary screw or as a salvage screw if the 3.5-mm cancellous screw strips. Cancellous screws are used in the lateral mass because of their greater pullout strength as compared to cortical screws. Screws of 26 mm and longer are subjected to significant bending forces in their locations in C2, T1, and T2 and are thus designed as 4.0-mm cortical screws with a heftier 2.9-mm core diameter compared to the 1.9-mm core diameter of the 3.5 mm and 4.0-mm cancellous screws. All screws have an increasing core diameter taper at the head to resist breakage at this high-stress location. The heads fit standard hexagonal screwdrivers.

All instruments used for insertion of the device were designed with safety in mind without sacrificing expeditious fixation. Figures 16–4 through 16–9 illustrate use of the cervical instrumentation for the Axis Fixation System. The awl has a retractable tip protector to prevent inadvertent injury to surgeons and operating room personnel. The drill, tap, and guide are well marked to allow for visualization of penetration depth. All instruments are long and slender, including the depth gauge, which fits the anatomic constraints of the posterior cervical approach. Plate benders and twisters allow for accurate plate contouring. Easily bendable trial tem-

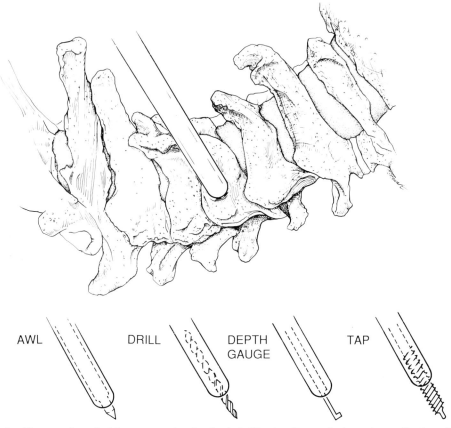

Figure 16–4. The use of cervical instrumentation for the Axis Fixation System is shown by application of a three-hole plate to the midcervical spine at C3 to C5. Plate design allows for a variety of insertion techniques including Roy-Camille, Magerl, and the Jonsson-Rauschning method of directing the screw tip toward the projection of the pedicle on lateral fluoroscopic image. The steps for screw hole preparation include use of an awl, drill, depth gauge, and tap. Unicortical or bicortical purchase may be obtained. The standard screw for use in C3 to C7 is a 3.5-mm cancellous screw. A 4.0-mm cancellous salvage screw is available. Longer screws (>26 mm) for placement into the anterior column of the cervical spine from the posterior approach (C2, T1, T2, and at times C7) are 4.0-mm cortical screws for improved rigidity and resistance to bending stress.

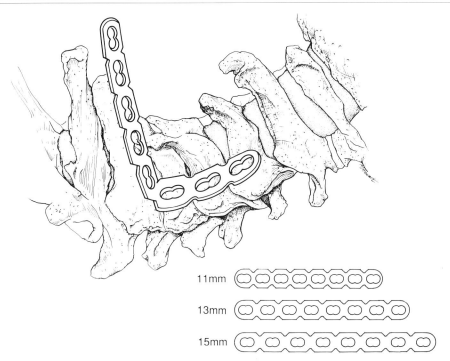

11mm
13mm
15mm

Figure 16–5.   Selection of the Axis plate with proper hole spacing is facilitated by use of lightweight, malleable aluminum templates. Intersegmental spacing options include 11-mm, 13-mm, and 15-mm size plates. Note that intrasegmental options for screw placement are also accommodated by the Axis plate design.

plates permit choosing of proper plate size and contour. The plate holder and screwdriver allow for quick, efficient insertion of the device. Titanium burrs and titanium or plastic sucker tips will minimize debris particles, which, when made of ferromagnetic materials, often interfere with the quality of subsequent MRI scans. Compact, well-organized, and clearly legible storage cases are provided for all implants and instruments.

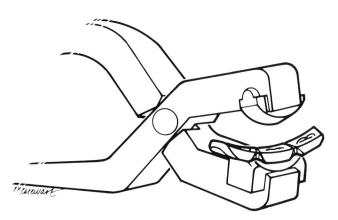

Figure 16–6.   Plates may be contoured into lordosis. Use of the specific lordotic plate bender included in the Axis Fixation System cervical instrument set is recommended so that proper limits of radius of curvature are not exceeded for the specific titanium plate design. Note that the plates are designed to bend at scored sections and not through screw holes. Plates may also be contoured by twisting and inducing medial-lateral bends.

Mechanical Test Results

Tests were conducted to determine the mechanical properties of the Axis fixation plates. Although there are no written standards outlining the required plate strength for application to the posterior cervical spine, clinical experience has determined which plates successfully withstand anatomic loading in the cervical region. Some of these plates were tested along with the new plates to determine whether the Axis plates will also be acceptable in similar applications.

Two styles of Axis fixation plates were tested. These were plates with 13-mm and 11-mm hole spacing. Although not tested, a 15-mm plate is also available. Because it is constructed of proportionately more material, it is presumed to be even stronger than the 13- and 11-mm plates. Both versions of the Axis fixation plate were machined to least material conditions (LMC), which should give worst-case results. Four styles of currently used plates were tested for comparison. These consisted of the Synthes 1/3 tubular small fragment plates made from both commercially pure titanium and stainless steel and the Synthes/Anderson plate (Synthes Spine, Paoli, Pa) made from commercially pure titanium (previously the 2.7-mm reconstruction plates). The two styles of Anderson plates were of 8- and 12-mm hole spacing. None of these comparative plates were at LMC; therefore, more nominal results are illustrated.

A four-point bend fixture in conjunction with an Instron testing machine (Instron Corporation, Canton, Mass) was used to apply both static and fatigue loads to failure (Fig. 16–10). All plates were oriented with the anterior surface facing the applied load. This would simulate flexing of the

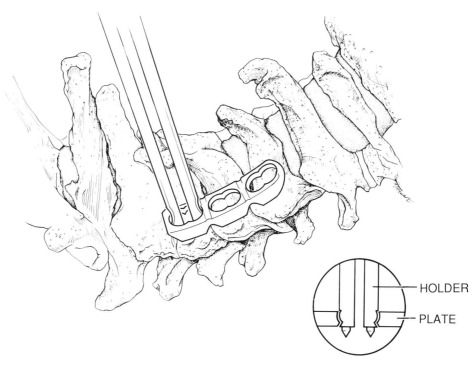

HOLDER

PLATE

Figure 16–7.   The plate holder grasps the implant securely through any hole for placement of the bone plate into the cervical spine. Subsequent screw-hole preparation and screw insertion at multiple levels may occur. Small prongs at the plate-holder tip interface with bone and minimize plate motion during screw-hole preparation. The plate holder is easily and quickly applied and removed by a simple mechanism.

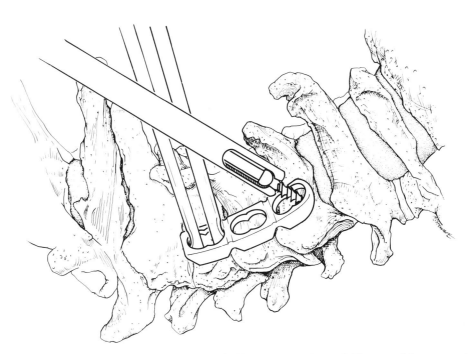

Figure 16–8.   While the plate is stabilized with the plate holder, screws are inserted. The screwdriver grasps the screw head firmly until the surgeon desires release. All instruments are designed with narrow, thin shafts for optimal visualization and all have proper shaft length to prevent instrument handles from entering the surgical wound.

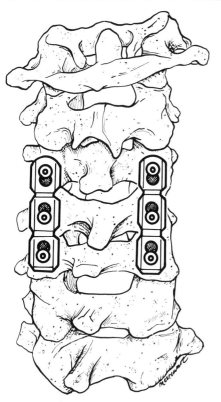

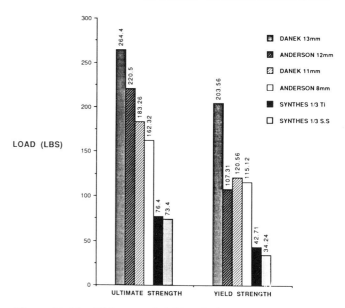

Figure 16–11. Ultimate and yield static flexural strength test results. Although not tested, it may be assumed that the 15-mm Axis plate would be even stronger than the 13-mm and 11-mm Axis plates.

Figure 16–9. Posterior view of Axis bone plates applied to the posterior cervical spine. Note screw head locations in figure-eight slots.

neck. The distance between supports was chosen such that a sufficient length of each plate type was contained between the two innermost supports, thus equally stressing all design features of each of the plates. A load versus cycles to failure curve was developed as a fatigue comparison for all the plates. All fatigue testing was run at 10 Hz.

The ultimate and yield static flexural strength using the four-point bend fixture was determined for all six plates (Fig. 16–11). Both the 13-mm and 11-mm Axis fixation

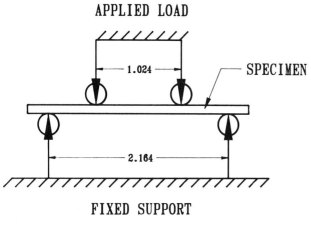

Figure 16–10. Schematic illustration of experimental setup used for comparison testing of plates. Plates were oriented to simulate flexion. Distances between load points are in inches.

plates showed higher yield strengths than the other four plates. The 13-mm Axis plate was higher in ultimate strength than the other five plates. The 11-mm Axis plate was third behind the 13-mm Axis plate and the 12-mm Anderson plate.

The load versus cycles to failure fatigue curves were determined (Fig. 16–12). The 13-mm Axis plate performed comparably to both the Anderson 12-mm and 8-mm plates. The 11-mm Axis plate performed slightly less well than the Synthes/Anderson plates in fatigue testing, although much better than both the titanium and stainless steel Synthes 1/3 tubular plates.

The fatigue data did not follow the same pattern as the static failure data. This is most likely due to the design of the Axis plates, which have scored, "necked down" sections, thus acting as areas of stress concentration. This design characteristic is an advantage to the surgeon when contouring the plate to match each individual patient's spinal curvature, and thus it allows for stabilizing and correcting highly complex spinal deformities. The bending occurs at these scored sections and not at the screw holes, therefore maintaining predictable plate failure characteristics and the required fit between screw and plate. In my clinical experience, breakage of even the weakest plates (Synthes titanium and stainless steel 1/3 tubular) has not occurred in over 5 years when such devices are used as a tension band in the posterior cervical spine. The more clinically relevant mode of failure of these constructs is screw pullout from the lateral mass bone, and this has been addressed in the Axis system by specific attention to screw design.

Reviewing both the static and fatigue data, it can be seen that the Axis 13-mm and 11-mm plates perform admirably when compared to other plates involved in this study.

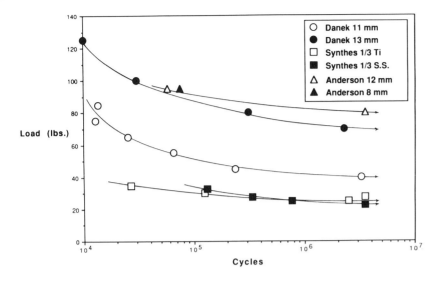

Figure 16–12. Load versus cycles-to-failure fatigue curves. Although not tested, it may be assumed that the 15-mm Axis plate would be even more resistant to fatigue than the 13-mm and 11-mm Axis plates.

Because these other plates have been shown clinically to withstand anatomic loading in the posterior cervical spine, it can be concluded that the Axis 13-mm and 11-mm plates can also withstand the same types of loading. In addition, because the 15-mm Axis plate has proportionately more material than the 13-mm or 11-mm Axis plates, it can be concluded that the 15-mm Axis plate should be even stronger.

CLINICAL APPLICATIONS

The Axis fixation plate has now been used as a custom device in 24 patients with a variety of clinical disorders including degenerative instability, congenital and acquired stenosis, trauma, ossification of the posterior longitudinal ligament, and others. A total of 196 screws have been used. Currently, with 1-year follow-up, there have been no plate failures, dislodgments, losses of reduction, or screw pullouts. When long 4.0-mm cancellous screws were utilized in situations where the 1.9-mm core diameters were exposed to cantilever bending forces (ie, C2, T1, and T2), they occasionally broke near midsection (3 of 196 screws). The system was then modified to include 4.0-mm cortical screws in lengths of 26 mm or more to improve fatigue resistance to bending forces. Reduction and stability were maintained in those few cases in which broken screws were noted.

Difficult and complicated cervical reconstructive procedures often involved anterior and posterior approaches, either at the same sitting or staged. The Axis plates were helpful in these cases by providing protection to long strut grafts when anterior plates could not be applied and by providing additional support and protection to anterior plates when they could be applied (Figs. 16–13A to H).

In my series there were no deaths. There were one radiculitis and no spinal cord injuries related to use of the device in the posterior cervical spine. One patient with an ossified posterior longitudinal ligament (OPLL) and severe myelopathy had posterior laminectomy and plate/screw fixation from C2 to T2. Six weeks later, anterior corpectomies

of C3 through C7 with excision of OPLL, extensive fascia lata dural grafting, and reconstruction of C2 to T1 with fibular graft were performed. Somatosensory evoked potential (SSEP) monitoring was normal throughout the case, but the patient awoke with worsened myelopathy. Slow recovery has occurred, and the anterior and posterior cervical reconstructions show no evidence of failure and have not required halo support. There have been no instances of vertebral artery compromise in this series.

All cases have had postoperative 2-mm section CT scans to assess lateral mass screw placement. All screws were analyzed according to angle of insertion and depth of penetration. Three zones of angulation can be identified from the screw entry point radiating out to the vertebral artery foramen in the C3 through C7 vertebral bodies (Fig. 16–14). The medial zone is unacceptable, the central or vertebral artery zone is risky but acceptable if depth of penetration is not excessive, and the lateral zone is optimal, resulting in strong bicortical screw purchase provided that penetration is not excessive and does not cause nerve root impingement. A total of 94 screws have been placed in the first 13 consecutive patients and analyzed by postoperative CT scanning. No screws were placed in the medial zone. Three screws were placed in the central vertebral artery zone, with no screws showing excessive penetration. There were no vertebral artery injuries. Ninety-one screws had optimal angular placement in the lateral zone. Two screws showed excessive penetration in the lateral zone, with one patient demonstrating symptoms of pain and numbness relating to the nearby nerve root. He had no motor deficit. Persistent symptoms prompted screw removal at 10 months postoperatively. No screws were placed too far laterally (which would result in fracture of the lateral mass by the screw).

One-year follow-up on this series of patients shows the grafts to be incorporating, without evidence of dislodgment of struts, and intact functioning implants with no loss of reduction in any case. The method and technique appears to be safe and effective, versatile, and able to be utilized in the most serious and difficult spinal reconstructive problems.

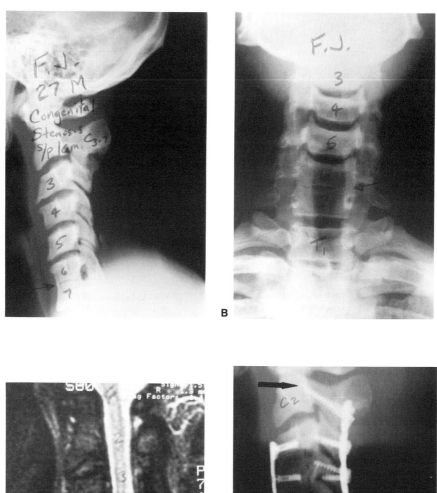

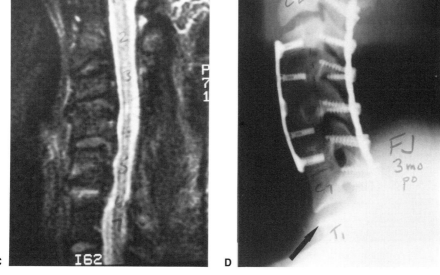

Figure 16–13.   History: F. J. is a 27-year-old male who fell through a mobile home floor, which gave way beneath his feet while he was carrying a four-burner kitchen range and oven. He had radicular and myelopathic findings. Nine years previously he had a C3 to C7 laminectomy for congenital stenosis and transient quadriplegia secondary to a football injury. (**A**). Lateral radiograph after fall demonstrates previous C3 to C7 laminectomies, Klippel-Feil C6 to C7, degenerative disk C3 to C4, and loss of cervical lordosis. Flexion/extension films failed to demonstrate gross instability. (**B**). AP radiograph shows Klippel-Feil at C6 to C7 and good cervical alignment. (**C**). MRI demonstrates kyphosis and C3 to C6 stenosis with evidence of acute spinal cord injury (increased signal intensity) at C3 to C4. (**D**). Lateral radiograph 3 months after two-stage procedure. Stabilization over all segments that were compromised by removal of laminae and interspinous ligaments was accomplished dorsally with fusion and instrumentation from C2 to T1. Lordosis was reestablished. Therefore, the factor of safety for proceeding with ventral decompression, fixation, and fusion was increased, and the patient has a stable, lordotic cervical spine. Note screw placement in C2 and T1 (arrows). A soft cervical collar only was utilized for comfort postoperatively. Most anterior plate systems currently available do not allow for reconstruction of more than three cervical segments (ie, plates are not long enough). Performing posterior plating prior to the anterior reconstructive procedure protects long strut grafts when anterior plating cannot be accomplished and halo vest support is avoided.

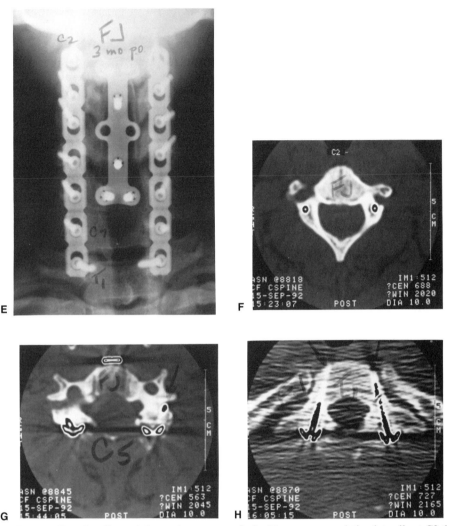

Figure 16–13. Cont. (**E**). AP radiograph 3 months postoperatively. Note screw angulation laterally at C3 through C7, medially at T1, and cephalad at C2. (**F**). Routine postoperative noncontrasted CT with 2-mm slices demonstrates screw placement in C2. The vertebral arteries must be avoided laterally as well as the spinal canal medially. (**G**). CT section at C5 level shows screw directed laterally to avoid the vertebral artery; controlled penetration avoids nerve root injury and enables a bicortical lateral mass purchase to be obtained. (**H**). CT section at T1 demonstrates medially directed screws through the pedicles of T1 to the ventral surface of the T1 corpus.

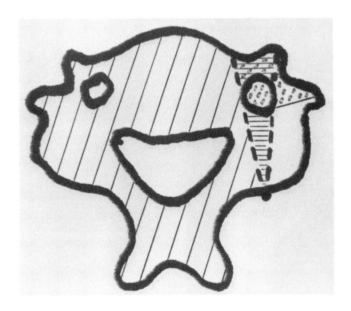

Figure 16–14. Zones identified as useful for analyzing screw placement in the lateral masses of the cervical spine from C3 to C7. Medial zone is crosshatched. Central vertebral artery zone is horizontally hatched. The lateral zone is without hash marks. Areas of excessive screw penetration in the central and lateral zones are identified with dots.

Indications and Contraindications

Indications for application of the Axis fixation system to the posterior cervical spine may be deduced from a clear understanding of the expected function of the implant (Table 16–1). Therefore, the surgeon may find the Axis system useful, and at times essential, in treating patients with an extensive variety of spinal disorders (Table 16–2). Indications for use of the implant may be found in any disease process that renders the spine unstable, malaligned, unreduced, or painful provided that the nature of the condition is improved by decreasing spinal motion with a rigid implant system.

Table 16–1. Functions of the Axis System when Applied to the Posterior Cervical Spine.

1. Effect reduction and restore alignment.
2. Maintain reduction and alignment.
3. Restore stability.
4. Promote fusion.
5. Relieve mechanical pain.
6. Protect neurovascular and other vital structures by attaining goals 1 through 4 above.
7. Improve outcome of, increase safety factor of, and/or salvage or supplement anterior procedures.

Table 16–2. Indications for Posterior Fixation with the Axis System.

1. Degeneration of the spine
   Spondylosis
   Degenerative disk disease
   Degenerative facet arthrosis
2. Inflammation and/or rheumatologic
   Rheumatoid arthritis
   Ankylosing spondylitis
3. Trauma to the spine
   Fractures
   Dislocations
   Subluxations
4. Neoplasia
   Benign
   Malignant
5. Congenital/developmental disorders
   Os odontoideum
   Aplastic dens
6. Iatrogenic instability
   Postlaminectomy
   Postfacetectomy
   Failed fusion
7. Deformity of the spine

Other spinal disorders may be included when the clinical situation warrants. Of course, successful outcome relies heavily on the surgeon's understanding of the basic disease process, its role in production of the patient's symptoms and signs, the natural history of the disease process both without and with surgical intervention, the mechanical nature of the spinal disorder, and how the Axis implant is expected to function to improve the clinical situation. Always keep in mind the basic functional capabilities of the Axis system, as discussed previously.

Relative contraindications to use of the Axis implant exist and should be assessed adequately prior to its use. Contraindications are listed in Table 16–3. This list, although not exhaustive or complete, may serve as a guide to assist the surgeon in analyzing those factors that may adversely affect eventual outcome.

Table 16–3. Contraindications to Posterior Lateral Mass Stabilization with the Axis System.

Active local or systemic infection
Significant risk of infection (immunocompromise)
Shortened life expectancy (malignant neoplasia)
Debility
Mental incompetence
Poor bone quality (osteoporosis, osteomalacia, osteodystrophy, etc)
Anatomic constraints (congenital anomaly, infancy and early childhood, etc)
Metal allergy
Inadequate hospital facilities and/or support personnel
Inadequate surgeon training and/or preparation

CONCLUSION

The Axis Fixation System is versatile and is particularly accommodating when applied to the posterior cervical spine for stabilization and promotion of fusion (Table 16–4). Axis screws and plates can be used for fixation to the cranium in occipitocervical procedures, for atlantoaxial fixation, for a variety of lateral mass techniques in the midcervical spine, and for fixation across the cervicothoracic junction. Utilization of the Axis Fixation System in the cervical spine is facilitated by instrumentation that is specifically designed for posterior cervical procedures and not simply adapted for cervical use from long bone or other instrumentation systems.

Table 16–4. Advantages of Axis Fixation System.

Occipitocervicothoracic fixation
Variety of lateral mass techniques C3 to C6 or C7 (ie, maximal screw angulations achievable)
Corporal fixation C2 and thoracic
Fixation compatible with laminectomy and foraminotomy
Titanium
Attachment and extension to thoracolumbar implants
Minimal interference with location of bone graft
Maximal versatility for screw placement
   Three plate sizes (11-, 13-, and 15-mm intersegmental spacing)
   Two screw locations per segment
Optimal static and fatigue mechanical characteristics compared to other available plate systems
Instrumentation designed specifically for use in anatomic area of application of implant
Cases and trays designed for organization and ease of use

REFERENCES

1. Sutterlin CE, McAfee PC, Warden KE, Rey RM, Farey ID. A biomechanical evaluation of cervical spine stabilization methods in a bovine model. *Spine.* 1988;13:795–802.
2. Coe JD, Warden KE, Sutterlin CE, McAfee PC. Biomechanical evaluation of cervical spinal stabilization methods in a human cadaveric model. *Spine.* 1989;14:1122–1131.
3. Sutterlin CE, Maxey JO. Biomechanics of cervical implants. In: Cotler H, ed. *Spinal Rehabilitation.* In press.
4. Sutterlin CE, Grogan DP, Ogden JA. Diagnosis of developmental pathology of the neuraxis by magnetic resonance imaging. *J Pediatr Orthop.* 1987;7:291–297.

than 1 mm to the normal disk spaces above or below the fusion because motion at the normal interspace may be transmitted to an encroaching plate, resulting in plate failure due to fatigue (Fig. 17–1). In addition, the vertebral endplate is less likely to be entered during screw placement if the plate is not too close to the adjacent disk space. Finally, plates close to normal disk spaces may promote fusion across that motion segment. Anterior osteophytes must be removed to optimize plate contact with the spine, but the anterior longitudinal ligament does not need to be stripped from the vertebral bodies. Carefully noting the midline, the plate is positioned centrally. Fluoroscopy is helpful for confirming proper plate position.

The plate is held firmly with either a hemostat or the specially designed plate clamp while drilling the vertebral body. The posterior cortex must be penetrated with the drill in preparation for bicortical screw placement (Fig. 17–2). It is mandatory that all drilling and screw placement be monitored with fluoroscopy. Attention to detail and careful technique are necessary to avoid entering the spinal canal.

Finely adjustable drill guides are available to ensure safety. These guides fit into the plate holes or slots and allow the depth of drilling to be selected to within a millimeter. The starting length of the guide hole is estimated by direct measurement of the interspace as well as appraisal of the preoperative radiographs. Initially, drilling should proceed through the vertebral body, stopping short of the posterior cortex. The ideal trajectory angles 15° medial and courses parallel to the endplate; if the double-armed drill guide is used, the proper medial trajectory is assured.[12,22] The blunt end of a Kirschner wire (K wire) is used to probe the guide hole under fluoroscopic guidance. Once the posterior cortex has been penetrated, the posterior longitudinal ligament is palpable. If firm cortical bone is encountered, the drill depth is increased by 1-mm increments until the posterior longitudinal ligament is felt.

If the level is difficult to visualize radiographically, such as T1 (and occasionally C7 or T2), the initial drill depth may be estimated as 1 mm less than the depth of the vertebral body above. Drilling continues as discussed earlier until the posterior cortex is penetrated.

Two holes are placed in each vertebral body to be stabilized. Vertebral body replacement grafts are fixed to the plate with one or two unicortical screws. If a partial corpectomy has been performed, screws should be placed through the graft and engage the posterior cortex of the remaining vertebral body (Fig. 17–3).

The plate must be held in the proper position during drilling. K wires may be placed through the plate into the drill holes to prevent plate motion while drilling is completed.[10] Alternatively, a unicortical screw may be placed into a bone strut if a corpectomy has been performed, or screws may be placed (but not tightened fully) after each hole is created.

Screws of sufficient length to penetrate the posterior cortex but not significantly violate the canal should be chosen for insertion. The number of times a screw must be placed and removed from any individual hole should be minimized. Screw size may be estimated by noting the length of exposed drill necessary to drill the hole or measuring the hole with a depth gauge or K wire. All measurements should be performed with the plate in place.

The screw selected should have a threaded shaft 1 mm less than the length of the guide hole.[10] This allows for settling of the plate against the vertebral body as the screw is tightened. Care must be taken to ensure the appropriate length of the threaded portion of the screw. The screw head length is included in the overall length recorded by the manufacturer. We believe it is best always to confirm the length of the threaded shaft by direct measurement prior to placement.

The drill hole must be tapped before placing any screw. The Caspar tapper has an adjustable sleeve to protect surrounding soft tissues and prevent overpenetration. Only the anterior cortex needs to be tapped; however, we prefer to tap about two thirds of the hole. The screw is then placed under fluoroscopic guidance. It should engage or just penetrate the posterior cortex (Fig. 17–3). If the screw size is inappro-

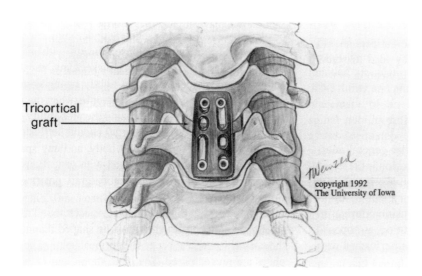

Tricortical graft

copyright 1992
The University of Iowa

Figure 17–1. One-level anterior plate. The plate should not encroach on either the rostral or caudal disk spaces.

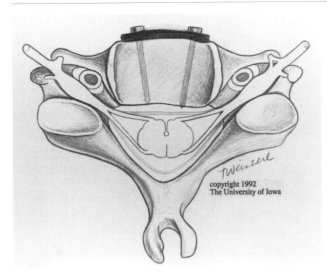

Figure 17–2. Axial view of an anterior plate. The screws are angled medially and must extend to or through the posterior cortex.

priate, it should be removed immediately and replaced. Repeated removal and reinsertion may result in suboptimal screw purchase and increases the risk of plate failure; therefore, every effort should be made to choose the correct screw length initially. The screw should not be secured fully until all are in position, after which they should be tightened gradually in a stepwise fashion. The central screws are tightened first when plating three vertebrae.[12] Although each screw should seat firmly into the vertebral body, care must be taken to avoid stripping the screw by overtightening.

If a screw does not tighten adequately, it may be removed, a new hole drilled, and a new screw inserted.[12,22] Alternatively, a second screw may be placed in a hole near the first screw.[10,12,26] Larger-diameter "rescue" screws are also available. The diameter of these screws is 4.5 mm (as opposed to the standard 3.5-mm screw), and they may be placed directly into the "stripped" hole without further tapping. Some surgeons have described replacing the original screw after packing the hole with bone chips or injecting a

small amount of methyl methacrylate.[10,12,22,26]

After the plate is secured, traction is discontinued and the neck flexed and extended while monitoring in real time with the image intensifier.[26] This is particularly useful when treating traumatic injuries to rule out ligamentous instability at levels that were not stabilized surgically. The wound is irrigated and closed. We prefer to obtain final permanent anteroposterior and lateral cervical radiographs while closing. Such studies may show a screw to be of improper length even though the fluoroscopic images suggested otherwise, although this occurs rarely. Detection of such a discrepancy in the operating room allows one to address the problem easily and replace the affected screw when appropriate.

Postoperatively, the risk of tracheal edema warrants close airway monitoring. Patients at risk for respiratory insufficiency should remain intubated overnight to allow adequate time for reversal of anesthesia and aggressive pulmonary toilet. If permanent radiographs were not obtained in the operating room, they should be taken in the recovery room to assess plate, screw, and graft position as well as cervical alignment. A neurological evaluation should be obtained shortly after the reversal of anesthesia and new deficits should be evaluated aggressively and treated.

The need for cervical immobilization following an anterior plating procedure is somewhat controversial. Although the use of postoperative immobilization is not universal, most surgeons recommend some type of external cervical support.[10,11,12,19,21,22,24,26,28,29] The need for postoperative external bracing is best addressed in a case-by-case manner. Young, healthy patients with only posterior instability probably need only wear a soft collar for 4 weeks, whereas older individuals and patients with severe preoperative instability may require a rigid collar for 2 to 3 months.[12] Halo immobilization should be considered for patients with osteoporosis, systemic disease (rheumatoid arthritis, diabetes mellitus, etc), or severe preoperative instability.[12,26]

Regardless of the underlying pathology, number of levels plated, or type of postoperative immobilization used, it is

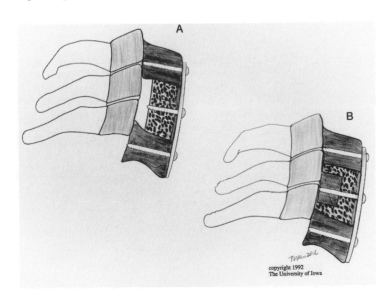

Figure 17–3. Lateral view of screw placement after complete or partial corpectomy. (**A**). The central vertebral body has been removed completely. The plate is secured to the spine with bicortical screws and the iliac crest graft is held with a unicortical screw. (**B**). When performing a partial corpectomy, the screw should traverse the graft and engage the remaining vertebral body.

important to follow each patient with frequent examinations and serial radiographs until fusion is achieved.

COMPLICATIONS AND RESULTS

Six hundred sixty-two reported cases of anterior plate fixation have been reviewed in sufficient detail to determine outcome.[30] Among these cases, there were no intraoperative deaths and the perioperative mortality was approximately 3%. All deaths were related to complications associated with quadriplegia, and no patient expired as a direct result of the plating procedure.

The risks of anterior cervical plate stabilization are similar to those of other anterior cervical procedures.[30] Esophageal perforations have occurred during the exposure, as have temporary vocal cord dysfunction and Horner's syndrome. Significant dysphagia may occur and is usually temporary.[30] Prominent graft and hardware was responsible for this complication in two patients, necessitating reoperation.[22,27] The incidence of wound infection is low, and most infections can be managed with antibiotics and drainage (without removal of plates, screws, or the graft).[30] It may be best, however, to remove the hardware if severe osteomyelitis develops.[19]

Iatrogenic spinal cord injury, the most feared complication of bicortical screw fixation, did not occur in this group of 662 patients.[30] One case of radicular pain secondary to poor screw placement has been reported.[21] This patient improved with screw removal.

The incidence of screw loosening is 3.5%.[30] Loosening of only one or two threads is usually of no consequence and requires only radiographic monitoring; more serious screw loosening resulted in an esophageal perforation in one patient.[12,19,22] Symptomatic screw loosening must be addressed surgically. The primary cause of screw loosening—improper screw placement—can often be prevented by meticulous surgical technique. Screws placed in a disk space are particularly prone to loosening.[22]

The overall fusion rate is 99%.[30] Minor graft resorption and collapse in the first several weeks following surgery (2 mm) does not lessen the likelihood of fusion.[12]

CONCLUSION

The Caspar trapezial plating system provides internal fixation with a high fusion rate. It may reduce the number of segments requiring fusion, decrease the need for postoperative immobilization, and it has an acceptably low complication rate when applied properly. These osteosynthetic plates provide an important option in the surgical management of cervical instability; therefore, surgeons interested in the management of cervical spinal pathology should become familiar with their application.

REFERENCES

1. Cloward RB. The anterior approach for removal of ruptured cervical disks. *J Neurosurg.* 1958;15:602–617.
2. Robinson RA, Smith GW. Anterolateral cervical disk removal and interbody fusion for cervical disk syndrome. *Bull Johns Hopkins Hosp.* 1955;96:223–224.
3. Smith GW, Robinson RA. Treatment of certain cervical spine disorders by anterior removal of the intervertebral disk and interbody fusion. *J Bone Joint Surg Am.* 1958;40A:607–624.
4. Cloward RB. Treatment of acute fractures and fracture-dislocations of the cervical spine by vertebral-body fusion. *J Neurosurg.* 1961;18:201–209.
5. Hoff JT, Wilson CB. Microsurgical approach to the anterior cervical spine and spinal cord. *Clin Neurosurg.* 1979;26:513–528.
6. Verbiest H. Anterior operative approach in cases of spinal cord compression by old irreducible displacement or fresh fracture of cervical spine. *J Neurosurg.* 1962;19:389–400.
7. Verbiest H. Anterolateral operations for fractures and dislocations in the middle and lower parts of the cervical spine. Report of a series of forty-seven cases. *J Bone Joint Surg Am.* 1969;51A:1489–1530.
8. Bailey RW, Badgley CE. Stabilization of the cervical spine by anterior fusion. *J Bone Joint Surg Am.* 1960;42A:565–624.
9. Van Peteghem PK, Schweigel JF. The fractured cervical spine rendered unstable by anterior cervical fusion. *J Trauma.* 1979;19:110–114.
10. Caspar W. *Anterior Cervical Fusion and Interbody Stabilization with the Trapezoidal Osteosynthetic Plate Technique.* Tuttlingen, Germany: Aesculap Scientific Information, Aesculap-Werke-AG; 1986.
11. Caspar W, Barbier DD, Klara PM. Anterior cervical fusion and Caspar plate stabilization for cervical trauma. *Neurosurgery.* 1989;25:491–502.
12. Caspar W, Harkey HL. Anterior cervical fusion. Caspar osteosynthetic stabilization. In: Young PH, ed. *Microsurgery of the Cervical Spine.* New York: Raven Press; 1991:109–142.
13. Ulrich C, Wörsdörfer O, Claes L, et al. Comparative study of the stability of anterior and posterior cervical spine fixation procedures. *Arch Orthop Trauma Surg.* 1987;106:226–231.
14. Ulrich C, Woersdoerfer O, Kalff R, et al. Biomechanics of fixation systems to the cervical spine. *Spine.* 1991;16:S4–S9.
15. Coe JD, Warden KE, Sutterlin CE III, et al. Biomechanical evaluation of cervical spinal stabilization methods in a human cadaveric model. *Spine.* 1989;14:1122–1131.
16. Schulte K, Clark CR, Goel VK. Kinematics of the cervical spine following discectomy and stabilization. *Spine.* 1989;14:1116–1121.
17. Traynelis VC, Donaher PA, Roach RM, Kojimoto H, Goel VK. Biomechanical comparison of anterior Caspar Plate and three-level posterior fixation techniques in a human cadaveric model. *J Neurosurg.* 1993;79:96–103.
18. Goffin J, Plets C, Van den Bergh R. Anterior cervical fusion and osteosynthetic stabilization according to Caspar: a prospective study of 41 patients with fractures and/or dislocations of the cervical spine. *Neurosurgery.* 1989;25:865–871.
19. Pentelényi T, Zsolczai S, Turóczy L, et al. Ventral spondylodesis: basic method in the treatment of cervical spine injuries. *Acta Chir Hung.* 1989;30:299–310.
20. Tuite GF, Papadopoulos SM, Sonntag VKH. Caspar plate fixation for the treatment of complex hangman's fractures. *Neurosurgery.* 1992;30:761–765.
21. de Oliveira JC. Anterior plate fixation of traumatic lesions of the lower cervical spine. *Spine.* 1987;12:324–329.

22. Ripa DR, Kowall MG, Meyer PR Jr, et al. Series of ninety-two traumatic cervical spine injuries stabilized with anterior ASIF plate fusion technique. *Spine.* 1991;16:S46–S55.
23. Böhler J, Gaudernak T. Anterior plate stabilization for fracture-dislocations of the lower cervical spine. *J Trauma.* 1980;20:203–205.
24. Boccanera L, Laus M. Osteosynthesis of the cervical spine with an anterior plate. *Ital J Orthop Traumatol.* 1989;15:287–294.
25. Hall DJ, Webb JK. Anterior plate fixation in spine tumor surgery. Indications, technique, and results. *Spine.* 1991;16:S80–S83.
26. Tippets RH, Apfelbaum RI. Anterior cervical fusion with the Caspar instrumentation system. *Neurosurgery.* 1988;22:1008–1013.
27. Brown JA, Havel P, Ebraheim N, et al. Cervical stabilization by plate and bone fusion. *Spine.* 1988;13:236–240.
28. Levi L, Wolf A, Rigamonti D, et al. Anterior decompression in cervical spine trauma: does the timing of surgery affect the outcome? *Neurosurgery.* 1991;29:216–222.
29. Randle MJ, Wolf A, Levi L, et al. The use of anterior Caspar plate fixation in acute cervical spine injury. *Surg Neurol.* 1991;36:181–189.
30. Traynelis VC. Anterior and posterior plate stabilization of the cervical spine. *Neurosurg Quarterly.* 1992;2:59–76.

18 Stabilization of the Cervical Spine with the Locking Plate System

Setti S. Rengachary, M.D., Derek A. Duke, M.D.

INTRODUCTION

The anterior approach to the cervical spine was devised and popularized in the early to mid-1950s by Bailey and Badgley,[1] Cloward,[2] Robinson and Smith,[3] and Dereymaeker and Mulier.[4] This approach was used initially to treat degenerative disk disease and spondylosis. Subsequently, the indications were extended to include trauma of the lower cervical spine. It became apparent that spondylotic disk disease at a single motion segment could be treated by diskectomy and fusion alone with no need for further stabilization. With multisegmental operations, however, the fusion rates were lower and the incidence of graft extrusion and delayed angular deformity were higher. This created the need for external stabilization. This was even more evident in patients with cervical spine trauma in whom, in addition to an anterior lesion, there was commonly posterior ligamentous instability. In such individuals anterior decompression and fusion alone did not render complete stability to the spine. Additional measures were needed that included prolonged bed rest with traction, application of rigid external orthosis, or a second posterior stabilization procedure. Rigid external orthosis is not well tolerated by patients, especially elderly individuals or quadriplegics. Pin-site complications remain a nuisance even in otherwise healthy individuals. Patients do not like the idea of prolonged rigid fixation of the head and neck for 3 months, hindering mobility and the ability to work in many occupations. Occasionally even after 3 months of rigid external fixation, the spine remains unstable, requiring additional stabilizing surgery at the end of that period. None of these measures designed to augment the stability of the spine are attractive; they cause considerable morbidity, patient dissatisfaction, and prolonged hospital stay. These factors led to the development of improved systems for rigid internal stabilization allowing a one-step anterior decompression with internal stabilization. The introduction of anterior plate stabilization techniques has dramatically reduced the morbidity, shortened hospital stay, reduced the number of motion segments to be fused, restored the normal curvature of the spine in the sagittal plane, and increased the likelihood of fusion.[5–20]

Viewed from a historic prospective, internal stabilization of the cervical spine has long been carried out only posteriorly using either interspinous or sublaminar wire and bone. Anterior internal fixation techniques have been developed in the past 3 decades. Early attempts consisted of makeshift devices that were originally intended for internal stabilization of the jaw or metacarpals. Bohler is credited as being the first to fixate the cervical spine anteriorly in 1964 using a heavy plate and large screws.[5] Other devices include a steel rod by Schurmann and Busch, which was inserted within a bone cylinder that reached into othe adjacent vertebral bodies.[21] Junghanns used a Kirschner wire in the shape of a staple to hold the Cloward bone dowel in place.[22] These latter two devices were intended primarily to keep the bone graft from dislodging rather than stabilizing the spine. Tscherne used the Association for the Study of Internal fixation (ASIF) plate or a cortical bone graft fixed with screws.[23] Orozco and Tapies in 1970 were the first to use an ASIF small-fragment plate for anterior cervical stabilization.[24] Subsequently in 1971 they modified their technique to include an oblique H-shaped plate,[25] and in 1975 they described single-H and double-H plates that are the forerunners of the contemporary locking plates. Simultaneously Senegas and Gauzere described the similar use of H-shaped ASIF plates.[26] Caspar popularized the plate and screw technique by devising a standardized protocol using specially designed instruments for the cervical spine.[11] He used a trapezoidal plate with bicortical screws placed under fluoroscopy. His technique brought into focus the potential role of plate and screw systems to stabilize the cervical spine instantly without the need for rigid external orthosis or other stabilizing procedures.

However, Caspar systems suffered a few major disadvantages. One was the potential for screw migration, which varied from series to series but nevertheless was significant in most hands. The second was the necessity to use the fluoroscope throughout the procedure, causing an increased cumulative radiation risk to the surgeon. Third was the necessity to include the posterior cortex of the vertebral body to ensure proper fixation of the plate. This required precise measurement and micrometer drilling. Recent biomechanical studies on the Caspar systems suggest that posterior cortical penetration may not be necessary,[27] but this observation requires further confirmation before it can be implemented clinically.

The development of the titanium-coated hollow screw reconstruction plate (THORP) system in the department of maxillofacial surgery at Berne by Raveh and his associates revolutionized instrumentation systems for bone fixation.

This new plate and screw system required only monocortical fixation.[28,29] Morscher, also from Switzerland, adapted this system for the cervical spine.[30] This system has virtually eliminated the screw pullout problem yet provides a comparable degree of stability to the bicortical screw and plate system. Although the titanium-coated hollow fenestrated screws are extremely stable, the removal of these screws is technically complicated and cumbersome. Additionally, when used in the cervical spine, there is a significant incidence of screw breakage. The recommendation now is to use solid-core rather than titanium-coated hollow screws. Recently this has been modified further by extending the thread depth, offering a more secure bone purchase. Thus, the locking plate system using titanium cancellous monocortical screws represents the state of the art in plate and screw fixation system for the lower cervical spine.

Some of the advantages of anterior stabilization are improved fusion rates, which approach 100%. Because of the high incidence of fusion with internal stabilization, one has an option of using allograft material, which takes longer to fuse. With internal stabilization, delayed fusion is not a disadvantage because the screw and plate system holds the graft in place for several months until fusion occurs. This eliminates the need for autogenous graft harvesting, which leaves behind a painful hip wound for several weeks. In fact, this is the most distressing postoperative symptom that patients have. Anterior plating gives the option to fuse only one unstable motion segment and thus eliminates the need for rigid external orthosis as compared to posterior fusions for instability. Another advantage of the anterior approach over the posterior approach is that the dissection is carried out in natural anatomic planes with minimal tissue disruption. Postoperative morbidity is less and recuperation is faster. All of these advantages represent a real advance in patient management with lower cervical disorders.

INSTRUMENTATION

Anterior plating of the cervical spine is probably one among the simplest of internal stabilization systems of the spine. In most instances, any available system that the surgeons are familiar with in their respective hospitals can be utilized for surgical exposure of the anterior cervical spine, disk resection, vertebral body decompression, and strut grafting. The only additional instruments required are those for plating, and they are few and straightforward. The plating itself in most instances requires only 30 to 45 minutes of additional operative time, depending on the number of levels to be stabilized. The components of the instrumentation are discussed next.

Plate

The plate is made of pure titanium and thus causes minimal artifact in either magnetic resonance imaging (MRI) or computed tomography (CT). This is particularly important in patients with cervical trauma who may require an MRI at a later date to rule out the possibility of syringomyelia. In patients with degenerative disk disease and spondylosis, this is an advantage as well because progressive degenerative disease at levels other than the operative site can be followed. Postoperative MRI scans to assess the completeness decompression are also possible.

The plates are either H or double H shaped depending on the length (Fig. 18–1A). The length varies from 24 to 92 mm. In a single H plate there are five screw holes, and in a double H plate there are eight screw holes. In the newer extra long H-plate system, there are double screw holes at either end to anchor to the vertebral bodies. In the center there is only a single row of holes that are designed to fall against the center of the vertebral bodies or against bone graft(s). This plate is thought to provide a better anchor to the vertebral bodies (Fig. 18–1B). An arrow at the end of the plate designates the superior end. At the superior end the screw holes are slanted 12 degrees cephalad to facilitate screw placement with a similar angulation (Fig. 18–1C). This is particularly useful in high cervical lesions where, because of the projection of the mandible, straight vertical placement of the screws may not be possible. At lower levels the 12-degree slant carries no advantage other than possibly improving the pullout strength. All screw holes are also slanted internally to allow the screws to enter in a towed-in position, which gives a superior pullout strength. The screw holes are cylindrical in shape to accommodate the screw heads. The plates are gently curved in the coronal plane to conform to the contour of the vertebral bodies. The plates, however, are straight in the sagittal plane, but they can be bent to conform to the contour of the cervical spine (Fig. 18–2). During plate bending the manufacturer recommends that the bends be placed between the holes such that the circular geometry of the holes is not distorted, preserving the good fit of the locking screw head in the screw hole. We have found, however, that the gentle curvature that is required to align the plate with the normal lordosis of the cervical spine does not alter the geometry of the hole enough to prevent proper placement of the screw head. The plate thickness is 2 mm.

Screws

PLASMA-COATED HOLLOW FENESTRATED SCREWS

This screw is now withdrawn from the market by the manufacturer because of the significant rate of screw breakage. The discussion that follows is of historic interest only. This is a hollow screw with fenestrations in the shaft of the screw (Fig. 18–3A). The screw is 14 mm long and 4.0 mm in diameter. The shaft of the screw is plasma coated with titanium. This plasma coating roughens the surface and is said to increase the surface area sixfold. This allows greater contact between the bone and the screw. The fenestrations are designed such that bone will grow through these fenestrations into the core of the screw. Thus the screw has been withdrawn from cervical spine applications. The screw head

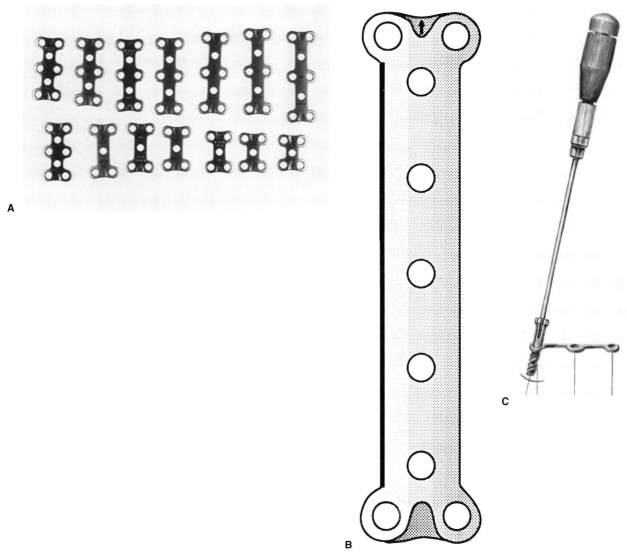

Figure 18–1. (**A**). A standard set of locking titanium plates. (**B**). The new extra long locking plate with a single H configuration and a central row of screw holes. (**C**). The 12-degree cephalad angulation of the superior screw.

is expansile because of its thin, soft metal shell and the presence of a cross-shaped slot in the screw head. This is designed to expand with the insertion of the locking screw. The tip of the screw is flat. Removal of the screw, if required, is difficult due to the solid incorporation of cancellous bone into the fenestrae. The screw head may be twisted off to allow removal of the plate. The screw head is designed such that it will break at the neck between the screw head and the shaft, and thus the plate can be removed and the screw shaft can be left in the bone. If one desires to remove the screw shaft, a special cutting tool is required to cut a core around the screw shaft to aid in extraction.

SOLID-CORE UNCOATED SCREW

An alternative screw is a solid-core screw that is not titanium coated (Fig. 18–3A). Recently the manufacturer has introduced a slight modification of this with a deeper thread design. This allows greater bone purchase. This screw can

be removed easily when compared to the titanium-coated hollow fenestrated screw. Other dimensions and configurations are identical to the titanium-coated screw.

LOCKING SCREWS

Locking screws are small, 1.2-mm screws that insert into the foundation screw (Fig. 18–3B). They have a conical head that is slightly larger than the diameter of the anchoring screw. Thus as the locking screws are tightened, they expand the head of the anchoring screw, locking it into the plate (Fig. 18–3C).

Plate Holder

The plate holder is designed to hold and position the plate while the drill holes are being made (Fig. 18–4A). It is has a prong in the center that fits into the screw hole. The prong has the same dimensions as the screw hole. A plate holder of

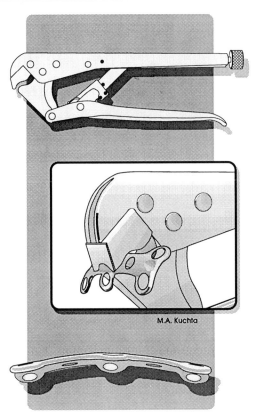

Figure 18–2. Technique of bending the plate in the sagittal plane.

improved design has been introduced (Fig. 18–4B). It has a ratcheted clamp that holds the plate at its edges.

Drill Guide and Drill

The drill is 3 mm in diameter and when inserted through the guide projects only 14 mm beyond the guide (Fig. 18–5A). Thus penetration of the posterior cervical cortex is avoided. The drilling can be done manually or with a power drill. Manual drilling is simpler and more expedient.

Tapping Screw

A tapping screw is available to tap the drill hole (Fig. 18–5B). It is 4 mm in diameter and has a sleeve that protects the soft tissue. The sleeve also guards against penetration beyond 14 mm.

Screwdrivers

The screwdrivers come in two sizes (Fig. 18–5C): one for the anchoring screw and the other for the locking screw. Both have their respective protective sleeves that hold the head of the screw during insertion. The protective sleeve on the screwdriver for the anchoring screw guards against expansion of the screw during its insertion. Once the screw head descends into the screw hole in the plate, the protective sleeve disengages automatically. The small screwdriver also has a protective sleeve to hold the screw in place. It also disengages as the screw is tightened. Both screws should be flush with the plate surface when tightened fully.

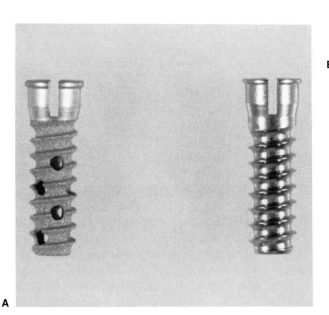

B

C

Figure 18–3. (**A**). Foundation screws. Left: Plasma-coated hollow fenestrated screw. Right: Solid-core uncoated screw. (**B**). Locking screw. (**C**). Top view showing locking screw in place within the head of the anchor screw causing expansion of the latter.

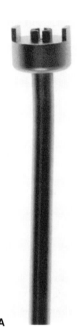

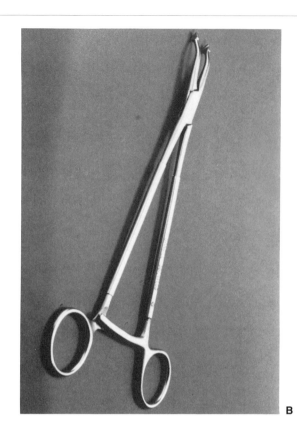

Figure 18–4. (**A**). Standard plate holder. (**B**). Plate holder of improved design.   **A**

B

COMPARISON OF THE LOCKING PLATE SYSTEM WITH THE CONVENTIONAL NONLOCKING PLATE SYSTEMS WITH BICORTICAL SCREWS

Compared to the conventional bicortical screw and plate system, the locking plate system is simple to use. It virtually eliminates the need for fluoroscopy because the length of the screw is designed to penetrate only 14 mm. Given that the average sagittal diameter of the vertebral body is 21 to 22 mm, there is a 4- to 5-mm safety factor. To the best of our knowledge, there has been no reported instance of penetration of the posterior cortex with this screw system. Given this advantage, there is no need for fluoroscopy. This is particularly useful in the lower cervical spine in heavy individuals with big shoulders, where fluoroscopy could be difficult. The absence of the need for fluoroscopy has eliminated the operative time and decreased the radiation exposure to the patient and the surgeon. In addition, the instrumentation is simpler because (1) there is no need for a depth gauge; (2) precise drilling to the posterior cortex is not required; and (3) there is no need for screws of differing lengths. Some have argued that fluoroscopy is still necessary for proper placement of screws with the locking plate system. They reason that the screw might penetrate the superior cortical endplate and may appear in the disk space, reducing the biomechanical stability of the system. However, we find that because of direct visualization of the disk space, one can

gauge the point of entry using the disk space as a reference point. With experience, one should able to place the screws precisely such that there is a minimal possibility of screw penetration through the cortical endplate. We believe that a single anteroposterior (AP) and lateral radiograph at the end of the plating, but before closure of the wound, will suffice.

Another major advantage of the locking plate system is that the screw migration rate is virtually zero. Screw migration has been a persistent problem with bicortical screw systems. Biomechanically, the stability of the nonlocking plate system requires the constant pressure of the screw head to hold the plate against the bone. If the plate is not flat against the bone, or if there is even minimal screw pullout, the stability of the construct is lost. In the locking plate system direct approximation of the plate against the bone is not a requirement (Fig. 18–6). Once the locking screw has been inserted into the anchor screw, the screw and plate function as a single unit. In the cervical spine this is especially advantageous; the anterior surface of the vertebral bodies have an undulating contour precluding direct bony contact through the entire length of the construct. Clinical experience so far indicates that the mechanical stability of the nonlocking bicortical screw plate system and the monocortical locking plate system is equal. The rate of fusion in both instances approximates 100%. Thus, we consider the monocortical locking plate system the latest-generation system rather than a mere alternative to the bicortical screw and plate system. The rapidly increasing popularity of this system supports this assertion.

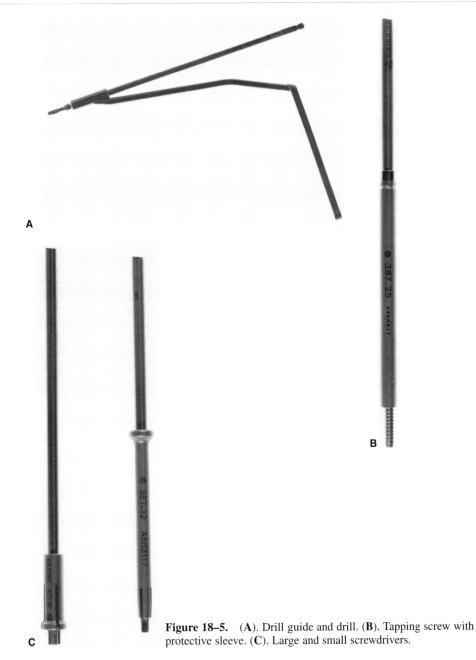

Figure 18–5. (**A**). Drill guide and drill. (**B**). Tapping screw with protective sleeve. (**C**). Large and small screwdrivers.

INDICATIONS AND CASE SELECTION FOR THE LOCKING PLATE STABILIZATION SYSTEM

The general indications for application of the anterior stabilization locking plate system are cervical spine instability, caused either by trauma or induced by surgical decompression such as multilevel diskectomy or corpectomy. Cervical spine trauma, diskogenic disease, and spondylosis are the most common indications for cervical spine stabilization. Less common indications include instability from step deformities and subluxations in rheumatoid arthritis, instability from resection of malignant neoplasms of the cervical vertebrae, and late kyphotic deformities of the spine from healed osteomyelitis of the cervical spine.

Trauma

Numerous classifications schemes exist to categorize various types of lower cervical spine trauma. It is beyond the scope of this chapter to discuss all of the various schemes. However, what is presented here is a modification of Allen's scheme.[31] This scheme, like others, classifies lower cervical spine injuries based on the vector forces that act on the spine.

FLEXION COMPRESSION INJURIES

In flexion compression injuries, there is axial loading with the head in the flexed position (Fig. 18–7A). With mild injuries, there is blunting of the anterosuperior cortical endplate without loss of stability. In more severe injuries, there

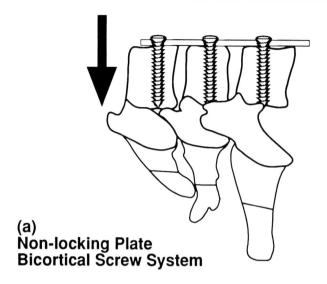

(a)
Non-locking Plate
Bicortical Screw System

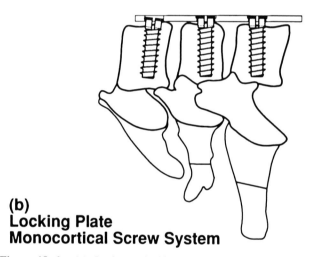

(b)
Locking Plate
Monocortical Screw System

Figure 18–6. (**a**). In the nonlocking plate bicortical screw system, the plate is held against the bone by the compressive force of the screw head against the plate (arrow). Thus, for the secure anchoring of the plate, the plate should be flush against the anterior surface of the vertebral bodies. (**b**). With the locking plate monocortical screw system, secure anchoring of the plate does not depend on the pressure of the screw head against the plate. Thus the plate does not have to sit flat against the bone.

is a "teardrop fracture" with varying degrees of retropulsion of the posterior part of the vertebral body into the spinal canal (Fig. 18–8A). These severe injuries are associated with posterior ligamentous instability and are amenable to corpectomy, removal of disk fragments above and below the fractured body, removal of the comminuted vertebral body, decompression of the canal, and strut grafting with plating. The operative goal is to decompress the spinal canal from anteriorly, where the compressive elements exist, and stabilize it during a single operation. Use of the strut graft under slight distraction and plating stabilizes the spine enough not to require postoperative halo immobilization or additional

fusion posteriorly (360° fusion) in most instances. Without the plating, however, the strut graft may not offer sufficient stability to the spine in the presence of posterior ligamentous injury. In addition, the need for a rigid external orthosis such as a halo is eliminated. With internal stabilization and a comfortable external orthosis such as a soft collar, the patient can be mobilized early.

VERTICAL COMPRESSION INJURIES

In mild cases, there is cupping of the superior or inferior endplate without significant instability (Fig. 18–7B). However, severe injury produces comminuted fractures of the vertebral body, with retropulsed fragments into the canal causing partial or complete cord injury (Fig. 18–8B). Such cases will require corpectomy and strut grafting similar to teardrop injuries. The same advantages apply with the anterior approach (namely, removal of the compressive element from anteriorly and stabilization).

FLEXION ROTATION INJURY

Flexion rotation injuries (Fig. 18–7C) may give rise to unilateral facet dislocation (Fig. 18–8C). Unilateral facet dislocations are treated conventionally with closed external reduction through Gardner tongs by gradually increasing the traction weight with serial x-ray monitoring. If closed reduction is not accomplished, then reduction is attempted with pharmacological muscle relaxation or general anesthesia. If this fails, open reduction may be performed through a posterior cervical approach followed by interspinous or sublaminar wire fusion or lateral mass plating. This injury may also be approached anteriorly. The dislocated site is exposed and the disk is removed from the involved intervertebral space. The vertebral space is distracted gradually under fluoroscopy, if necessary, and the upper vertebrae at the level of the dislocation is gently tapped back into place (Fig. 18–9). After drilling the cortical plates, an interbody graft is inserted and the plating is completed. With this technique, there is quick reduction, instant stabilization, nearly a 100% probability of fusion, and the need for only simple orthosis. The advantages over the posterior approach are as follows:

1. Only a single involved segment needs to be fused. By the posterior approach, the fusion is generally done to include levels above the dislocation if sublaminar or interspinous wiring is used.
2. With the anterior approach, the graft is placed between the vertebral bodies under some degree of axial load, which promotes more rapid fusion than if the graft had been placed under minimal pressure on the laminar surface.
3. Posterior fusion constructs generally act as tension bands and generally are not preferable for lesions that are likely to lead to kyphotic deformity. Anterior fusions restore physiological lordosis.
4. Open reduction by the anterior approach is simpler, done

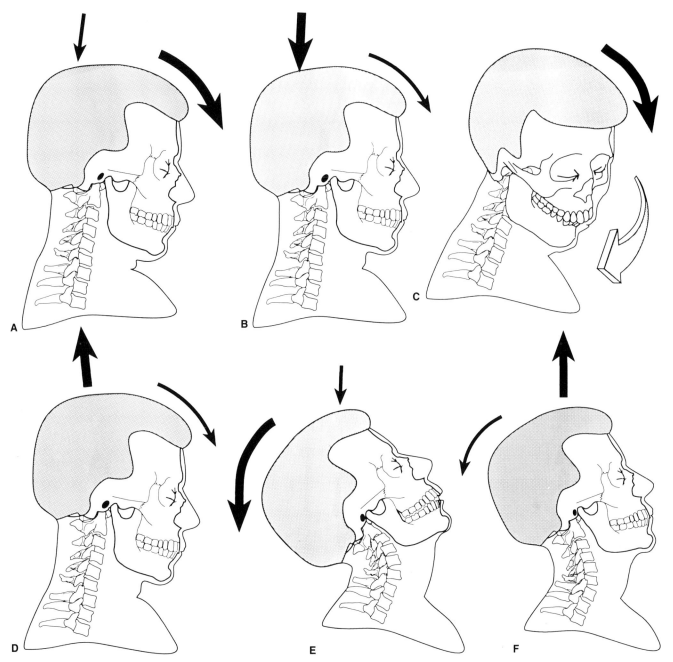

Figure 18–7.   (**A**). Flexion-compression injury. The arrows represent the vector forces acting on the head. (**B**). Vertical compression injury. (**C**). Flexion-rotation injury. (**D**). Distraction-flexion injury. (**E**). Compression-extension injury. (**F**). Distractive-extension injury.

in a single step and as a prelude to definitive internal stabilization.

5. The anterior approach allows anterior decompression of the canal if associated extruded disk fragments are present. There is a potential risk of worsening of neurological deficit if posterior reduction and fusion is performed without removing an unrecognized extruded disk fragment.

DISTRACTION FLEXION INJURIES

With distractive flexion (Fig. 18–7D) there is disruption of the posterior ligaments, including the interspinous

supraspinous ligaments, ligamentum flavum, and capsule of the facet joint. There may be minimal or no injury to the vertebral body. The upper vertebral body glides over the lower, resulting in bilateral facet dislocation (Fig. 18–8D). These injuries generally result in complete cord injury. The major goal is early rehabilitation. Reduction and internal fixation can be accomplished by a single-step anterior procedure in a manner described earlier. The vertebral bodies are distracted gently under direct vision and tapped back in place, the intervertebral disk is removed, and an interbody graft is applied and plated. The disadvantage of closed traction reduction with this injury mechanism is that if the patient has a partial cord injury, there is a risk of worsening the deficit

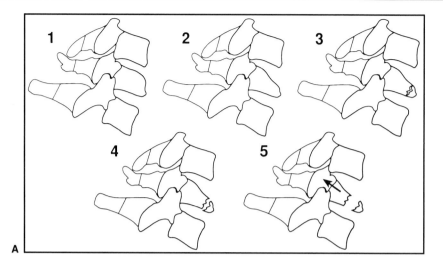

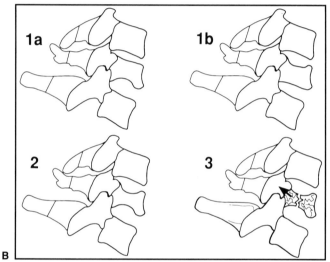

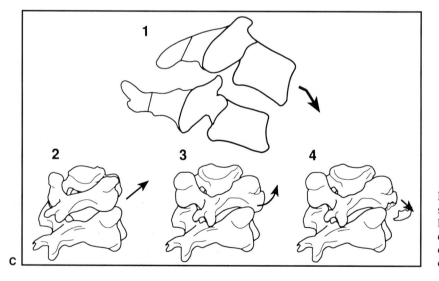

Figure 18–8. (**A**). Sequentially increasing severity of injury with flexion-compression loading of the spine. (**B**). Sequentially increasing severity of injury with axial loading of the spine. (**C**). Unilateral facet dislocation of varying severity.

with overdistraction. This is eliminated by open reduction under direct fluoroscopic guidance. In patients with cord injuries, early mobilization is possible.

A word of caution, however, is necessary when depending on anterior plate fixation alone in the management of severe dislocations that may occur with distractive injuries. In ex-

treme distraction flexion injuries, the involved motion segment is very unstable due to the disruption of all the ligamentous structures that support the vertebrae, including the anterior longitudinal ligament, annulus fibrosis, nucleus pulposus, capsular ligaments, posterior longitudinal ligament, ligamentum flavum, interspinous ligament, and supraspin-

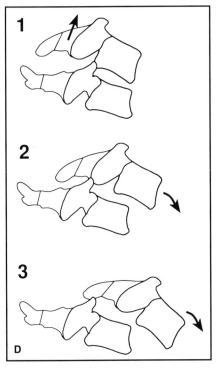

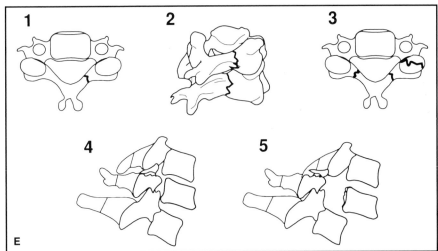

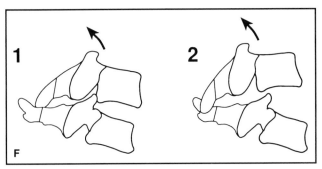

Figure 18–8. Cont. (**D**). Sequentially increasing severity of injury with distractive flexion of the spine. (**E**). Sequentially increasing severity of injury with compression extension of the spine. (**F**). Sequentially increasing severity of injury with distractive extension of the spine.

ous ligament. In these instances, plate stabilization in itself may be insufficient to confer adequate stability. If instability is inferred from postoperative radiographs, one must depend on rigid external orthosis, or preferably an additional posterior stabilization procedure.

Another caveat in the technique of treating extreme distraction flexion injuries is that one should resist the temptation to distract maximally the intervertebral space with a large graft (which is easy to do because of total ligamentous disruption). With hyperdistraction of the intervertebral space, the natural locking mechanism of the reduced facets is lost, allowing redislocation to occur with relative ease.

COMPRESSIVE EXTENSION INJURY

With a compressive extension injury (Fig. 18–7E) there is fracture of the posterior bony elements without disruption of the intervertebral disk, annulus, or the anterior or posterior ligaments. These fractures are stable and thus require no internal fixation. With severe injury there is complete separa-

tion of the vertebral body from the posterior elements, with varying degrees of dislocation of the vertebral body (Fig. 18–8E). Such cases will benefit from closed reduction and anterior stabilization with a diskectomy and interbody grafting.

DISTRACTIVE EXTENSION INJURY

This injury (Fig. 18–7F) produces disruption of the anterior longitudinal ligament, disruption of the disk, and widening of the disk space with a tiny teardrop fracture (Fig. 18–8F). One should do an MRI to see whether the disk is disrupted and displaced posteriorly, causing either cord or root compression. If this is the case, diskectomy is performed and stabilization is necessary. In the absence of cord or root compression, the dislocation can be reduced and treated with simple external orthosis if the posterior ligamentous structures are intact.

From the foregoing discussion, one can see that the locking plate system can be utilized in lower cervical spine

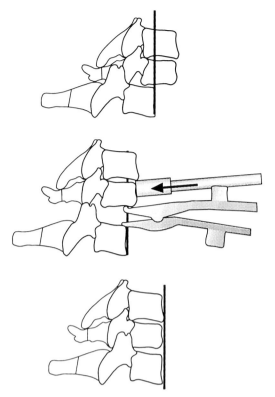

Figure 18–9. Technique of open reduction of unilateral facet dislocation by the anterior approach.

trauma (C2 to T1) regardless of the mechanism of injury. Thus, a single standardized procedure is helpful in internally stabilizing almost all unstable lower cervical spine injuries. Exceptions to this rule are as follows:

1. A laminar fracture with direct compression of the cord by a fragment of the lamina. This injury is rare and is seen only with direct trauma to the lamina. A posterior approach is obviously necessary to treat this problem.
2. With complete disruption of all ligaments, as may happen with extreme distractive injuries, one should not depend solely on anterior plating; careful postoperative assessment of stability is needed and, if indicated, a posterior stabilization procedure may have to be done as well.

Disk Disease

With soft cervical disk disease, anterior diskectomy with interbody grafting (without plating) at a single level is curative in most instances. However, the fusion rate varies from 70% to 90%. One may question the need for plating after single-level diskectomy and fusion. The advantages are that (1) the fusion rate approaches 100%, (2) delayed angular deformity from collapse of the graft is prevented, and (3) the plate holds the spine in physiological alignment until fusion occurs and thus acts as an internal splint. Additionally, with secure plate fixation, anterior graft extrusion cannot occur.

Cervical Spondylosis

The operative approach to cervical spondylotic radiculopathy is no different than the approach to cervical disk disease, which was discussed in the previous section. However, in cervical spondylotic myelopathy a more radical surgical technique is needed to obtain optimal results. It is beyond the scope of this chapter to discuss the mechanism of myelopathy and the rationale for selecting the optimal surgical procedure to treat the myelopathy. Suffice it to say that any procedure intended to alleviate the symptoms of myelopathy should confer stability to the spine in addition to decompressing the spinal canal. In patients with spondylotic disease with superimposed congenital spinal stenosis, multilevel partial median corpectomy with strut grafting offers the best chance of alleviating the symptoms. With this procedure, stabilization is required using either an external halo orthosis or an internal plate. Internal stabilization with plating is more comfortable to the patient. In addition, one can use a tricortical iliac crest graft because the axial load is shared in part by the plate, and thus there is less risk of fracture of the graft. This procedure thus reduces the need for the use of the fibula, which is slow to heal.

Rheumatoid Arthritis

Rheumatoid arthritis affecting the cervical spine causes three major types of instability: (1) anterior atlantoaxial subluxation, (2) cranial settling with cranial migration of the odontoid, and (3) multilevel lower cervical spine subluxation causing a step deformity. The anterior plate stabilization is well suited for multilevel anterior step deformity due to subluxation. This should be carried out only in patients with advanced subluxation with impending or actual cord compression. Patients with only neck pain should be followed to assess whether the subluxation will become severe enough to cause neurological abnormality. Mere demonstration of subluxation without the onset or progression of a neurological deficit is not an indication for anterior plate stabilization. If stabilization is contemplated, the involved segments should be stabilized by resection of the rheumatoid granulation tissue involving the disk space, interbody grafting, and plate stabilization at the involved levels. The technique is not different from the one used for multilevel disk disease or spondylosis.

Tumors

With malignant primary or metastatic tumors of the cervical spine that are limited to the vertebral body, one can do a corpectomy. Following corpectomy, a surgical option is to fill the gap with methacrylate and stabilize it with a Steinman pin driven axially through the vertebral bodies. Plate and screw systems work well, but Steinman pin fixation is an acceptable alternative.

Infection

In patients with active ongoing osteomyelitis, implantation of plates and screws is not recommended. We prefer to curette and debride the infected tissue, obtain appropriate cultures, treat the patient in a halo device, and use appropriate long-term antibiotics. In most instances, this regimen alone will suffice. If there is angular kyphotic deformity, it can be corrected with corpectomy at the appropriate level, with strut grafting and plating at a later date.

OPERATIVE APPROACH

In patients with unstable cervical spine injuries, the patient is moved carefully from the cart to the operating table with the cervical collar in place. Awake fiberoptic intubation is preferred. A tracheostomy should be deferred, whenever possible, for up to 2 weeks to allow time for the cervical wound to heal and the prevertebral space to seal off.

The patient is positioned supine and a silastic gel roll is placed behind the neck to maintain the physiological curvature of the cervical spine. Cervical traction is maintained throughout the procedure. Overdistraction should be avoided in trauma cases. The cervical spine is exposed in the usual manner as with any anterior procedure and will not be discussed further.

Constructs

Several constructs are possible. In patients with a single-level ruptured disk or spondylotic disease, diskectomy is carried out by sharply excising the annulus. The nucleus pulposus and the remainder of the disk material is removed using a combination of pituitary rongeurs and up-biting curettes. Distraction is then applied with an intervertebral distracter. Additional distraction may be obtained by adding more weight on the traction device. Some prefer distracters that utilize screws placed in the midportion of the vertebral bodies. Although such a system gives an unobstructed view of the intervertebral disk space, the screw hole that is used for the distracter cannot be used for the placement of permanent screws for the plate. Using a high-speed drill, the cortical plates of the superior and inferior vertebral bodies are drilled out and osteophytes are removed. A sharp nerve hook is used to make a longitudinal incision in the posterior longitudinal ligament by sliding the hook up and down between the fibers. Using a small Kerrison rongeur, the posterior longitudinal ligament is excised. Attention is then directed to the hip, and through a curvilinear incision the iliac crest is exposed and tricortical bone graft is harvested using an oscillating saw. The graft should be 1 mm longer than the measured length of the recipient space and gently impacted in place. We generally prefer to insert the cortical end facing posteriorly, which gives maximal strength at the middle pillar, the site of maximal axial load. Any gaps that are left on the sides of the graft are filled with cancellous mush. Before filling with cancellous mush, the gaps are packed gently with a small, thin layer of gel foam such that the cancellous mush does not drop into the epidural space.

Multilevel Diskectomy and Fusion

Multilevel diskectomy and fusion is carried out in a manner analogous to the single-level fusion but is done at more than one level (Fig. 18–10A).

Partial Median Corpectomy

Corpectomy is carried out by removing the intervertebral disk in a manner described earlier, and then removing the intervening vertebral bodies through the use of both Leksell rongeurs and a high-speed drill. A strut graft made of either iliac crest or fibula is then tapped into place under distraction (Fig. 18–10B).

Plating

It is important to prepare the vertebral bodies properly for the plate. After placing the graft, it will be apparent that the anterior vertebral body surface will be undulating, with concave surfaces at the midvertebral body level and convex ridges near the anterior osteophytes. In addition, the sharp corners of the graft may be projecting as well. Using a high-speed drill, the osteophytes and anterior beaks are drilled out as well as any part of the graft that is projecting out. However, one should be careful not to drill extensively at the superior and inferior ends of the host vertebral bodies because overaggressive drilling to remove osteophytes may actually thin out the cortical bone and thus limit the purchase for the foundation screws at these critical sites. In choosing the appropriate length of the plate, one must make sure that the plate extends well into the vertebral body above and the vertebral body below. It is better not to anchor the plate in the midvertebral body because the waistlike constrictive dimensions of the vertebral body are at its midpoint. The plates have the largest diameter with an H-shaped configuration at this point, and the horizontal dimension of the plate may extend beyond the waist of the midvertebral body, precluding good screw purchase.

Once a plate of appropriate length has been chosen, it is bent gently in the sagittal plane with a plate bender (Fig. 18–2) to fit the contour of the C curve of the cervical spine. In most instances it is only a gentle curve that is needed. Sometimes a sharper curve may be needed at the upper and lower ends of the plate where the plate seats on the vertebral body. The manufacturer recommends that the screw hole at the apex of the maximal curvature not be used because it may alter the hole geometry and thus the expansive screw head may not lock into the screw hole. In creating a gentle curvature of the plate, we do not find this to be true. The plate is bent in small increments with repeated checking rather than in a single move. This is far superior than having to go back and reduce the curvature. The plate is then seated over the proposed site, using the guidelines stated earlier. The plate should be in direct contact with the bone without intervening soft tissues. We prefer to anchor the plate with a screw near the center of the plate first so that it is used as an anchor. We take an anteroposterior radiograph to make sure

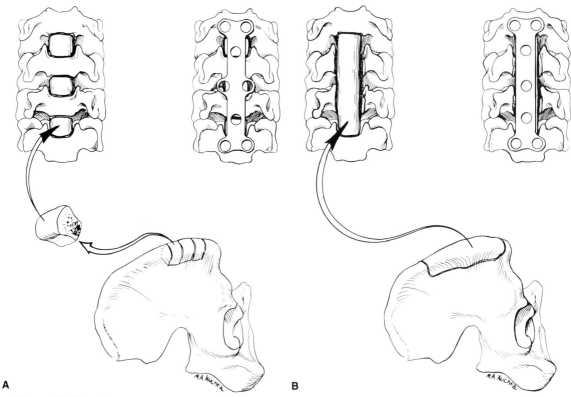

A   B

Figure 18–10.   (**A**). Multilevel diskectomy and fusion followed by internal stabilization and plating. (**B**). Multilevel partial median corpectomy, strut grafting with tricortical iliac crest bone and plating.

it is oriented vertically and then apply the rest of the screws.

A drill hole is first placed using a drill guide to a constant depth of 14 mm (Fig. 18–11A). The drilling can either be done by hand or with a power attachment. In most instances manual drilling is expedient. The drill guide with a depth stop prevents drilling beyond 14 mm. This obviates the need for lateral fluoroscopy during drilling. After drilling, the screw holes are tapped. It is necessary to tap through the entire depth of the screw hole. The tap has a protective sleeve that prevents the sharp edges of the tapping screw from catching soft tissue (Fig. 18–11B). After the tapping is completed, the foundation screw is inserted. The foundation screw is held on the screwdriver by a sleeve that protects the screw head from expanding during the insertion. Once the screw head enters the plate, the protective sleeve retracts automatically (Fig. 18–11C). The remainder of the screw holes are then made in the same sequence (namely, drilling to the constant depth of 14 mm using the drill guide, tapping, and then application of a foundation screw). In each instance, it is important to make sure that the screw head is flush with the plate. We prefer first to finger tighten the screw gently and then retighten after all of the screws have been inserted. If by chance a screw strips, one can try to pack the screw hole with cancellous mush and then apply the screw again. If that fails, we simply disregard that screw hole because every hole does not have to be utilized due to the redundant number of holes. "Rescue" screws are not available at present. The screws are only one length regardless of whether they go through the vertebral body or into the graft. After the

foundation screws are applied, the small locking screws are placed snugly to ensure expansion of the foundation screw head and locking (Fig. 18–11D). After all of the locking screws are applied, an anteroposterior and lateral radiograph are taken to confirm proper positioning of the screws and plate. We leave a 10 French Blake drain in the prevertebral space attached to a suction bag. Only the platysma layer requires closure, and the skin is always closed in a subcuticular fashion.

COMPLICATIONS

Postoperative complications may be divided into general complications that are inherent in any anterior cervical exposure and those that are specific to plate application.

The general complications include wound hematoma, injury to the carotid artery or jugular vein, perforation of the pharynx, injury to the recurrent laryngeal or superior laryngeal nerves, infection, and spinal cord or root injury. These complications are better avoided than treated.

Specific complications include screw migration and plate failure. In our series of 50 anterior plating procedures with a follow-up of up to 22 months, we have not encountered a single instance of screw migration. We have had two complications. In one patient with a severe distractive injury, despite anterior plating, the spine was unstable; the patient had to be returned to surgery for further stabilization through the posterior approach. Another patient who underwent partial median corpectomy refused to have a banked bone graft. A

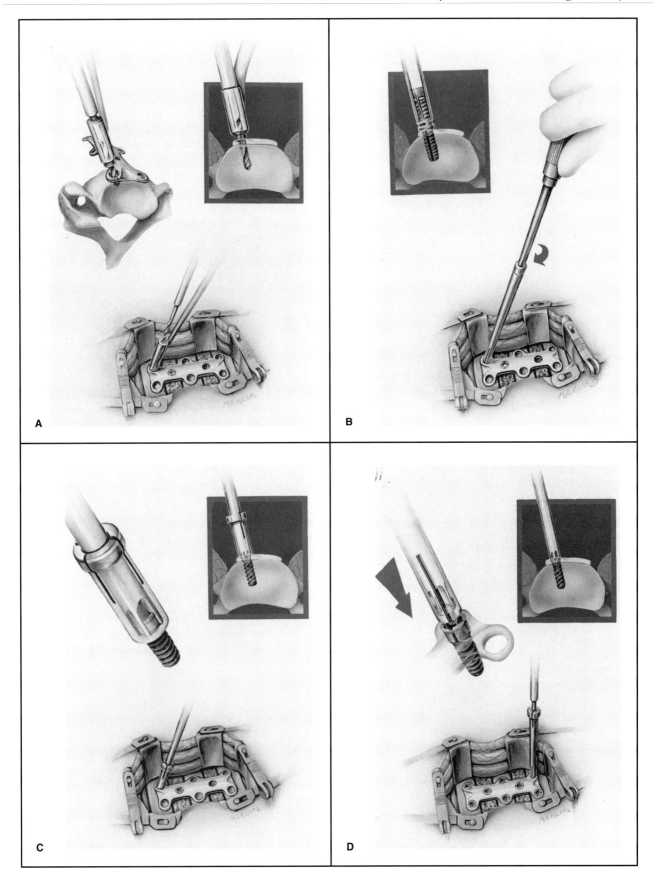

Figure 18–11. (**A**). Technique of drilling with a drill guide in place. (**B**). Tapping. (**C**). Insertion of anchor screw. (**D**). Insertion of locking screw.

long tricortical autologous strut graft was used, but because of the curvature of the graft and insecure seating, it migrated forward and displaced the plate and screws. The patient was then willing to have an allograft placed. The patient underwent a second operation to remove the iliac crest graft and to place a fibula strut graft. The patient was placed in a halo postoperatively and did well following the procedure.

REFERENCES

1. Bailey R, Badgley C. Stabilization of the cervical spine by anterior fusion. *J Bone Joint Surg Am.* 1960;42:565–594.
2. Cloward R. The anterior approach for removal of ruptured cervical disks. *J Neurosurg.* 1958;15:602–617.
3. Robinson R, Smith G. Anterolateral cervical disc removal and interbody fusion for cervical disc syndrome. *Bull Johns Hopkins Hosp.* 1955;96:223–224.
4. Dereymaeker A, Mulier J. Nouvelle cure chirurgicale des discopathies cervicales. La meniscectomie par voie ventrale, suivie d'arthrodese par greffe intercorporeale. *Neurochirurgie.* 1956;2:233–234.
5. Bohler J, Gaudernak T. Anterior plate stabilization for fracture-dislocations of the lower cervical spine. *J Trauma.* 1980;20:203–205.
6. Aebi M, Zuber K, Marchesi D. Treatment of cervical spine injuries with anterior plating. Indications, techniques, and results. *Spine.* 1991;16(suppl):38–45.
7. Suh PB, Kostuik JP, Esses SI. Anterior cervical plate fixation with the titanium hollow screw plate system. A preliminary report. *Spine.* 1990;15:1079–1081.
8. Goffin J, Plets C, Van den Bergh R. Anterior cervical fusion and osteosynthetic stabilization according to Caspar: a prospective study of 41 patients with fractures and/or dislocations of the cervical spine. *Neurosurgery.* 1989;25:865–871.
9. Gassman J, Seligson D. The anterior cervical plate. *Spine.* 1983;8:700–707.
10. Bremer AM, Nguyen TQ. Internal metal plate fixation combined with anterior interbody fusion in cases of cervical spine injury. *Neurosurgery.* 1983;12:649–653.
11. Caspar W, Barbier DD, Klara PM. Anterior cervical fusion and Caspar plate stabilization for cervical trauma. *Neurosurgery.* 1989;25:491–502.
12. Traynelis VC. Plate stabilization following anterior cervical spine surgery. *Contemp Neurosurg.* 1992;14:1–6.
13. Traynelis VC. Anterior and posterior plate stabilization of the cervical spine. *Neurosurg Quarterly.* 1992;2:59–76.
14. Brown JA, Havel P, Ebraheim N, et al. Cervical stabilization by plate and bone fusion. *Spine.* 1988;13:236–240.
15. Tippets RH, Apfelbaum RI. Anterior cervical fusion with the Caspar instrumentation system. *Neurosurgery.* 1988;22:1008–1013.
16. Ripa DR, Kowall MG, Meyer PR, et al. Series of ninety-two traumatic cervical spine injuries stabilized with anterior ASIF plate fusion technique. *Spine.* 1991;16(suppl):46–55.
17. Oliveira JC. Anterior plate fixation of traumatic lesions of the lower cervical spine. *Spine.* 1987;12:324–329.
18. Cabanela ME, Ebersold MJ. Anterior plate stabilization for bursting teardrop fractures of the cervical spine. *Spine.* 1988;13:888–891.
19. Randle MJ, Wolf A, Levi L, et al. The use of anterior Caspar plate fixation in acute cervical spine injury. *Surg Neurol.* 1991;36:181–189.
20. Lesoin F, Cama A, Lozes G, et al. The anterior approach and plates in lower cervical posttraumatic lesions. *Surg Neurol.* 1984;21:581–587.
21. Schurmann K, Busch G. Die Behandlung der cervicalen Luxationsfrakturen durch die ventrale fusion. *Der Chirurg.* 1970;41:225–228.
22. Junghanns H. Metallfixation von knochenblacks an der halswirbelsaule. *Der Chirurg.* 1973;44:87–90.
23. Tscherne H, Hiebler W, Muhr G. Zur operativen behandlung von frakturen und luxationen der halswirbelsaule. *Heft Unfallheik.* 1971;108:142–145.
24. Orozco Delclos R, Llovet Tapies J. Osteosintesis en las fractures de raquis cervical. *Revista Ortop Traumatol.* 1970;14:285–288.
25. Orozco Delclos R, Llovet Tapies J. Osteosintesis en las lesiones traumaticas y degeneracion de la columna cervical. *Revista Traumatol Cirurg Rhabil.* 1971;1:45–52.
26. Senegas J, Gauzere JM. Plaidoyer pour la chirurgie anterieure dans le traitement des traumatismes graves des cinq dernieres vertebres cervicales. *Rev Chirurg Orthop.* 1976;62:123–128.
27. Maiman DJ, Pintar FA, Yoganandan N, et al. Pull-out strength of Caspar cervical screws. *Neurosurgery.* 1992;31:1097–1101.
28. Raveh J, Sutter F, Hellem S. Surgical procedures for reconstruction of the lower jaw using the titanium-coated hoolow screw reconstruction plate system: bridging defects. *Otolaryngol Clin N Am.* 1987;20:535–558.
29. Raveh J, Stesh M, Stutter F, et al. Use of titanium-coated hollow screw and reconstruction plate system in bridging of lower jaw defects. *J Oral Maxillofac Surg.* 1984;42:281–294.
30. Morscher E, Sutter F, Jennis M, et al. Die Vordere verplattung der halswirbelsaule mit dem hohlschrauben-plattensystem. *Der Chirurg.* 1986;57:702–707.
31. Allen BL, Fergusion RL, Lehman TR, et al. A mechanistic classification of closed indirect fractures and dislocations of the lower cervical spine. *Spine.* 1982;7:1–27.

19 Anterior Cervical Osteosynthesis: Orion™ Anterior Cervical Plate System

Gary L. Lowery, M.D., Ph.D.

INTRODUCTION

The primary indication for anterior cervical osteosynthesis is to provide internal stability. Anterior cervical plating can provide sufficient stability, especially in degenerative conditions, to obviate the need for external immobilization (halo, hard collar, etc). Anterior cervical plating provides selective vertebral immobilization while allowing all remaining vertebral motion segments to be functionally mobile. A halo or an orthosis can only provide overall immobilization and cannot selectively immobilize any cervical segment(s).

Anterior cervical plates are reported to be stable enough for reconstruction after acute trauma or corpectomy. Essentially, any patients requiring decompression and reconstruction would be candidates for anterior cervical osteosynthesis and plating. This would include patients with acute trauma, posttraumatic deformities, tumors, ossification of the posterior longitudinal ligament, and multilevel cervical spondylosis with osteophytosis, to name a few examples. Severe osteoporosis is a relative contraindication to anterior plate fixation.

We feel that anterior cervical plating enhances fusion rates, especially in cases of multilevel fusions. Anterior instrumentation helps provide a stable local environment for vascular ingrowth that is necessary to promote bony fusion, especially when using allograft. Anterior cervical plates can provide the needed stability, can be applied safely, and can remain securely fixed, either with adequate bicortical screw purchase or locked unicortical screws (locked to the plates). The history and rationale for anterior cervical plating were addressed in Chapters 17 and 18. The biomechanics of anterior plating as well as the indications for such stabilization devices were also reviewed in those chapters.

Since anterior plating was first performed in 1964, a variety of devices has been attached to the anterior cervical vertebral bodies in an effort to impart stability to the spine.[1] The Orion™ Anterior Cervical Plate System (Danek Medical, Inc., Memphis, Tenn) for anterior cervical osteosynthesis is one of the most recently developed systems. The rationale for the design of the Orion™ plate and its use are described in this chapter.

ORION™ ANTERIOR CERVICAL PLATE SYSTEM

The Orion™ plate is constructed of titanium alloy, which minimizes both computerized tomography (CT) and magnetic resonance (MR) scanning artifacts (Fig. 19–1). The smallest plate is 25 mm long. Plate lengths increase by 2.5-mm increments up to 90 mm and then by 5-mm increments up to 110 mm. Each plate has a predetermined lordotic curve that was derived from an average lordosis (C3-C7) taken from multiple lateral cervical spine x-rays. Although the plate contour is preset, it is possible to contour them further if necessary.

The mechanical properties of the Orion™ plate as well as the Morscher plate [Cervical Spine Locking Plate System (Synthes Spine, Paoli, Pa)], the Orozco plate [Cervical Vertebrae Plate (Synthes Spine, Paoli, Pa)], and the Caspar ACF Plate [Aesculap, Inc., South San Francisco, Calif] have been evaluated by securing the ends of the individual plates into artificial vertebral bodies constructed of ultrahigh-molecular-weight polyethylene (UHMWPE). The UHMWPE test pieces were loaded axially 0.516 in from the bone plate/UHMWPE interface using an Instron servohydraulic test machine. Both static and fatigue testing were performed; the fatigue testing was conducted at 8 Hz (Fig. 19–2).

The Orion™ plate had an ultimate strength of 87.36 lb and a yield strength of 77 lb (Fig. 19–3). Four plates were fatigue tested with a limit of about 55 lb. Failure occurred through the notched-down region of one Orion™ plate or through the screw holes for the other three plates. The Orozco plate had an ultimate strength of 10.9 lb and a yield strength of 7.05 lb. Three plates were fatigue tested with a limit near 10 lb and none of the specimens fractured, but failure occurred by permanent bending through the center screw hole. The ultimate strength of the Caspar plates was 22 lb, and the yield strength was 13.6 lb. Three plates were tested with a fatigue limit near 15 lb and, as in the Orozco plates, failure occurred secondary to permanent bending. The Morscher plate had an ultimate strength of 32.4 lb and a yield strength of 22.68 lb. Four plates were fatigue tested

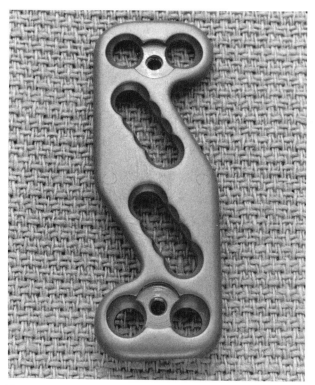

Figure 19–1. Orion™ Anterior Cervical Plate System.

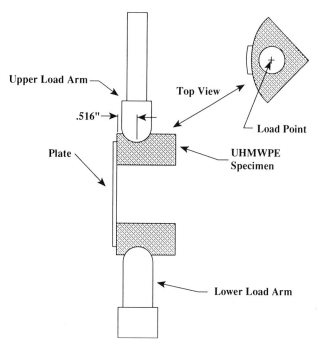

Figure 19–2. The setup for mechanical testing of the Orion™ Anterior Cervical Plate System (Danek Medical, Inc., Memphis, Tenn), Morscher plate [Cervical Spine Locking Plate System (Synthes Spine, Paoli, Pa)], the Orozco plate [Cervical Vertebrae Plate (Synthes Spine, Paoli, Pa)], and the Caspar ACF Plate (Aesculap, Inc., South San Francisco, Calif).

with a fatigue limit near 22.5 lb. During fatigue, these plates fractured through the single hole away from the end of the plate.

During both the fatigue and static testing of the Orion™ plate, no failure occurred due to the bone screws or locking screws. In conclusion, the Orion™ plate had an ultimate strength ranging from 2.7 to 8 times, a yield strength ranging from 3.4 to 10.9 times, and a fatigue limit ranging from 2.4 to 5.5 times that of the other plates tested (Fig. 19–4).

Two different types of Orion™ plates are available. Similar to other anterior plating systems, one set of plates may be secured with converging screws (Fig. 19–5). The screws angle 6° medially and, additionally, the superior screws are angled 15° rostrally and the inferior screws angle 15° caudally. The second type of plate is secured with screws that diverge 10° (Fig. 19–6). There are theoretical reasons to believe that diverging screws may be stronger than converging screws: The lateral posterior cortex is thicker than the midline posterior cortex, and longer screws may be used, which would increase the area of bone-screw interface. Placement of diverging screws requires less soft-tissue retraction than during the placement of converging screws because the direction of the drill, tap, and screws centers from the midline of the wound. The diverging screws also angle rostrally and caudally 15° (Fig. 19–7).

Intervening scalloped diagonal slots allow two screws to be placed in each vertebral body, as is necessary for multi-level interbody fusions, as well as for screws to be secured to long strut grafts. The intervening screws can be directed medially, laterally, rostrally, or caudally and are not locked to the plate (Fig. 19–8).

The plates are secured to the vertebral bodies with 4.0-mm diameter screws. The minor diameter is 2.4 mm, and the threads are pitched at 1.75 mm. In essence, the screws carry a cancellous thread design that results in improved vertebral purchase. The screws vary in length from 10 to 26 mm (thread in bone) in 1.0-mm increments. A smaller locking screw secured over each pair of cancellous screws prevents backout of the bone screws.

The plates may be secured with either unicortical or bicortical screws. The ability to have unicortical and–or bicortical purchase of the vertebral body allows for significant flexibility in difficult reconstructive procedures. This can be appreciated especially in cases of osteoporotic bone and in long strut reconstructions, where the forces on the plate-strut construct may best be counteracted through bicortical purchase. The end-locking screws can be locked to the plate, whether unicortical or bicortical.

IMPLANTATION TECHNIQUE

The pathologic lesion is approached through a standard exposure to the anterior cervical spine. The decompression or tumor resection is performed, and an intervertebral wedge graft or strut is placed. As accurately as possible, a normal cervical lordotic curve should be achieved.

Ultimate and Yield Strength
For Anterior Cervical Plates

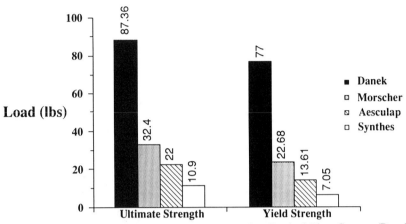

Figure 19–3. Ultimate and yield strengths for the Orion™ Anterior Cervical Plate System (Danek Medical, Inc., Memphis, Tenn), Morscher plate [Cervical Spine Locking Plate System (Synthes Spine, Paoli, Pa)], the Orozco plate [Cervical Vertebrae Plate (Synthes Spine, Paoli, Pa)], and the Caspar ACF Plate (Aesculap, Inc., South San Francisco, Calif).

Anterior Cervical Plates

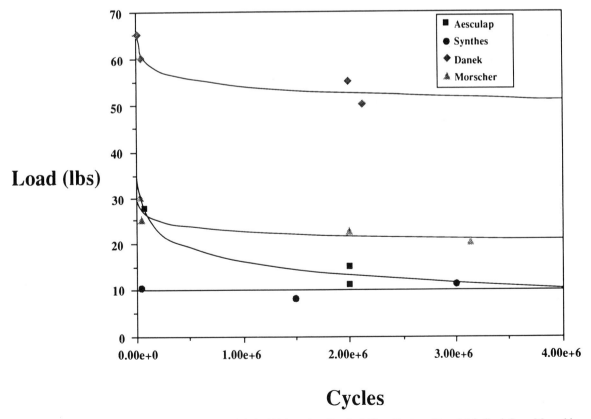

Figure 19–4. Fatigue strengths of the tested Orion™ Anterior Cervical Plate System (Danek Medical, Inc., Memphis, Tenn), Morscher plate [Cervical Spine Locking Plate System (Synthes Spine, Paoli, Pa)], the Orozco plate [Cervical Vertebrae Plate (Synthes Spine, Paoli, Pa)], and the Caspar ACF Plate (Aesculap, Inc., South San Francisco, Calif).

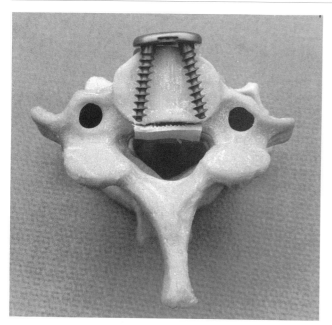

Figure 19–5. Orion™ plate with converging screws.

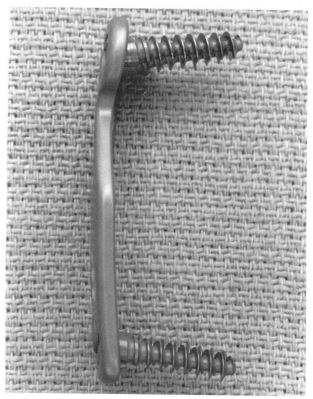

Figure 19–7. Lateral view of Orion™ plate demonstrating rostral and caudal angulation of the screws.

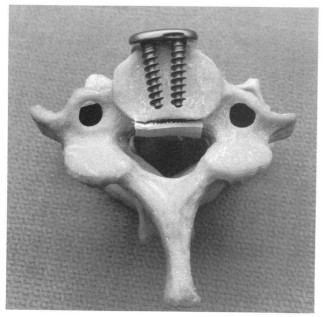

Figure 19–6. Orion™ plate with diverging screws.

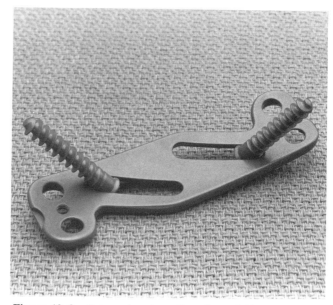

Figure 19–8. Intervening slots allow for variable screw placement.

A plate of appropriate size is selected. The plate should cover the levels to be stabilized but not be so long that it impinges on other levels or that the screws enter the disk space above or below. It should be kept in mind that the superior and inferior screws will be angled 15° rostral and caudal to the plate, respectively. Care should be taken to place the plate exactly in the midline. This is particularly important when using divergent screws because if the plate is off center, the screws may not engage the vertebral body adequately. If necessary, the plate may be contoured further.

Once a plate is selected, it is placed in the plate holder (Fig. 19–9). There are two plate holders: one each for the converging and diverging plates. Each plate holder spans the

varied length of the plates (25 to 110 mm). The rigid plate-holder attachment allows for precise and controlled positioning of the plate with one hand. The surgeon's other hand is free to drill and tap through the drill sleeve and then place the screw through the plate holder (and plate) without frustration. The plate holder (with the Orion™ plate) can be positioned easily by the surgeon with one hand.

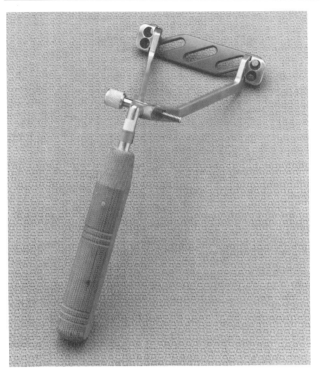

Figure 19–9. Plate held with plate holder.

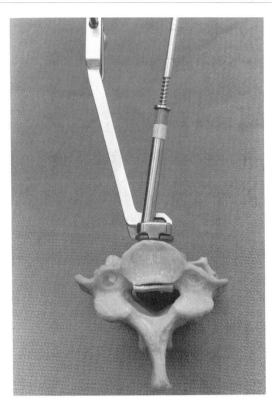

Figure 19–11. Tapping is performed through the drill-guide sleeve. Note that there is not a stop on the tap, which allows for penetration of the posterior cortex if necessary.

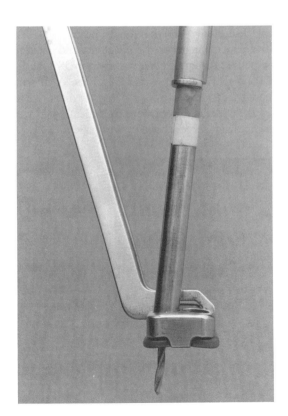

Figure 19–10. The plate is held with the plate holder and the drill sleeve is in place. Note the fixed drill stop, allowing penetration of drill bit only to 16 mm (adjustable drill stop also available, 15–29 mm).

A drill sleeve fits into the plate holder, allowing for proper angulation of the drill and bone tap and soft-tissue protection (Fig. 19–10). It is important to fit the drill sleeve snugly.

At this point, one must decide whether unicortical or bicortical screw purchase is desired. A drill with a predetermined stop at 13 mm (under the plate) may be used for unicortical screw placement. A separate drill has finely adjustable stops (depths 10 to 26 mm at 1-mm increments), and this may be used for bicortical screw placement or for placing unicortical screws other than 13 mm. Bicortical drilling should be monitored with fluoroscopy.

After drilling the hole, the bone tap is inserted through the drill sleeve, and the bone is tapped (Fig. 19–11). It is best to tap the entire length of the drilled hole. The bone tap has a protective stop to indicate the correct depth of penetration. Tapping of the posterior cortex for bicortical purchase should be performed under fluoroscopic guidance.

After drilling and tapping the hole, the screw length is measured with the depth gauge unless a standard 13-mm screw is implanted. A cancellous screw of appropriate length is inserted through the plate holder and tightened securely (Fig. 19–12). Although the screw should not be tightened fully, it must be placed securely enough that the head does not sit so high that it hampers removal of the plate holder.

A screw is placed in the hole that is diagonal from the first hole, and then the other screws are placed sequentially. The

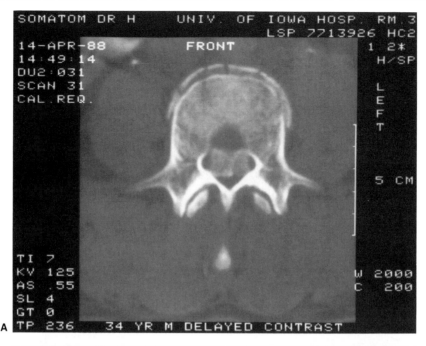

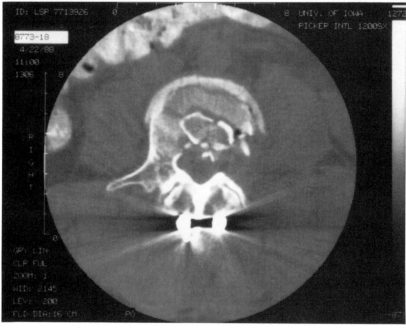

Figure 20–3.   (**A**). Burst fracture of L4 with cauda equina compression secondary to retropulsion of bone. (**B**). Lateral extracavitary approach on the more symptomatic side with decompression and ventral interbody fusion with iliac crest bone grafts.

tomy is performed at the site of suspected canal compromise for the assessment of the canal with intraoperative ultrasonography. The extent of bone removal should be minimized and the bone fragments saved to use for grafting at the end of the procedure. Once the site of maximal canal compromise has been identified, a partial facetectomy on one or both sides as necessary with partial pediculectomy as indicated is undertaken. This allows inspection of the spinal canal through a posterolateral exposure. An air drill with a

4-mm bit or equivalent is utilized to undermine the retropulsed bone fragment. Any retraction on the spinal cord must be avoided and is poorly tolerated. The retropulsed bone can usually be impacted (Redmond Impactors, Redmond, Lake Zurich, Ill) to reestablish the normal caliber of the canal (Figs. 20–2A and B). If the posterior longitudinal ligament is still intact and has not been disrupted by the fracture, this impaction of the canal can be accomplished while still preserving the integrity of that ligament. A similar decompression of the canal can also be accomplished through a costotransversectomy or lateral extracavitary approach. The latter procedure in addition to decompression can provide for eventual interbody fusion with rib or iliac crest bone[6,7] (Figs. 20–3A and B).

Once the canal has been reconstituted, the stabilization can be accomplished with correction of the spinal deformity. The process of decompression by either the transpedicular or lateral extracavitary approach provides for greater ease in the correction of the spinal deformity or angulation. Stabilization to include two levels rostral and two levels caudal to the fracture site is usually sufficient. In cases of severe angulation of 30° or more, or vertebral body collapse in excess of 50%, stabilization may be needed for three levels rostral to the site of injury.[8] An air drill or appropriate 45° rongeur is used to enlarge each interlaminar space, creating a window for the passage of the sublaminar wire. This window need not be larger than 5 to 7 mm in diameter. The underlying ligamentum flavum is incised and excised to expose the dura (Fig. 20–4). Eighteen-gauge ball-tipped Luque wires (Zimmer, Warsaw, Ind) are then bent 1 to 1¼ in from the main stem of the wire. The tip is angled to allow it to engage in the rostral interlaminar defect previously created. The wires are usually advanced from caudal to rostral with digital pressure only. The wire loops should not be forced into the epidural space but should slide gently without cross-

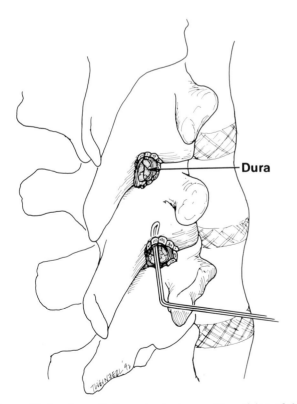

Figure 20–4. A small, 5-mm laminotomy with excision of the ligamentum flavum exposes the underlying dura, allowing the passage of the Luque wire.

ing the midline. The short end of the wire should be long enough to span the lamina and is thus longer in the lumbar than in the thoracic spine. Songer cables (Danek Medical Inc., Memphis, Tenn) may be used and are passed in the same fashion.

The necessary length of the Luque rod is then estimated by utilizing a malleable rod that should be present always in the spinal tray. An appropriate length of ¼-in L-shaped Luque rod is then cut and bent with a rod bender to conform to the normal spinal curvature. In case a ³/₁₆-in Luque rectangle of appropriate length is available, it may be used with equal efficacy.[9] The closed ends of the Luque rectangle provide rigid crossbracing, which prevents migration and rotation that can occur with the L-shaped Luque rods. The bend in the rods is concave anteriorly in the thoracic spine, S-shaped at the thoracolumbar junction, and convex anteriorly in the lumbar spine. The curvature of the Luque rod must be estimated carefully so that it will correct the angulation of the spine yet remain in contact with each lamina. The short limb of the L-shaped rod must be underneath the long limb of the contralateral rod, as shown in Figure 20–5. The long limb of each rod must be cut appropriately to avoid excessive length beyond the area of stabilization. At the level where the short limb crosses from one to the other side, this may be accomplished underneath the interspinous ligament without sacrificing the latter. The wires are then tightened around each rod using the appropriate wire twister for Luque loops (Zimmer, Warsaw, Ind). Because the laminae usually traverse in an upward direction from the spinous process to the facet joint, the wires are usually tightened such that the rostral end of the wire is medial and the caudal end of the wire lateral to the rod, as shown in Figure 20–5. Exceptions to this rule may occur at either end. All attempts should be undertaken to have the least amount of wire exposed and the rod abutting against the underlying laminae. An extra wire loop at the point of intersection of the two rods may further strengthen that junction and reduce the chances of rotation.

Having accomplished the decompression and stabilization, attention should be directed to the bone fusion in case of fracture. The transverse processes and facets are eburnated for three or more levels at the site of fracture. This can be done with rongeurs or an air drill. Once cancellous bone is exposed, the harvested bone fragments from the laminectomy or iliac crest are applied on either side, avoiding the spinal canal. The retractors on the muscles are then released and further bleeding points from the muscle coagulated. A medium-sized suction drain is brought out laterally to facilitate withdrawal postoperatively. The perforations of the drain usually span the entire length of the spinal exposure. Where the spinous processes have been removed, the muscle is usually approximated in the midline using 2-0 absorbable sutures. The same suture material is used to approximate the fascia and subcutaneous tissue. The skin may be closed with 3-0 nylon or staples. When preoperative ra-

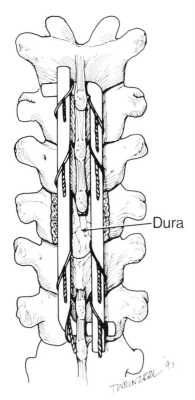

Dura

Figure 20–5. The L-shaped Luque rods in place with fixation accomplished using sublaminar wires bilaterally two levels above and two levels below the site of instability and decompression. The wires are passed lateral to the rods caudally and medial to them rostrally.

diation has been delivered in case of tumors of the spine or is anticipated postoperatively, 2-0 nonabsorbable sutures are used. To prevent postoperative discomfort while lying supine, a bulky dressing over the incision is to be avoided.

In cases of ventral spinal compression by tumor, at least one pedicle is usually involved and will dictate the side of the transpedicular approach. The pedicle may be identified by careful probing of the lateral recess after the laminectomy has been completed. The tumor-involved pedicle is usually soft and removed easily with curettes. If the pedicle is still bony, the air drill should be used to core the center, leaving a thin shell of cortical bone to protect the thecal sac. This cortical shell may then be removed with curettes to provide lateral access to the ventral canal. Stabilization is as described earlier. Bony fusions are unlikely to take due to pre- or postoperative radiation.

Postoperatively, intravenous patient-controlled analgesia is usually indicated and is well appreciated. Two or three days following surgery when the pain has subsided, the patient may be measured for thoracolumbar acrylic shells or Jewett brace. The patient is only mobilized out of bed when pain has abated and the patient is ready. It is important to monitor the patient's blood count postoperatively because a transfusion may be necessary for up to 3 days following surgery.

RESULTS

In cases of fracture, Luque rods have thus far been used in two cases of flexion compression, five of fracture dislocation, ten of burst, and one of slice distraction. Seven patients underwent a lateral extracavitary, seven a transpedicular decompression of the canal, and four underwent neither. Only one case was operated emergently. This patient with a flexion compression fracture of T7 to T8 underwent a transpedicular decompression and Luque stabilization for increasing paraparesis. Postoperatively, the patient showed gradual recovery. The rest of the cases were operated on at the earliest opportunity when medically stable. The average blood loss was estimated at 1000 cc. Eight patients required transfusion, with the average overall transfusion requirement being 1.3 units. No patient demonstrated an increase in neurological deficit following surgery. At the time of discharge, within 1 month after surgery, the postoperative angulation improved an average of 1° when compared to preoperative angulation. At a mean follow-up of 18 months, angulation had increased, however, by an average of 9°. Rod removal was performed in five patients due to discomfort from rigidity of the system and in one case due to fracture of the wires and twisting of the rods (Fig. 20–6).

In cases of tumor, most patients had disease confined to a single level and underwent one or two laminectomies, with transpedicular decompression and stabilization two levels

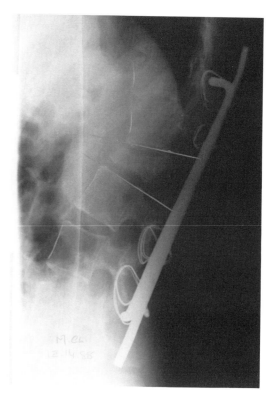

Figure 20–6. Progressive angulation at L1 secondary to wire fracture and twisting of the Luque rods. Three-level stabilization rostral to the fracture may have obviated this occurrence.

above and below the laminectomies. Six patients had improvement in neurological function postoperatively. One was worse in the immediate postoperative period. One patient had a pulmonary embolus. No other complications occurred. Because the stabilization procedure requires only modest additional dissection and operating time, patients tolerated the procedures well and could usually be mobilized within 48° after the operation. All patients received external beam radiation therapy postoperatively if they had not been treated previously. No patient developed evidence of progressive instability postoperatively. No patients required removal of the hardware.

SUMMARY

The Luque system is intended for the correction of scoliosis, and unlike early distraction devices it provides for segmental fixation. It does require the passage of sublaminar wires, which may be dangerous (particularly in the presence of a narrow, compromised canal). Furthermore, this system does not lend itself to the application of compressive or distractive forces. It lacks the rigidity required to provide and maintain a lordotic curvature to the lumbar spine. Newer, more versatile devices have obviated the need for sublaminar wires by resorting to facet or transverse process hooks that provide for compression and distraction, as the case may be. Pedicular screws with plates or rods are more effective in maintaining the necessary fixation for the lumbar spine and the normal lordotic curvature.[10]

Acknowledgments. The authors acknowledge the assistance of Susan Piper, Gatana Stoner, and Karen VanDenBosch in the collation and analysis of the data. They also thank Linda Shalla and Judy Huston for the preparation of this manuscript.

REFERENCES

1. Luque ER. The anatomic basis and development of segmental spinal instrumentation. *Spine.* 1982;7:256–259.
2. Luque ER, Cassis N, Ramirez-Wiella G. Segmental spinal instrumentation in the treatment of fractures of the thoracolumbar spine. *Spine.* 1982;7:312–317.
3. Denis F. The three column spine and its significance in the classification of acute thoracolumbar spinal injuries. *Spine.* 1983;8:817–831.
4. Panjabi MM, Thibodeau LL, Crisco JJ III, White AA III. What constitutes spinal instability. *Clin Neurosurg.* 1986;34:313–339.
5. Hardaker WT Jr, Cook WA Jr, Friedman AH, Fitch RD. Bilateral transpedicular decompression and Harrington rod stabilization in the management of severe thoracolumbar burst fractures. *Spine.* 1992;17:162–171.
6. Larson SJ, Holst RA, Hemmy DC, Sances A Jr. Lateral extracavitary approach to traumatic lesions of the thoracic and lumbar spine. *J Neurosurg.* 1976;45:628–637.
7. Maiman DJ, Sypert GW. Management of trauma of thoracolumbar junction—part II. *Contemp Neurosurg.* 1989;11:1–6.
8. Purcell GA, Markolf KL, Dawson EG. Twelfth thoracic-first lumbar vertebral mechanical stability of fractures after Harrington-rod instrumentation. *J Bone Joint Surg.* 1981;63A:71–78.
9. Panjabi MM, Abumi K, Duranceau J, Crisco JJ. Biomechanical evaluation of spinal fixation devices: II. stability provided by eight internal fixation devices. *Spine.* 1988;13:1135–1140.
10. An HS, Vaccaro A, Cotler JM, Lin S. Low lumbar burst fractures comparison among body cast, Harrington rod, Luque rod, and Steffee plate. *Spine.* 1991;16(suppl 8):S440–S444.

21 Harrington Distraction Rods for Thoracic and Lumbar Fractures

Patrick W. Hitchon, M.D.

INDICATIONS

Like most techniques of spinal instrumentation, Harrington compression and distraction rods were first developed for the treatment of scoliotic deformities of the thoracic and lumbar spine.[1] This technique was later advocated for the treatment of thoracic and lumbar fractures[2] and adopted and advocated by spinal surgeons thereafter.[3-8] The tensile forces applied by the distraction rods were ideally suited for fractures associated with loss in height, as in burst fractures or fracture dislocations (Figs. 21–1A and B). It was recognized early on that for this system to function properly, the anterior and posterior longitudinal ligament needed to be intact. The integrity of these ligaments would contribute to bony reduction and the prevention of overdistraction. The mechanism whereby the distraction rods achieved the desired ends was through the rostral caudal forces generated by the hooks and the ventral pressure applied at the kyphos generated by the rods on the neural arches. This mechanical construct consisting of a three-point fixation device[1,2,5] created the foundation for the development of future spinal implants. Through the implantation of Harrington rods, spinal surgeons were able to achieve stability of the spine, reduction of dislocations, and early mobilization of patients.

TECHNIQUES

It is generally accepted that surgical intervention in the treatment of thoracic and lumbar fractures should be undertaken at the earliest opportunity when the patient is medically stable. Emergent surgery is indicated, however, in the face of progressive neurological loss. In the face of a partial neurological deficit with an unstable fracture, it may be judicious to intubate and position the patient while still awake. This may prevent neural compression arising from positioning alone prior to decompression and stabilization. Intra-operative positioning is usually on laminectomy rolls, with the table horizontal and the knees flexed. The preparation of the operative site is usually wide and should include one iliac crest for potential harvesting of bone. An early intraoperative film will help confirm alignment and identify the ap-

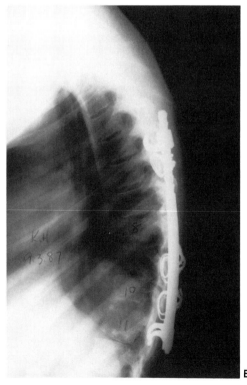

Figure 21–1. (**A**). Fracture dislocation at T7 to T8 with paraplegia. (**B**). Reduction and stabilization performed with Harrington distraction rods and sublaminar wiring from T5 to T11.

204

propriate level. The dissection is carried out laterally to include the facets and transverse processes, four levels rostral to the site of fracture, and three levels caudal. The dissection is carried out with dispatch using electrocautery while keeping the blood loss at a minimum. The surgeon and assistant are both equipped with suction, electrocautery, and bipolar coagulation. It is important to identify fractures of the neural arch to prevent further neural damage secondary to exposure. Although distraction alone may contribute to partial reduction of the neural canal,[9] the posterior longitudinal ligament is often disrupted.[10] Hence the reduction of retropulsed bone by distraction alone is only partial, and overdistraction may result.[11] It is important to expose the cord or cauda equina at the site of fracture and assess the extent of canal compromise using intraoperative ultrasonography. Where neurological deficit is partial, the neural elements must be decompressed by either a transpedicular approach[6,7] or through a costotransversectomy or extracavitary approach.[12,13] The advantages of the former are in its ability to expose the dura and repair lacerations with ease. The latter technique, on the other hand, allows the ability to perform an interbody fusion transversing the fractured vertebral body. The hockey-stick incision mandated by the extracavitary approach requires a wide lateral exposure of at least 4 in from midline. The short limb is chosen on the side of increased neurological deficit. If the posterior longitudinal ligament is found to be intact, every attempt should be taken to safeguard its integrity. Disimpaction of retropulsed bone into the vertebral body can be achieved when surgical intervention is undertaken early within the first week (Redmond Impactors, Redmond Surgical Instruments, Lake Zurich, Ill). Otherwise, the retropulsed bone must be undermined with a 4-mm air drill. The adequacy of decompression of the neural elements can be confirmed using either laryngeal mirrors or intraoperative ultrasonography.

The inferior facets of the third vertebra rostral to the fracture site are exposed and cleared of their capsule and synovium. They are amputated caudally (Fig. 21–2) to accommodate the rostral number 1253 ratchet hooks (Zimmer, Warsaw, Ind). Careful seating of the rostral hook beneath the inferior facet is mandatory to prevent fracture or splitting of the latter. Caudally, the leading edge of the lamina belonging to the second vertebra below the fracture site is prepared to accommodate the 1254 collar hook. This preparation requires enlarging the interlaminar space and excision of the ligamentum flavum with exposure of the underlying dura. The seating should be confirmed such that the blade of the hook is entirely beneath the lamina (Fig. 21–2). In vitro studies have shown that with caudal hooks inserted two levels below the site of instability, advancing the rostral hooks from two to three levels above results in a significant improvement in both threshold and bending moments of the instrumented spine.[14] The incorporation of sublaminar wiring with Harrington rods has been advocated for greater stability and contributes to earlier mobilization.[3–5,7] The interlam-

inar spaces are widened using either a Hardy 40° rongeur or an air drill. The ligamentum flavum is excised, exposing the dura through a window measuring 5 to 7 mm. Through these openings, sublaminar 18-gauge Luque loops are advanced in a rostral-caudal direction. The advancement of the wire should be gentle and performed with digital pressure alone without the need of a hemostat forcing the wire ahead. Two sublaminar wires are needed on each side rostral to the fracture site and one caudal. The placement of the hooks and passage of the wires can be performed bilaterally at this time.

Attention is then directed toward distraction for the reduction of the dislocation. This can generally be performed by a carefully contoured seven-ratchet Harrington rod; otherwise the 1248 outrigger device can be used. The appropriate length Harrington rod is contoured with the spinal rod bender such that following reduction, the rod will be in close apposition to the laminae. To facilitate engagement of the collar end into the caudal hook, the lamina of the vertebra rostral to the hook may need to be shaved with a Leksell rongeur. All bone harvested must be saved for the purpose of the bony fusion. If the 1254 hook proves too short to allow engagement of the rod, the longer-throated 1201-053 hook may be utilized. The process of distraction can be accom-

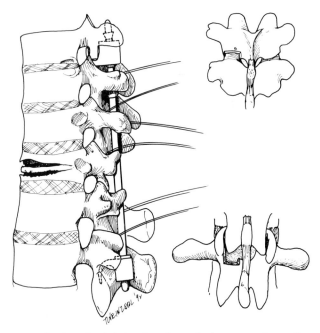

Figure 21–2. The inferior facet is notched transversely to allow for engagement of the rostral hook as shown in the upper inset on the right. The leading edge of the lamina is also notched for proper engagement of the collar-end hook, as shown in the lower inset on the right. Instrumentation should extend three levels rostral and two levels caudal to the site of instability. Stability provided by Harrington rods is further improved by the use of sublaminar wires. Wires are to be utilized wherever the laminae are intact. Caution is mandatory to prevent overdistraction.

plished easily by advancing the rostral hooks on the ratchets. This must be performed with caution to avoid overdistraction, particularly in the case of lacerated anterior and–or posterior longitudinal ligaments. Once the distraction has been accomplished and intraoperative films have confirmed the adequacy of reduction, C washers are applied beneath

the ratchet hooks. The wires are twisted down to bring the lamina in closer apposition to the rods for further correction of the deformity and stability (Fig. 21–2). Because the ratchet portion of the rods is narrower and less rigid than the smooth portion, seven ratchet rods should be used in preference to those with 13 ratchets.

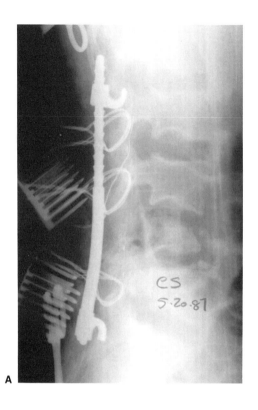

A

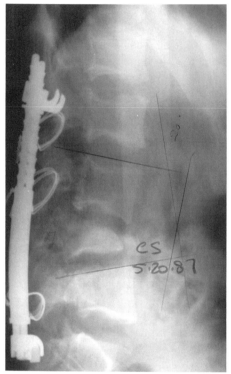

B

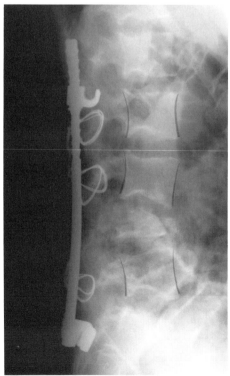

C

Figure 21–3. (**A**). Burst fracture of L4. Bilateral transpedicular decompression with Harrington rod stabilization from L1 to S1 with Harrington rods. (**B**). Postoperative mobilization to 45° reveals twisting of the Harrington rods with reversal of the lordotic curvature in spite of sublaminar wires. (**C**). Improved alignment and lordosis of the lumbar spine accomplished with square-ended Moe rods and sublaminar Andre hooks at S1.

The transverse processes and facets at the level of the fracture and one level rostral and caudal are eburnated with rongeurs or an air drill until vascular cancellous bone is exposed. Bone harvested from the decompression or the iliac crest is then laid on either side of the rods overlying the decorticated bone but not on the exposed dura. The ½-in twisted-wire stems are bent over the bone grafts for a low profile using a Schlein clamp or other instrument of personal choice. Gelfoam is applied over the exposed dura, and a medium-sized suction drain is brought out through a lateral stab wound. The muscles are approximated in the midline where the spinous processes have been removed. The fascia is closed with 2-0 absorbable sutures, and the subcutaneous tissue and skin are approximated with 3-0 absorbable and nonabsorbable sutures, respectively. A small dressing is applied to prevent discomfort to the patient when in the supine position. The patient is maintained at bed rest until the thoracolumbar shells or other orthosis are made available. Careful attention to the blood count is necessary because a transfusion may be in order 1 or 2 days postoperatively. The drain is usually removed on the second postoperative day. Passive or active exercises of the legs are mandatory to prevent deep vein thrombosis postoperatively. Intermittent pneumatic compression stockings have been recommended by some but are not accepted universally. Sequential x-rays at 45° and 90° are obtained at the time of mobilization to confirm the stability of the spine. Physical therapy and rehabilitation begin at the earliest time possible.

RESULTS

The authors have undertaken Harrington distraction instrumentation for the treatment of 30 thoracic and lumbar fractures since 1987. Sixteen of these fractures were burst, and 14 were fracture dislocations. The average blood loss during surgery was estimated at 1200 cc. The average transfusion requirements were 1.5 units. Ten of these patients did not undergo decompression due to total neurological loss. Decompression of the canal was achieved in 13 patients via the transpedicular approach and via the costotransversectomy in seven. The mean ± standard deviation (SD) angulation on admission was 17 ± 9°, and immediately following surgery the kyphotic angulation measured 10 ± 6°. At latest follow-up of a median of 18 months, angulation had increased to 15 ± 7°. This improvement in angular deformity is similar to that encountered by others.[3,5–8,13] When the correction of angular deformity is analyzed in terms of the fracture type, burst fractures had an admission angulation of 14 ± 7° and at latest follow-up measured 16 ± 8°. Fracture dislocations, on the other hand, an admission angulation of 20 ± 10°, which measured only 14 ± 6° at latest follow-up. It would appear that the angular deformity of burst fractures is not as great as that of fracture dislocations, and due to the greater maintenance of body height in the latter, the correction in angulation is sustained. These findings are again similar to those encountered in similar retrospective studies.[15]

Our patients with partial neurological deficits demonstrated improvement in neurological function following surgery. Whether this improvement exceeds that encountered in patients treated with recumbency remains controversial, particularly because the two groups are incomparable in terms of their deficits, type of fracture, residual canal, and spinal angulation. The average hospital stay of our 30 patients that underwent surgery was 37 days, only 3 days shorter than that of patients treated with recumbency. On the other hand, surgical patients were confined to bed rest for 1 week less than those treated with recumbency (26 versus 33, P = .0020).

COMPLICATIONS

Due to the tensile force that can be applied by Harrington distraction rods, it is easy to overdistract a patient with disruption of the anterior and posterior longitudinal ligaments. Careful analysis of preoperative imaging studies, including magnetic resonance imaging, is necessary to identify the fracture type and avoid this complication. Round-ended Harrington rods are incapable of maintaining lordotic curvatures in the lumbar spine in spite of sublaminar wires (Figs. 21–3A, B, and C). To achieve and maintain such a contour, square-ended Moe rods with appropriate hooks are necessary. Careful examination of the spinal canal with an intraoperative ultrasound is necessary prior to distraction in the presence of a retropulsed bony spicule or a medially displaced pedicle. Distraction under such circumstances can be harmful to the cord or roots tethered by the displaced bone. Such complications can be avoided by first decompressing the canal and then resorting to the correction of alignment. In spite of sublaminar fixation of the rods to the neural arches, dislodgement of the rostral hooks can occur in the face of major moments. This has occurred in one of our cases, necessitating the removal of the hardware because it had been over 1 year from the time of implantation. Other miscellaneous complications, including wound infection, deep-vein thrombosis, and pulmonary embolism, were also noted and comparable in incidence to those of other series.[2,3,7,11,15]

SUMMARY

The Harrington distraction device is ideally suited for fracture dislocations and burst fractures where the anterior and posterior longitudinal ligaments are intact. This device provides for the reduction of dislocations, spinal stabilization, and early mobilization. In the absence of a claw configuration, as can be obtained with newer devices, Harrington distraction rods have no compressive component. Sublaminar wires do contribute to improvement in stability yet are associated with risks involved in the passage of these wires in the face of a compromised canal. The assortment of hooks is limited, and hooks with different throat sizes for a low profile are unavailable. In spite of square-ended rods for the maintenance of lordosis in the lumbar spine, these devices have now been replaced by newer techniques using transpedicular screw and plate fixation.[16]

Acknowledgments. The authors would like to thank Susan Piper, Gatana Stoner, and Karen VanDenbosch for the collation of data.

REFERENCES

1. Harrington PR. Treatment of scoliosis. *J Bone Joint Surg.* 1962;44A:591–610.
2. Dickson JH, Harrington MD, Erwin WD. Results of reduction and stabilization of the severely fractured thoracic and lumbar spine. *J Bone Joint Surg.* 1978;60A:799–805.
3. Akbarnia BA, Fogarty JP, Tayob AA. Contoured Harrington instrumentation in the treatment of unstable spinal fractures. The effect of supplementary sublaminar wires. *Clin Orthop.* 1984;189:186–194.
4. Bryant CE, Sullivan JA. Management of thoracic and lumbar spine fractures with Harrington distraction rods supplemented with segmental wiring. *Spine.* 1983;8:532–537.
5. Cotler JM, Vernace JV, Michalski JA. The use of Harrington rods in thoracolumbar fractures. *Orthop Clin N Am.* 1986;17:87–103.
6. Flesch JR, Leider LL, Erickson DL, Chou SN, Bradford DS. Harrington instrumentation and spine fusion for unstable fractures and fracture dislocations of the thoracic and lumbar spine. *J Bone Joint Surg.* 1977;59A:143–153.
7. Hardaker WT, Cook WA, Friedman AH, Fitch RD. Bilateral transpedicular decompression and Harrington rod stabilization in the management of severe thoracolumbar burst fractures. *Spine.* 1992;17:162–171.
8. Willen J, Lindahl S, Nordwall A. Unstable thoracolumbar fractures. A comparative clinical study of conservative treatment and Harrington instrumentation. *Spine.* 1985;10:111–122.
9. Willen J, Lindahl S, Irstam L, Nordwall A. Unstable thoracolumbar fractures. A study by CT and conventional roentgenology of the reduction effect of Harrington instrumentation. *Spine.* 1984;9:214–219.
10. Willen JAG, Gaekwad UH, Kakulas BA. Burst fractures in the thoracic and lumbar spine. *Spine.* 1989;14:1316–1323.
11. McAfee PC, Bohlman HH. Complications following Harrington instrumentation for fractures of the thoracolumbar spine. *J Bone Joint Surg.* 1985;67A:672–686.
12. Larson SJ, Holst RA, Hemmy DC, Sances A Jr. Lateral extracavitary approach to traumatic lesions of the thoracic and lumbar spine. *J Neurosurg.* 1976;45:628–637.
13. Maiman DJ, Sypert GW. Management of trauma of the thoracolumbar junction—part II. *Contemp Neurosurg.* 1989;11:1–6.
14. Purcell GA, Markolf KL, Dawson EG. Twelfth thoracic-first lumbar vertebral mechanical stability of fractures after Harrington-rod instrumentation. *J Bone Joint Surg.* 1981;63A:71–78.
15. Gertzbein SD, MacMichael D, Tile M. Harrington instrumentation as a method of fixation in fractures of the spine. A critical analysis of deficiencies. *J Bone Joint Surg.* 1982;64B:526–529.
16. An HS, Vaccaro A, Cotler JM, Lin S. Low lumbar burst fractures. Comparison among body cast, Harrington rod, Luque rod, and Steffee plate. *Spine.* 1991;16(suppl 8):S440–S444.

22 Cotrel-Dubousset Instrumentation for Thoracolumbar Instability

Gregory J. Bennett, M.D.

INTRODUCTION

Cotrel-Dubousset instrumentation (CDI) is a versatile system that provides excellent fixation for the great majority of thoracolumbar instability disorders. Indications for posterior spinal stabilization with CDI include deformities, unstable fractures, tumors, and degenerative disease. The CD system was developed and used initially for spinal deformities (eg, scoliosis). Many of its design features, such as the set-screw mechanism of linkage between the hooks, screws, and rods, reflect its original intended use.[1]

COTREL-DUBOUSSET FOR SPINAL DEFORMITIES

For spinal deformities, CDI represented a significant improvement in fixation over previous instrumentation systems (eg, Harrington and Luque). Those systems have corrective capabilities, but they are different from CD. Harrington rods with laminar hooks can distract the spine and thereby treat pure axial instability (Y-axis translation). For scoliosis, the distraction rod was placed on the concavity of the curve and the spine distracted until an apparently maximal tension was reached, beyond which the spinal cord could be damaged from overdistraction. Somatosensory evoked potential (SSEP) monitoring can be helpful in preventing this complication, but distraction alone has significant other limitations when treating scoliosis.

A threaded compression rod was subsequently added to the Harrington system with hooks on the transverse processes in the thoracic spine. This enabled some additional side-to-side (coronal plane) correction, but the inferior laminar hook and transverse process hook were not used on the same spinal segment. A notched hook with the intent of pedicle fixation was also developed for the Harrington system, but because this hook was not linked rigidly to the rod, no translational or derotational forces could be applied other than Y-axis distraction. Its effect was to decrease the bulk of the hook in the relatively small thoracic spinal canal.

In contrast to Harrington instrumentation, the Luque system is more versatile and can be used to apply corrective forces to the spine in several directions simultaneously. Luque instrumentation utilizes sublaminar wires that are placed segmentally over multiple levels. The rod is then secured to the posterior laminar surface by tightening the wires and acts as a neutral splint in the spine, which eliminates motion. Tightening the wires can correct both coronal and sagittal plane deformities with great success. The system is limited, however, by the need to dissect beneath the lamina at multiple levels and pass the wires without damaging the spinal cord.

Compared to existing techniques, CDI accomplished a revolutionary change in fixation principles. By using both a transverse process and pedicle hook on the same spinal segment (Fig. 22–1), a secure grip on the spine was achieved. By rigidly linking the hooks at that segment to the spine, forces could be applied to that segment in many different directions, including distraction, compression, translation, and rotation.

For scoliosis, this provides the ability to correct rotational deformity by applying appropriate corrective forces rather than simply stretching the spine to the limits of the spinal cord distraction. Typical idiopathic thoracolumbar curves,

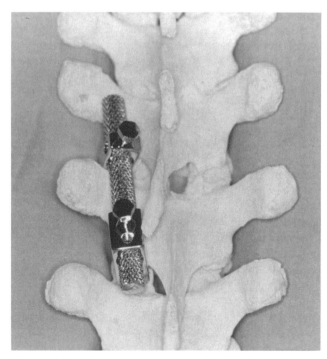

Figure 22–1. The transverse process and pedicle hook claw.

209

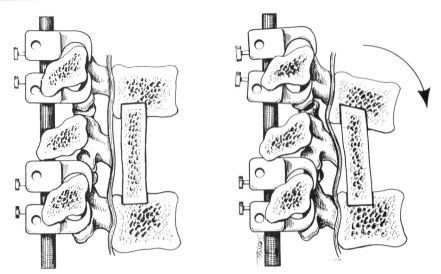

Figure 22–5. Postsurgical deformity with hook and rod construct caused by inadequate anterior graft, which is positioned posteriorly within the intervertebral space, and the limited stiffness of laminar hooks in flexion.

puterized tomographic (CT) scan with attention to the transverse diameter, which is the usual limiting dimension. Using the screws, some distraction force can be applied to the spine, which can assist in the reduction of retropulsed bone. However, the screws can be overloaded in flexion if the anterior column is still significantly weak in axial loading, resulting in screw fracture (Fig. 22–6).

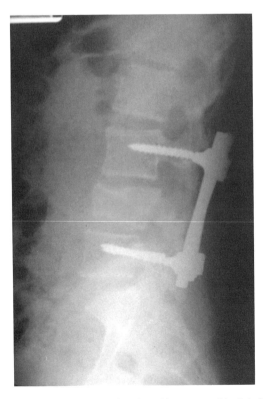

Figure 22–6. An obese female with an unstable L4 fracture treated with posterior fixation and fusion using CD noted increased back pain 3 months postoperatively. Note fractured screws in L3 and L5.

The limits of CD hook fixation when the anterior graft fails are further shown by the case of a 13-year-old female (Fig. 22–7). This patient sustained an L4 burst fracture and was in good alignment after incomplete excision of the L4 vertebral body and stabilization. She recovered neurological function but developed a painless L4 to L5 spondylolisthesis. Upon reoperation, the graft was found to be inadequately contacting the L5 level. Seventeen months after the initial surgery, the patient underwent an L4 to L5 interbody fusion with allograft and autograft; the construct was further stabilized in flexion by the addition of pedicle fixation at L5 (Figs. 22–7A through D).

Despite the complications discussed earlier, the reality of using CD for fixation of spinal trauma is that the system is generally successful and safe. It offers an excellent array of hooks for a variety of specialized anatomic sites, screw fixation, crosslinks, sacral fixation, offset linkage for lumbar pedicle screws, and recently an occpital-cervical fixation device. These numerous components can present a challenge when learning to use the system but can be helpful when dealing with variations in the normal anatomy.

COTREL-DUBOUSSET FOR TUMORS

When tumor surgery results in spinal instability, the CD system can provide fixation. In the thoracic spine, the usual surgical patient has vertebral body disease with varying degrees of kyphosis. If there is no kyphosis and the posterior elements are intact, an anterior resection using either a bone fusion alone or, in patients with a shorter life expectancy, using polymethyl methacrylate (PMMA) and Steinmann pins may provide adequate stability. If a significant kyphosis with posterior disease is also present, then posterior instrumentation should be considered for additional early spinal stability. However, previous radiotherapy does increase the incidence of wound infection, skin necrosis, and

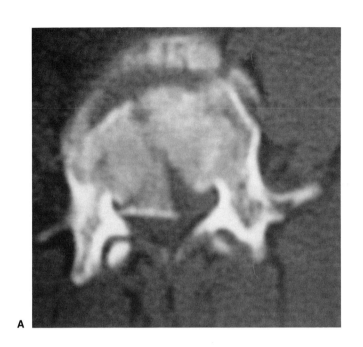

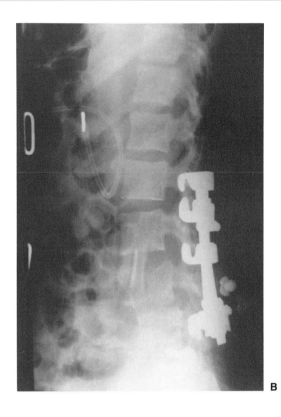

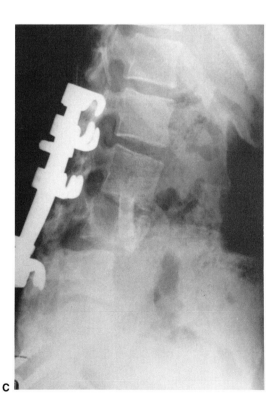

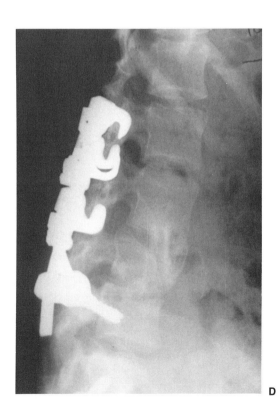

Figure 22–7. (**A**). L4 burst fracture in a 13-year-old female. (**B**). Immediate postoperative result with good spinal alignment. (**C**). L4 to L5 spondylolisthesis. (**D**). L4 to L5 interbody fusion with pedicle fixation and subsequent stability.

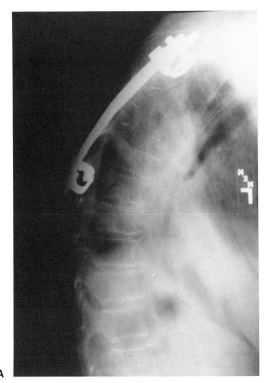

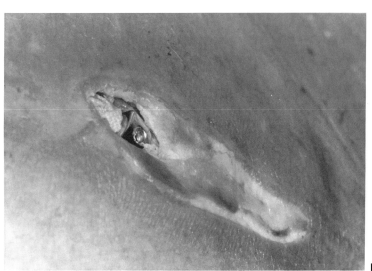

A   B

Figure 22–8. (**A**). Sixty-year-old female whose metastatic lung tumor at T4 has been resected. Note the lower hooks at the apex of the round-back kyphotic deformity. (**B**). Skin erosion over the lower hook in the same patient, radiated after surgery, now bedridden and hypercalcemic 5 months later.

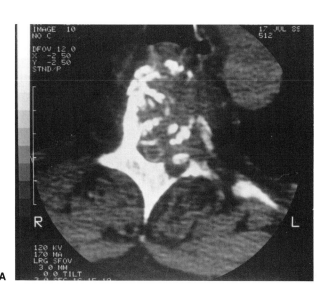

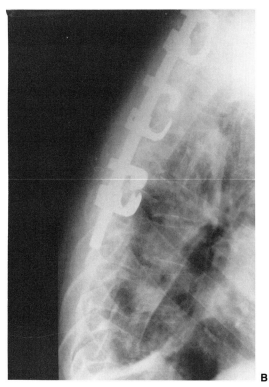

A   B

Figure 22–9. (**A**). Paraplegic 46-year-old male with a solitary lytic lesion at T4. (**B**). Note anterior intervertebral graft hooks at T1, T3, and T5 with no crosslink.

other soft-tissue complications and should be considered when treating patients with circumferential disease. In addition, patients with metastatic tumors tend to be older and more debilitated than those with unstable thoracolumbar fractures, which also increases the risk of complications. Yet surgery can be successful for patients with both metastatic and primary tumors, and CD fixation is frequently helpful.

When planning surgery for spinal tumors, the quality and quantity of the posterior soft tissues is my primary concern. In large and previously healthy individuals, the posterior approach can be identical to that used for fracture cases. In the midthoracic spine, the clawed hooks can be positioned two above and two below without difficulty. If there has been previous radiotherapy, and particularly if a significant kyphosis is also present, the hooks and crosslink must not be positioned near the apex of the kyphosis. There is a significant risk of skin erosion over the hooks when they are positioned at the kyphosis. This area is the posterior contact point when the patient is supine and, as shown in Figure 22–8B, the skin may not sustain the direct pressure.

The rod should be applied with direct contact to the lamina, which keeps it within tissues where it will not erode the skin. In elderly female patients, frequently there is a stiff "round-back" deformity. In these cases, the deformity need not be corrected, and the rod should simply follow the curve and attach at hooks positioned further caudally. An angular kyphotic deformity over a short segment is unstable, and when associated with a pathologic vertebral body fracture the kyphosis should be corrected if possible after an anterior decompression. The CD system permits the use of many posterior hooks, which should be used for distributing the three-point loads applied to correct thoracic kyphosis.

A large, otherwise healthy 46-year-old male with a solitary lytic lesion at T4 is shown in Figure 22–9. He was completely paraplegic but retained partial posterior column function. He underwent a combined vertebrectomy for solitary plasmacytoma using a lateral approach and posterior CD stabilization, resulting in complete neurological recovery and fusion. His hook position at T1 and T3 above and T5 below was well tolerated but imbalanced vertically. In addition, the construct lacked crosslinks. His ultimately successful fusion may be explained by the high intrinsic stability of the thoracic spine and his relatively young age and good health associated with rapid incorporation of the graft and the large size and anterior position of the graft. Nevertheless, a better construct would have extended to T6 and included a crosslink.

COTREL-DUBOUSSET COMPONENTS AND ASSEMBLY

CDI has a variety of components that can make the assembly of a construct easier and less traumatic for both the surgeon and the patient. In the upper thoracic spine, the T1 and T2 transverse processes originate more laterally than the lower levels. For the patient in Figure 22–9, the rod was con-

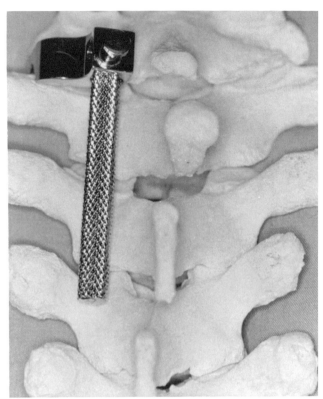

Figure 22–10. The offset lumbar laminar hook (number 84148L and R, Stuart Inc., Greensboro, Pa) provides fixation above the T1 or T2 transverse process without rod contouring.

toured laterally and hooks with longer blades compensated partially. Threading the contoured CD rod through closed hooks is the most difficult part of the assembly of the instrumentation, and any technique of preparation of the hook site or use of a specialized hook with a better fit facilitates the surgical procedure. The offset lumbar hook (Fig. 22–10) is frequently helpful when used as a transverse process hook at T1 or T2. The pedicle hook at T1 should be used cautiously because of the large size and neurological significance of the T1 root in the arm. If the hook is somewhat ventral in the foramen, it may damage the T1 nerve root, resulting in neurological symptoms.

In the lumbar spine, the narrow-blade lumbar laminar hooks can be helpful (Figs. 22–11A and B). The narrow-blade hook is useful in smaller individuals when the lumbar canal is too small to accommodate the conventional lumbar laminar hook (Fig. 22–11C). Forcing the large hook in bilaterally will lessen the contact between both hooks and the adjacent lamina and may result in severe iatrogenic stenosis as the hooks overlap at the midline. The high-profile lumbar laminar hook (Fig. 22–11B) is helpful as the superior laminar hook at L3, L4, and L5, particularly when there is a prominent lumbar lordosis. In this instance, the rod must be angled acutely between the superior and inferior hooks to run parallel with the laminar surface and fit the entry site of the closed hook and to permit the blocker to enter the open hook. The angulation of the rod is lessened or eliminated by

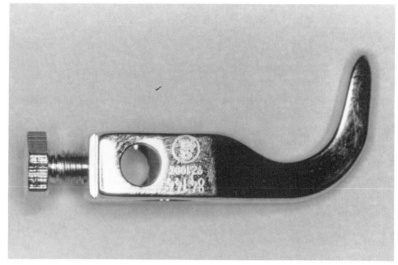

A

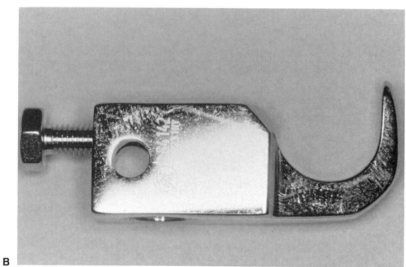

B

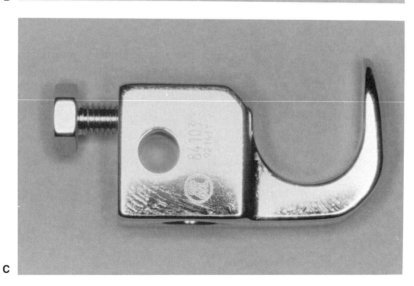

C

Figure 22–11.   (**A**). Narrow blade lumbar laminar hook (number 84144, Stuart Inc., Greensboro, Pa). (**B**). High-profile lumbar laminar hook (number 84142, Stuart Inc., Greensboro, Pa). (**C**). Conventional lumbar laminar hook (number 84103, Stuart Inc., Greensboro, Pa).

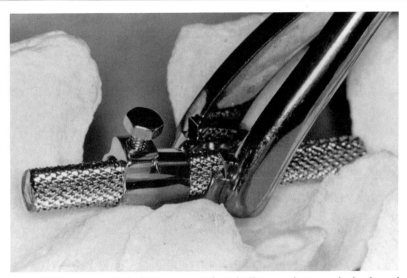

Figure 22–12.   The open hook shown can help compensate for misalignment between the hooks and rod. The blocker is used to secure the rod into the hook.

using the high-profile hook, which brings the rod up to the level of the inferior hook.

The open lumbar laminar hook and open pedicle hook are sometimes easier to align with the rod using the wider body of the hook and top entry to offset misalignment when applying corrective forces. The blocker can then secure the assembled claw, which is compressed for maximum fixation (Fig. 22–12).

SUMMARY

The CD system has many advantages for thoracolumbar stabilization, including the transverse process and pedicle hook claw, varied hook configurations for specialized anatomic situations, and linkage with pedicle screw fixation. The CD system has a stiff and precise assembly that requires that anatomic constraints be considered carefully during the exposure of hook sites and the alignment and orientation of the components. For appropriate patients, the CD system provides excellent posterior fixation.

REFERENCE

1. Cotrel Y, Dubousset J, Guillaumat M. New universal instrumentation in spinal surgery. *Clin Orthop.* 1988;227:10.

23 ISOLA Instrumentation

Eric Flores, M.D., Setti S. Rengachary, M.D., Patrick W. Hitchon, M.D.

HISTORY AND DEVELOPMENT

Initial efforts at spinal fusion and subsequent instrumentation had their origins in 1891 with the use of cervical interspinous wiring for Pott's disease.[1] Subsequently in 1911, Hibbs[2] split the spinous processes, whereas Albee[3] used tibial bone grafts for posterior spinal fusions in Pott's disease. The invention by Harrington in the 1950s of a rod and hook system to stabilize instantaneously the scoliotic deformities of the spine resulting from poliomyelitis represented a major breakthrough in the annals of spinal surgery.[4–6] The initial system consisted of rods threaded through sublaminar hooks positioned at the vertebra at the ends of the deformity. Positioning of the hooks allowed for both distraction and compression forces to be applied for the correction of scoliotic curves (thus the conception of dynamic correction of spinal deformity). With increasing experience with this system, substantial incidences of failures of the construct were observed. These consisted of failure to correct the original deformity, high rate of rod breakage (specifically at the ratchet-rod junction), and hook pullout from osseous failure either from fractures or osteoporosis. From the initial failures of this construct, it became evident that spinal fusion in conjunction with dynamic correction of deformity was necessary to maintain the spine in the reduced position. Multiple revisions to the Harrington system included strengthening of the rod components and redesigning the hooks to reduce the incidence of hook disengagement and to allow the hooks to fit better the contours of the laminae.[7] The evolution of a notched hook occurred as an adaptation to allow engagement of the pedicle. Multiple hook constructs were also used as a means of diffusing the stress among several hooks to lessen the chances of hook failure.[8]

The concept of segmental fixation was forwarded by Fritz Lang in 1910 with wiring of the spinous processes to a rod for the correction of kyphotic deformities due to Pott's disease.[9] Luque achieved spinal fixation at multiple levels by developing a technique employing sublaminar wires at multiple levels anchored to L-shaped rods.[10] Multiple fixation points allow for corrective forces to be distributed widely among the elements of the construct, providing for good correction of spinal deformity, increasing axial rigidity, and reducing the incidence of construct failure. Luque was likewise able to achieve a high rate of fusion with this construct.[11] Sequential rod application and wire tightening

of the convex side of the scoliosis followed by an opposite sequence of the concave side were used for curve correction. In 1982, Allen and Ferguson[12] described the Galveston technique of extending the construct into the pelvis by driving a segment of transversely angulated rods through the ilium for lumbo-sacral fixation. Panjabi,[13] using a thoracolumbar model, showed that the Luque system was biomechanically more stable through flexion, extension, and lateral bending compared to the Harrington system. Various ways of combining the advantages of the Luque and Harrington systems have been devised, such as the combination of multilevel sublaminar wire fixation with Harrington rods.[14] Significant neurological complications from improper technique in the application of sublaminar wires have been reported.[15] Likewise, reports of paraparesis have arisen from multiple sublaminar wire fixation in spines with marginal lumens, usually in the context of a kyphotic thoracic deformity.

The anatomy of the pedicle as a bridge between the posterior spinal elements and the vertebral body had been a point of interest in the 1950s, when Boucher in 1959[16] reported the initial use of a screw passed through the lamina and pedicle and anchored into the vertebral body. Thereafter several authors, including Wiltse, Kostuik, Roy-Camille, Harrington, and Steffee, reported on pedicle screw-rod and pedicle screw-plate constructs mostly for short-segment lower thoracic and lumbar spine fixation.

The introduction of a hook or screw and rod construct by Cotrel and Dubousset (CD system) in 1984 allowed for multilevel fixation and the application of multiple corrective forces on the rods while reducing the risk of spinal cord compromise intrinsic to sublaminar wiring.[17] The CD system incorporates a knurled rod, which affords a more stable hook and screw interface and helps prevent rod rotation. Hooks in this system are designed for laminar, pedicle, or transverse process fixation with which distraction or compression along the length of the rods can be applied. A stable rod-hook or rod-screw interface is accomplished with a bolt either through the body of the closed hooks or through a blocker in the case of open hooks. Biomechanically, Farcy (using a two-level CD hook and rod construct) demonstrated four to five times greater axial stability than the Harrington system; Farcy showed that the CD system was far more resistant to torsional stress than either the Luque or the Harrington systems.[18] Likewise, Gurr showed similar advantages of CD instrumentation.[19] The Scoliosis Research

Society reported in 1988 after 1-year follow-up of CD instrumentation an incidence of 0.2% for major neurological deficits, 1.7% for minor neurological deficits, an implant failure of 2.2%, and a 3.1% rate of reoperation. Aside from hardware failure, other complications arose from osseous failure likely due to stress generated by a relatively rigid system.

With further development along the principles of the Cotrel-Dubousset system, a universal spinal instrumentation system (ie, one that could be applied for the correction and stabilization at any spinal level and for any spine pathology) was developed at the Texas Scottish Rite Hospital (TSRH).[20] Virtually simultaneously the ISOLA system was developed by Asher and associates. In the TSRH system, a set of hook-rod and screw-rod constructs of various lengths was devised for multisegmental fixation as well as for the application of dynamic corrective forces. Vertebral anchoring devices are composed of contoured laminar hooks, notched pedicle hooks, transverse process hooks, and "fracture" hooks with narrow shoes and pedicle screws. These are attached to smooth rods by top- or side-loading eyebolts. Variable angle eyebolts, multispan topped, and half-topped hooks further increase the versatility of this system. Crosslinks between parallel segments of rods are integral to this system and add torsional rigidity to the construct. Screws with cancellous threads allow this system to be used for anterior fixation as well, although it may not be as rigid as other implants specifically devised for anterior fixation. Improvements in design and component composition provide some biomechanical advantages over other systems' components. Magnetic resonance imaging (MRI) of the spine is now possible with the recent addition of titanium alloy components. Lower-profile components for pediatric spine fixation are also available.

THE ISOLA SYSTEM

The ISOLA system (ACROMED Corporation, Cleveland, Ohio) draws its name from the butterfly species *Isola*, denoting its origins as a butterfly-shaped sacral fixation system that, with further development, evolved into a system of implants for reduction of deformity and/or stabilization at any level of the thoracic, lumbar, or sacral spine.[21] The design of the system is based on Harrington's principles of understanding the anatomy of the deformity and of maintaining the balance of the spine. The approach to correction of deformities adheres to the concept of a three-dimensional analysis of the deformity for 6 degrees of freedom of motion. Asher and associates[21] define the goals of the ISOLA system briefly as correcting constrictive, translational, or angular spine deformity; maximizing access to anchoring sites and allowing the use of supplemental devices necessary for the management of deformity; minimizing or obviating the need for external supports by providing adequate construct rigidity; and preserving motion segments.

The indications for the ISOLA system, not unlike other systems of spine instrumentation, are (1) to address the basic issues of spinal deformity either congenital or secondary to pathologic spine processes; and (2) to correct spinal instability resulting from pathologic processes or previous surgery. It is designed as a posterior spinal instrumentation system composed of anchors (screws, hooks, and wires) that are attached to smooth longitudinal members by a versatile anchor-to-rod connector system for instrumentation along the thoracic vertebrae to the sacrum. Hook anchors replace screws when the latter cannot be used due to size, fracture, or disease. ISOLA is compatible with the variable screw placement (VSP) system and the use of Steffee plates.

IMPLANTS

ISOLA implants are divided into four major categories: anchor, longitudinal members, connectors, and accessories. A brief description of each category follows.

Anchors

The most commonly used anchors are bone screws, hooks, and wires.

BONE SCREWS

Bone screws are approved by the Food and Drug Administration (FDA) for implantation in the sacrum or ilium. Approval for transpedicular usage is pending, but most spine surgeons use bone screws in the pedicle if such an application is in the best interest of the patient. ISOLA screws are the same as those used with the VSP system (Fig. 23–1). These pedicle screws have a bolt-type structure and share biomechanical properties with the ISOLA sacral and iliac screws. These screws have a 7.0 mm standard outer diameter, with 6.25-mm and 5.55-mm diameters also available. The cancellous threaded portion ranges from 25 to 50 mm at 5-mm increments, with 16 mm, 19 mm, or 30 mm for the machine-threaded portion. These screws are used with the ISOLA slotted connectors for rod attachment. Variability in the sagittal displacement of the rod construct is possible with the use of washers. A hex nut holds the slotted connectors on the threaded portion of the screw.

Iliac screws are designed for placement between the iliac cortices as anchors. Special rods with eyes slip over the threaded portion of these iliac screws and can be fixed in place with a washer and an 8.0-mm ($\frac{5}{16}$-in) hex nut. These screws come in 80-mm and 100-mm lengths with 6.25-mm and 7.0-mm diameters, respectively. Sacral screws for S1 and S2 fixation come in 30- to 40-mm sizes in increments of 5 mm and a uniform diameter of 8.5 mm. These screws are to be used with a special 8.5-mm tap, which one must remember not to use for tapping the pedicles. Sacral screws have a 23-mm machine-thread-length connector segment. Both iliac and sacral screws have a bolt-type construction (ie, the rod is sandwiched between an integral nut and the hex nut used for tightening, allowing for the containment of

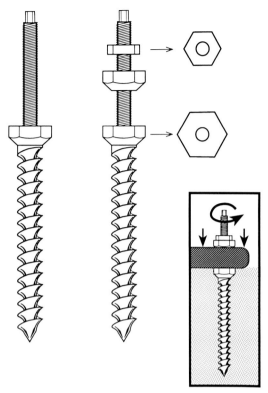

Figure 23–1. Pedicle screw. Note the lower integral hex nut, the upper hex nut that threads on the machine-threaded part of the screw, and the locking nut. Inset: Bolt construct showing the plate sandwiched securely between the two hex nuts. The bolt-type construct is mechanically more rigid and stable than the conventional screw.

translational forces within the implant component and avoiding force transmission to the bony pelvis). The bolt-type connector system has been biomechanically designed to eliminate the claw hammer pullout effect on the screw, and it decreases shearing of the screw threads on the osseous surface. The tapered thread root also improves pullout resistance and resistance to bending fatigue.

HOOKS

Drop-entry or closed-body hooks (Fig. 23–2) are available for anchoring to the laminae or the transverse processes. Drop-entry hooks are available in four hook heights with a shortened body and sublaminar blade to minimize canal impingement. Holes on the hook body are designed to mate with the rod diameters of 6.35 mm ($\frac{1}{4}$ in) and 4.76 mm ($\frac{3}{16}$ in). Hook throat sizes for 6.35-mm rods are 6.5 mm, 8 mm, 9.5 mm, and 11 mm. For the 4.76-mm rod 5-mm, 6.5-mm, 8.0-mm, and 9.5-mm hook throat sizes are available. Hooks with larger throat sizes (9.5 or 11 mm) are used for anchoring transverse processes, and smaller throat sizes (6.5 or 8 mm) are used for placement under the lamina. No hooks are specifically designated as pedicular hooks. There has been some debate on whether the forked ends of a pedicular hook in other systems actually encircle the pedicle without having to remove enough lamina, which in itself

may weaken the construct. Insertion of the drop-entry hook in the sublaminar or transverse process position can be accomplished with the hooks already threaded onto the rods. Alternatively, closed-end hooks may be placed at one end of the construct over transverse processes or under the lamina and the contoured rod may be entered into them.

Drop-entry hooks incorporate an oval-shaped rod hole that is slightly larger at one end than the other such that when loose on the rod, it rests at 15° to the axis of the rod. The hook is tightened on the rod with a 6.35-mm set screw that, when tightened, will cause the hook to rest at 5° to the rod. This system allows the placement of multiple closed-end hooks with the hooks already threaded on the rod, minimizing the use of open-body hooks. In addition, tightening the set screw on the closed hook causes the hook blade to grip the undersurface of the laminae better, thus achieving tighter hook-osseous interface. The hook-rod interface with the ISOLA system incorporates a V-groove hollow ground (VHG) design (Fig. 23–3). The rod hole on the body of the hook incorporates a groove corresponding in diameter to the diameter of the rods. With tightening of the set screw, the rod is driven against the edges of this groove at the waistline of the rods, thus increasing the surface and the force with which the hook grips the rod. The increased stability of the rod on the groove of the hook body also allows for lesser hook-rod motion and thereby less chances of loosening of the set screw. Tests of axial and torsional gripping strength of the VHG connection increase rapidly even at low set-screw torques. Set-screw torques at 6.8 Nm (60 in/lb) are recommended. It is important to note that this hook-rod interface can be maintained only when the rod size corresponds to the hook hole size. When the construct is viewed axially, light should be able to pass between the rod and the

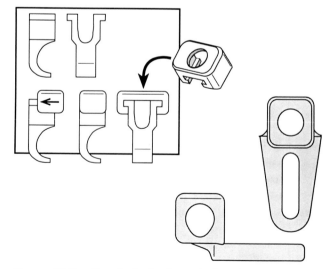

Figure 23–2. Open-body hooks and slotted connectors. The open-body hook is in two parts: the hook and the cap. The cap slides only in one direction (indicated by arrow). When the cap is in place, it is difficult to slide it off manually, except with a specially designed cap remover. The open-body hook, when capped, has virtually the same biomechanical properties as the closed hook.

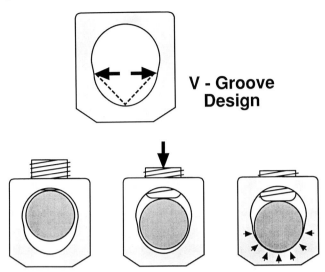

V - Groove Design

Figure 23–3. V-groove hollow ground (VHG) design. The hole for the rod is in two dimensions. When the rod is slid through the closed-body hooks, the rod glides easily in the upper roomier part of the hole. Once the rod is placed optimally, it is driven down into the snug-fitting lower half of the hole. This increases the area of contact of the rod and increases the biomechanical stability of the construct.

depth of the groove. In addition, applying the hook on a highly curved portion of the rod should be avoided because this may interfere with the strength of the hook-rod interface.

Open-body or top-entry hooks allow fixation of the hooks on the laminae or the transverse processes prior to positioning the rod. Once the rods are seated properly on the hooks, the gap at the top of the body of the hooks is closed with a cap whose grooves slip over the hook bodies and is fixed in place by a 6.35-mm set screw. The cap can be slid only in one direction as indicated by arrows on the top of the cap. Throat size and configuration are similar to those of the closed hooks.

WIRES

Sixteen-gauge wires are available for sublaminar or spinous process multisegmental fixation usually used for scoliosis and other spine deformity correction. Wires are provided as double-performed, double-with-button, and single-strand beaded wire. One may use multistranded braided cables with crimp instead of monofilamentous wires.

Longitudinal Members

ISOLA rods are smooth and can be contoured as necessary. Rods with eyes at one end are provided for iliac screw fixation. Rod diameters are 4.76 mm ($\frac{3}{16}$ in) and 6.35 mm ($\frac{1}{4}$ in) at a standard length of 46 cm (18 in). Sixty-one-centimeter (24-in) rods are available upon request. Rods can be cut to size and the remaining rod used at another time. Smooth rods were chosen for this system due to the biomechanical advantages of increased bending rigidity and strength as well as better resistance to fatigue compared to rods with

threads, knurls, or rachets. A set of six rod and plate benders, including two in situ benders, is part of the ISOLA set for angulation of the rods at almost any radius in three dimensions.

Connectors

SLOTTED CONNECTORS

Closed slotted connectors (Fig. 23–2) bridge the longitudinal construct members to the screw anchors. As in the hooks, the VHG design is used in the rod-connector interface. Connectors are slipped on the rods prior to rod fixation and are secured to the rod with a set screw. The slotted ends of the connectors are attached to the threaded portion of the screws and fixed in place by a hex nut. This allows a stable, user-friendly rod-connector-screw system that can conform to the three-dimensional morphological requirement of the construct. Connector sizes correspond to rod diameters (ie, 6.35 mm and 4.76 mm). The slotted connector blades are straight or angled 20° (to avoid the sacral alae) relative to the body of the connector and are available in the standard 16-mm length or the extended 24-mm length.

SPLIT CONNECTORS

These function like the closed connectors but can be applied at any time. Split connectors are composed of two unthreaded jaws gripping the rod with a VHG design and are squeezed and held together by an 8-mm hex nut torqued to a recommended 7.3 Nm (65 in/lb). Biomechanically, the split connectors have significantly less axial and torsional loosening strengths compared to the closed connectors and thus are not recommended for withstanding flexion-extension loads, especially in the absence of load sharing.

TRANSVERSE ROD CONNECTORS

Transverse rod connectors[22] (Fig. 23–4) are composed of two sets of split connector jaws with jaw diameters of 4.76 mm and 6.36 mm corresponding to the respective rod diameter. These split jaws are connected with a 4.76-mm 10-cm-long threaded rod and fixed in place by 8.0-mm ($\frac{5}{16}$ in) hex nuts on the lateral (external) or medial end of the transverse rod construct, depending on the span between the rods. Biomechanically, the bending moment of the transverse rod construct can be strengthened by threading nuts or stacking nuts on both sides of each pair of split connector jaws.

DUAL (BYPASS) CONNECTORS

Dual connectors allow side-to-side, rod-to-rod, or rod-to-plate connections. These connectors make it possible to splice broken rods or to connect two rod systems. Dual bypass connectors are composed of half of a threaded transverse connector rod, through which a dual connector jaw has been threaded, and the corresponding halves of a transverse connector jaw mated to each side of the dual connector jaw.

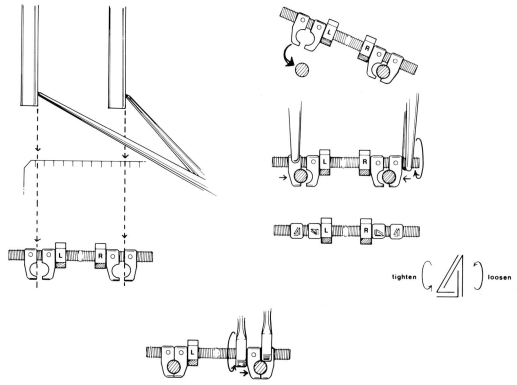

Figure 23–4.   Transverse rod connectors and the step-by-step technique of applying it.

Dual connector jaws come in three bore sizes, making it possible to connect any combination of rod sizes. Dual connectors should be used in pairs and are tightened with hex nuts.

TANDEM CONNECTORS

Tandem connectors are used to connect rods end to end. Three different sizes are available to allow connection of any combination of rod diameters.

Accessories

Washers are used as spacers to increase the dorsal height of a construct, to avoid contact with osseous structures, and to provide more space under the rods for bone grafts. When plates are used, washers strengthen the connection between plates and screws. Washers have 11-mm outer diameters and are either 3 mm or 5 mm in height. A washer with a 12.7-mm diameter and a 15° angulation is available for providing angular adjustments when using the sacral screws. Set screws used with the VHG system of connectors are 6.35 mm in diameter.

TECHNIQUES OF IMPLANTATION

Spinal instrumentation is carried out under appropriate general anesthesia. Muscle relaxation that does not abolish muscle reflexes accompanying nerve root irritation is preferred. Provisions to do a wake-up test and/or test for spinal reflexes during the procedure influence the choice of anesthetic tech-

nique and should be discussed preoperatively with the anesthesiology team. Because spinal instrumentation entails a certain degree of blood loss, preparations should be made for blood replacement such as antecedent autologous blood donations and the use of cell savers. Perioperative erythropoietin is also being utilized to minimize the need for blood transfusion. Hypotensive anesthetic techniques for the purpose of minimizing blood loss are favored by some but run the risk of complications in those who have some potential for vascular or cardiac compromise.

The patient is positioned prone on rolls, posts, or a spine frame. Some extension of the hip is recommended to approximate normal sagittal alignment. A spine radiograph, in anteroposterior and lateral views, helps determine alignment of the vertebral elements prior to fusion. Radiographic equipment for intraoperative studies should be placed after positioning the patient, and details of draping these items should be addressed. Antibiotic prophylaxis is suggested due to the length and extent of the instrumentation procedure. Careful handling of tissue and the avoidance of tissue devascularization, especially with the prolonged use of self-retaining retractor systems in conjunction with copious irrigation and debridement of dead tissue, are steps that prevent microorganisms from seeding the operative site. Neurological status can be monitored by somatosensory or motor evoked potentials, wake-up tests, and testing for clonus. Muscle activity related to the irritation of nerve roots is also helpful, particularly when in the foraminal area or during insertion of pedicle screws or dissection around the transverse processes.

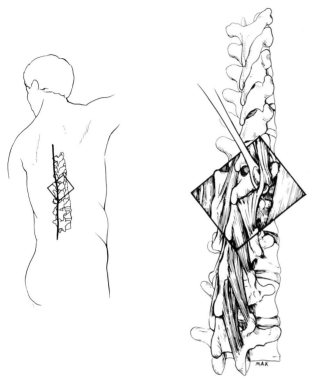

Figure 23–5. Exposure of the spine through midline incision. The paraspinal muscles are separated from the spinous processes, laminae, and transverse processes.

The spine is most commonly exposed through a midline incision (Fig. 23–5), although on occasion a paramedian incision may do as well. A generous incision to allow retraction of the soft tissue for access to the transverse processes is needed particularly in patients with thick layers of subcutaneous tissue. Dissection along tissue planes to expose the spine is then carried out with attention to hemostasis. Soft tissue and ligaments adherent to the bony surfaces, particularly those involved with arthrodesis, can be scaped off with curettes or rongeurs. In the preparation of the bony surfaces, care should be observed to preserve articular facets and capsules adjacent to the instrumented segments to minimize spine destabilization consequent to the procedure. Careful preservation of the elements of the motion segments above and below the instrumented levels is important during exposure. Decompressive spinal procedures can either be done before or after instrumentation depending on the extent of destabilization that may be entailed. Preoperative planning is necessary to avoid the apparent technical difficulties with decompression once implants are in place (particularly rods or plates overlying the laminae and pedicle screws).

The choice of construct with the ISOLA system depends on the level of the spine one is dealing with. In the high- and midthoracic regions, hooks are utilized as primary anchors. The hook sites are prepared initially. An 11-mm throat size hook is placed on the superior border of the transverse process and the second superiorly directed 8-mm hook under the lamina and facet. For proper placement of this hook, a part of the inferior articular process is removed with

a ¼-in osteotome (Fig. 23–6). The claw construct may include the transverse process and lamina of the same vertebra (intrasegmental claw) or of adjacent vertebrae (intersegmental claw). Staggering of the hooks on the vertebrae is helpful in minimizing stress on the posterior pillar of a given vertebrae. After creating the claw construct for two or three segments above and two segments below the site of instability, the required rod length is determined with a silk suture held on hemostats. The appropriate-diameter rod is then cut to the appropriate length using the tabletop ISOLA rod cutter. The rod is then contoured appropriately, not just to match but actually to correct the deformity when it is secured in place. Most prefer closed hooks at the ends of the construct or the upper half of the construct. The rod is then threaded through the closed hooks and laid on the surface of open hooks. The claws are temporarily approximated over the rod so that they will not dislodge from their anchoring sites. The caps for the open-ended hooks are then applied, and thus all the hooks and rods are in place. The rod is ready to be secured after applying appropriate distraction or compression of the construct as the clinical situation demands (Fig. 23–7). Generally one end of the rod is secured first with set screws. Using appropriate-sized rod holders and distractor, the hook immediately above the area of instability is distracted, secured with set screw, and the claw is compressed and secured as well. This process is repeated start-

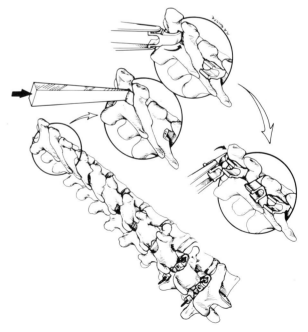

Figure 23–6. Technique of preparation of a claw construct: The lower end of the inferior articular facet and the lateral part of lamina is removed with a ¼-in straight osteotome. The laminar hook starter is then passed into the facet joint toward the pedicle. The hook (open or closed) is then grasped with a hook holder and wedged into the facet joint. Firm tapping with a hook driver may be necessary. Likewise, the soft tissues from the transverse process is separated with a transverse process hook starter and a hook is placed over the top of the transverse process. The two hooks together constitute a claw.

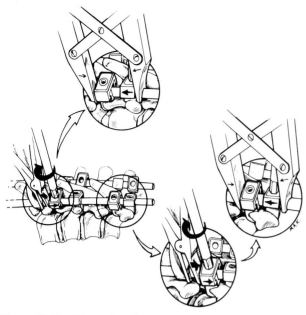

Figure 23–7.   Distraction of the construct and compression of the claw. The long-set screw wrench is used to tighten the set screws after these maneuvers.

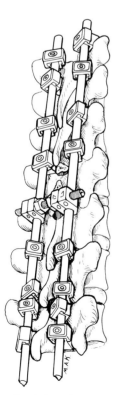

Figure 23–8.   A completed thoracic construct utilizing multiple transverse process laminar claws. Note the transverse connector in the middle of the construct.

ing at the site of deformity and moving cranialward. Hooks and rods are seated appropriately on the opposite site. Crosslinks are then placed ideally at the cranial and caudal ends of the construct (Fig. 23–8). If the construct is not sufficiently long, a single transverse connector at the middle of the construct may suffice. The cortical bone over the spinous processes, laminae, and transverse processes is eburnated using a high-speed drill, and autologous cortical cancellous bone is packed over these areas. It cannot be emphasized enough that one depends on solid bony fusion for long-term stabilization, not on hardware alone.

For the thoracolumbar region, a hybrid construct is generally utilized, with claws as anchors in the thoracic area and pedicle screws as anchors for the lumbar areas (Fig. 23–9). The rod is anchored to the pedicle screws either through slotted connectors or split connectors. For lumbar applications, pedicle screws are utilized exclusively as anchors.

Sublaminar wires provide better dorsal rigidity than hooks and better resist flexion (sagittal) moments. Although they provide some strength against translation in the coronal plane, wires do not add much to axial rigidity compared to hooks. Sublaminar wire fixation in the past has been associated with some morbidity, likely arising from the wire-passage technique as well as subsequent kyphotic deformity. Recent experience with sublaminar wires emphasizing patient selection and attention to technique has resulted in lower morbidity.

For sublaminar wire passage, the laminae must be cleared of soft tissue. In addition, the ligamentum flavum is excised, exposing the epidural fat and vessels. Excision of a small part of the edge of the lamina may be needed to allow unobstructed passage of the wire under the lamina. The soft tissue on the undersurface of the lamina is then carefully lifted off the bony surface, usually with Penfield dissectors or another similar curved, narrow, blunt-bladed instrument. Hemostasis of any violated epidural vein is carried out, which often improves the sublaminar exposure. Wire pas-

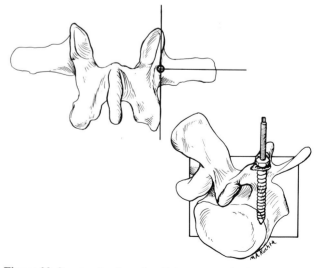

Figure 23–9.   Application of pedicle screw to the lumbar spine.

sage is usually done before the longitudinal members of the construct are applied. Double wire is biomechanically stronger than single wire, except when wire passage occurs after rod fixation (wherein a single strand is recommended). After the creation of a passage underneath the lamina, a semicircular arc of the desired radius is formed at the end of the wire loop. The wire is usually passed from a caudal to cranial direction so that the caudal end eventually lies lateral to the rod with the cranial end medial to the rod. When sublaminar wires are passed with the rods already in place, a single wire is used, usually passing the wire medial to the rod caudally, with wire exit cranially lateral to the rod. The wire is passed carefully under the lamina by following the arc of the wire such that the wire hugs the undersurface of the lamina at all times. The leading end of the wire is retrieved at the superior edge of the lamina with the help of a blunt nerve hook and carefully pulled out of the interspace by a hemostat or wire holder while constantly maintaining upward tension on the wire. The wire is then crimped tightly against the bony surface of the lamina to prevent the migration of the loose intracanalicular portion into the spinal cord. Wire passage through a hole drilled at the base of the spinous processes may also be done for constructs when a dorsally directed moment is desired.

Pedicle screw fixation with the ISOLA system is accomplished with the use of lumbar and S1 pedicular screws from the VSP system (Fig. 23–9). After exposure of the lamina, dissection is carried laterally to the dorsal aspects of the transverse processes. The facet capsule and the intertransverse-process soft tissue dorsal to the intertransverse ligament are excised. The bony landmark for pedicular screw insertion—the mamaillary process at the junction of the lamina, the transverse process, and the superior articular facet—is identified.

Evaluation of intraoperative radiographs and axial cut computed tomography (CT) scans is helpful in determining the axial and sagittal angulations necessary to cannulate the pedicle. The direction of the probe varies with the vertebral level and may further vary with existing deformities. Decisions regarding the direction of the screw, either straight down parallel to the sagittal axis of the pedicle or angulated ventromedially into the medial vertebral body, influence the entry point of the screw. Biomechanically, the anteromedially directed screw has a better pullout strength. A small bite with the rongeurs is made to decorticate the area over the entry point. A 3-0 straight curette or VSP pedicle probe is used to create a tract through the pedicle. Radiographic guidance with a C-arm image intensifier or similar means may be employed to view the pedicle and to monitor the advancement of the probe. The probe or "gear shift" is advanced carefully under proprioceptive control, ensuring that the tract remains within the cancellous core of the pedicle until the cancellous bone of the vertebral body is entered. The probe is advanced by successive rotations from side to side with very little downward pressure along the path of least resistance. Proprioceptively, in normal bone, the cancellous portion has a somewhat firm but yielding quality, whereas cortical bone will feel hard and resist advancement. A sudden "give" may indicate penetration of the cortical rim of the pedicle. Some slow cancellous bleeding is expected, and often fat globules drip out of the probe tract. The sides of the tract are then explored with a sound or feeler for breaks in the cortex. Markers such as different-sized Steinmann pins may be inserted at this time for confirmatory radiographs after all the other pedicles for instrumentation have been marked similarly with pins of different lengths. A depth gauge then determines screw length, and the tract is tapped with a tap of the appropriate diameter. The pedicle screw is advanced with the cannulated locking wrenches. Slotted connectors connect the screws to the rods and are tightened with a hex nut.

Biomechanically, transpedicular fixation provides excellent posterior stabilization and adds support to the middle and anterior columns as well. Zindrick, studying transpedicular fixation in lumbar spines, noted that transpedicular screws with the largest diameter have higher pullout strengths and that osteoporosis significantly reduces screw pullout resistance.[23] Krag noted that screw depths of over 50% of the vertebral body are needed for optimal fixation.[24]

RESULTS AND COMPLICATIONS

Most recently, the authors have used ISOLA rods and hooks alone or in combination with pedicular screws in 19 patients. Of these, 12 had fractures and 7 cancer of the spine (2 breast, 2 bronchogenic, 2 renal cell, and 1 chordoma). Recovery was generally unremarkable, and most patients were maintained postoperatively in thoracolumbar shells. There was one case of a superficial wound dehiscence in a 75-year-old woman with ankylosing spondylitis and paralysis, complicating a slice fracture of T10. Another 59-year-old man, who had received preoperative radiation for metastatic renal cell cancer to L2, developed a wound infection.

In cases of severe instability or multiple fractures, it may be necessary to extend the instrumentation two levels below the site of pathology and up to three levels rostral. In addition, the site of attachment of the implants must consist of solid and intact bone. Figure 23–10 shows a 28-year-old woman with a burst fracture of L1. Stabilization was attempted with pedicular screws at L2 and L3, with a claw configuration at T11 and sublaminar wires at T12. Mobilization and weight bearing resulted in bilateral, transverse process fractures at T11 with progressive angulation. This necessitated reoperation with ventral decompression, fibular strut grafting, and posterior pedicular screw fixation at T11 and T12, in addition to L2 and L3. The transverse processes of T10, T11, and T12 are of insufficient caliber for hook engagement when significant flexion loads are anticipated. The junction between the prosthesis and spine is selected to withstand the severe loads often created by the instability secondary to either fracture or cancer.

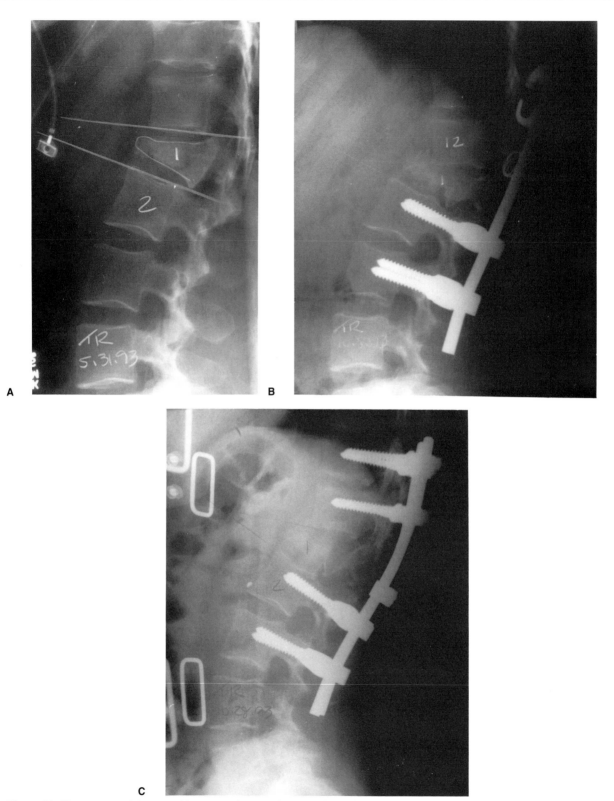

Figure 23–10. Twenty-eight-year-old woman with burst fracture of L1. (**A**). Preoperative lateral projection shows the burst fracture of L1 with angulation and retropulsion of bone. (**B**). Three months following surgery, progressive angulation is encountered due to bilateral transverse process fractures of T11. This progression occurred in spite of an attempted posterolateral fusion with iliac crest bone and thoracolumbar orthosis since surgery. (**C**). Reoperation for stabilization was undertaken using a fibular strut graft for an interbody fusion, pedicular screw fixation at T11 and T12, and revision of the posteriolateral transverse process and facet fusion.

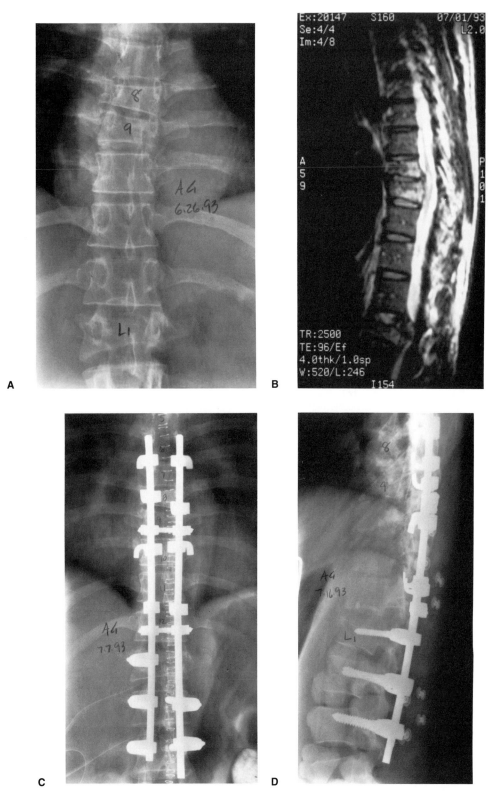

Figure 23–11.   Forty-six-year-old man sustaining closed head injury, with burst fracture at L1 and flexion-compression fractures at T8 and T9. Anterior posterior plain film (**A**) and T2-weighted sagittal MRI (**B**) reveal the spinal angulation and canal compromise. ISOLA hooks and pedicular screws were used for spinal stabilization following transpedicular decompression at L1. This extensive construct seen on anteroposterior (**C**) and lateral (**D**) projections was mandated by the occurrence of multiple spinal fractures. Multiple sites of fixation were necessary to resist significant moments of force at either end of this construct.

Multisegmental fixation with either VSP screws or ISOLA hooks is mandatory for load sharing. Limited fixation rostral and caudal to the site of instability may be responsible for construct failure. This occurrence was noted earlier with Harrington distraction rods, for which purpose sublaminar wires were incorporated. The extent of segmentation may frequently bridge more than one fracture. Figure 23–11 shows a 46-year-old paraplegic man sustaining a significant burst fracture at L1 and a lesser one at T9. Following decompression of the canal at L1, spinal stabilization was accomplished using both hooks and screws. To span both fractures, an intrasegmental claw was applied at T7 with pedicular screws bilaterally at L2 and L3. To consolidate this construct, additional hooks were interspersed for stress distribution between the aforementioned two levels. Crosslinks are imperative for further stability under torsional forces.

REFERENCES

1. Hadra BE. Wiring of the spinous processes in Pott's disease. *TransAmer Orthop Assoc.* 1891;4:206–210.
2. Hibbs RA. An operation for progressive spinal deformities. *NY J Med.* 1911;93:1013–1016.
3. Albee FH. Transplantation of a portion of the tibia into the spine for Pott's disease. *JAMA.* 1911;57:885–887.
4. Harrington PR. The history and development of Harrington instrumentation. *Clin Orthop.* 1988;227:3.
5. Harrington PR. Surgical instrumentation for the management of scoliosis. *JBJS.* 1960;42A:1448.
6. Irwin WD, Dixon JH, Harrington PR. Clinical review of patients with broken Harrington rods. *JBJS.* 1980;62A:1302–1307.
7. Jacobs RR, Montesano PX. Development of the locking hook spinal rod system. *Orthopedics.* 1988;11:1415.
8. Edwards CL, Levine AM. Early rod-sleeve stabilization of the injured thoracic and lumbar spine. *Orthop Clin N Am.* 1986;17:121–145.
9. Lange F. Support for the spondylotic spine by means of buried steel bars attached to the vertebrae. *Am J Orthop Surg.* 1910;8:344–361.
10. Luque E. The anatomical basis and development of segmental spinal instrumentation. *Spine.* 1982;7:256–259.
11. Luque E. Segmental spinal instrumentation for correction of scoliosis. *Clin Orthop.* 1982;163:192–198.
12. Allen B Jr, Ferguson R. L-rod instrumentation for scoliosis in cerebral palsy. *J Ped Orthop.* 1982;2:87–96.
13. Panjabi M, Abumi K, Duranceau J, Crisco J. Biomechanical evaluation of spinal fixation devices KK: stability provided by eight internal fixation devices. *Spine.* 1988;13:1135–1140.
14. Winter R, Lonstein J. Adult idiopathic scoliosis treated with Luque and Harrington rods and sublaminar wiring. *JBJS.* 1989;71A:1308–1313.
15. Zindrick MR, Knight GW, Bunch WH, et al. Factors influencing the penetration of wires into the neural canal during segmental wiring. *JBJS.* 1989;71A:742–750.
16. Boucher HH. A method of spinal fusion. *JBJS.* 1959;41B:248.
17. Cotrel Y, Dubousset J, Guillaumat M. New universal instrumentation for spinal surgery. *Clin Orthop.* 1988;227:10–23.
18. Farcy JP, Wiedenbaum M, Michelsen CB, et al. A comparative biomechanical study of spinal fixation using Cotrel-Dubousset instrumentation. *Spine.* 1987;12:877–881.
19. Gurr KR, McAfee PC. Cotrel-Dubousset instrumentation in adults. *Spine.* 1988;13:510–520.
20. Johnston CE II, Herring A, Ashman R. Texas Scottish Rite Hospital (TSRH) universal spinal instrumentation system. In: An HS, Cotler JM, eds. *Spinal Instrumentation.* Baltimore, Md: Williams & Wilkins; 1992:127–165.
21. Asher MA, Strippgen WE, Heinig CF, Carson WL. Isola spinal implant system: principles, design and application. In: An HS, Cotler JM, eds. *Spinal Instrumentation.* Baltimore, Md: Williams & Wilkins; 1992:325–351.
22. Asher M, Carson W, Heinig C, et al. A modular spinal rod linkage system to provide rotational stability. *Spine.* 1988;13:272–277.
23. Zindrick MR, Wiltse LL, Widell EH, et al. A biomechanical study of intrapeduncular screw fixation in the lumbosacral spine. *Clin Orthop.* 1986;203:99–112.
24. Krag MH, Beynnon BD, Pope MH, et al. An internal fixator for posterior application to short segments of the thoracic, lumbar, or lumbosacral spine: design and testing. *Clin Orthop.* 1986;203:75–98.

24 Texas Scottish Rite Hospital Hook–Rod Spinal Fixation

Edward C. Benzel, M.D., F.A.C.S., Nevan G. Baldwin, M.D., Perry A. Ball, M.D.

INTRODUCTION

Universal spinal instrumentation (USI) applies to those spinal implant systems that offer numerous options for spinal manipulation and fixation. Such systems allow significant latitude with regard to both the number of implant/bone interfaces available (multisegmental points of fixation) and the orientation of implants (rostral or caudal). This flexibility allows for controlled application of forces in compression, distraction, or neutral modes. This, in turn, provides the ability for spinal fixation and deformity correction.

Traditional systems have offered only simple compression or distraction at both extremes of the implant without the option of intermediate points of fixation. This limits the spine surgeon in both security of fixation and the variety of force applications available. The need for greater security of the implant and for the ability to utilize more complex constructs led to the design of systems that are more user friendly and more functional. Hence, USI systems were developed.

Perhaps the first USI system utilized clinically (in the most rudimentary sense of the term) was the Harrington compression rod system. It allowed for multiple hook placement as well as the placement of hooks in either a rostral or caudal orientation. The system, however, was difficult to apply, particularly when multiple hooks were utilized.

USI was introduced into the era of modern spine surgery by the development and implementation of the Cotrel-Dubousset (CD) instrumentation system.[1] The application of USI techniques allows for the relatively easy application of multiple hooks, in a rostral or caudal orientation and in either a compression or distraction mode. Furthermore, such techniques allow for the simultaneous utilization of pedicle screw fixation points and the crossfixation of one longitudinal member (rod) to the other. The attachment of the rod on one side to its companion on the other side creates a quadrilateral frame construct. A quadrilateral frame construct provides greater torsional stability and improves security of fixation at the hook/bone interface.[2] Finally, derotation of the spine utilizing universal spinal instrumentation techniques can be used to correct scoliotic deformities.

Other USI systems followed on the heels of CD. One of the first of these was the Texas Scottish Rite Hospital (TSRH) system.[3] It differed from the CD system in the attachment mechanism of the hooks to the rod, the surface characteristics of the rods, and the metallurgical properties of the implants.

The utilization of the TSRH USI system has indications similar to other USI systems. Specific indications that are unique to the TSRH system are described in this chapter (sequential hook insertion application and the crossed-rod deformity reduction technique).

TSRH IMPLANT ATTRIBUTES AND CHARACTERISTICS

The Three-Point Shear Clamp

A fundamental difference between all USI systems is the method of hook fixation to the rod. The TSRH system utilizes the three-point shear clamp mechanism, which employs an eyebolt/rod fixation method for all hooks, screws, and crossmembers (Fig. 24–1).[4] If applied appropriately, this mechanism provides 600 lb of axial resistance and 60 in-lb of torsional resistance, thereby making it the strongest hook-to-rod connection available currently.

The hooks can be attached to the rod with varying degrees of tightness. If the eyebolt is too loose, it will simply dislodge from the hook (loose). If the eyebolt is tightened slightly, it cannot dislodge but will allow movement of the hook/eyebolt assembly along the rod if a compression or distraction force is applied (friction-slide tight). If the eyebolt is tightened maximally, it offers a secure hook/rod fixation (tight).

Three-point shear clamp hook/rod fixation requires that the rod fit into a groove on the hook structure. Tightening the eyebolt ensures that the rod fits securely into this groove. The surface area of contact between the rod and the hook is increased by the matching contours of the rod surface and the groove in the hook.

With the TSRH drop-in technique, the full-top hooks (Fig. 24–2; left) may be placed in appropriate bony sites, whether they are transverse process, sublaminar, or pedicle (facet) hooks. After this is accomplished, the rod is contoured and dropped into the trough hook/rod attachment site (drop-in). The sequential hook insertion (SHI) technique is facilitated by the central-post hook/rod attachment configuration (Fig. 24–2; right). Both techniques are described in

229

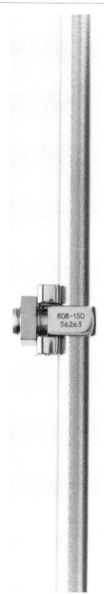

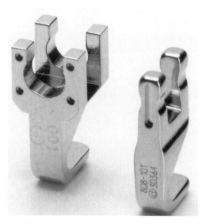

Figure 24–2. The two fundamental hook designs of the TSRH system. Left: The full top hook used with the traditional drop-in technique. Right: The central-post hook used with the SHI technique.

Figure 24–1. The three-point shear clamp mechanism of hook/rod attachment, observed from above.

this chapter; both use the three-point shear clamp method of hook/rod fixation.

The Hooks

Other (non-TSRH) systems have both open and closed hooks available for insertion. The open hooks of these systems (eg, CD and ISOLA) are less structurally sound than their closed counterparts, and thus the closed hooks are recommended for those segments of the system that require greater security of attachment of the hook to the rod (ie, the terminal hooks). The closed hooks are, by their nature, more difficult to affix to the rod. Complex manipulations are most often required to thread the rod through the eye of the closed hooks.

The TSRH system does not require closed hooks because of the substantial security of the three-point shear clamp fixation. The need for closed hooks, with their associated complexities and risks, is thus eliminated.

A variety of hook configurations are available with the TSRH system (Fig. 24–3). In addition to the full-top and central-post systems, both pediatric and adult sizes for most

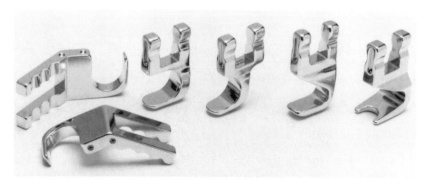

Figure 24–3. The variety of TSRH hooks available (adult sizes). Left and left foreground: The right and left offset hooks. Proceeding from left to right: The laminar hook, transverse process hook, thoracic laminar hook, and pedicle (facet) hook.

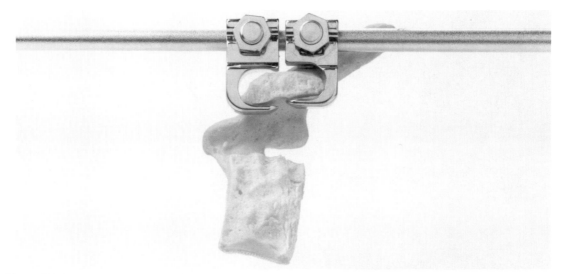

Figure 24–4. A large and small laminar hook are applied to achieve a single-level claw configuration. A wide lamina (rostral-caudal dimension) is necessary to eliminate the "kissing" of the two hooks.

hooks are available. The width of the TSRH hook/rod attachment site (in the rostral-caudal dimension) in the sagittal plane is 14 mm for all hooks, whereas the hooks of the ISOLA and CD systems are substantially smaller in this dimension (9 to 10 mm). In this regard, the hooks of the TSRH system are larger and more substantial, thus allowing for greater security. The increased width of the hooks, however, results in a greater degree of difficulty in securing a single level in the claw configuration of either the laminar or transverse process pedicle type (Fig. 24–4).

Several hooks are available with the TSRH system that are unique to this system. Of note are the cranial and caudal lumbar hooks (Fig. 24–5). These hooks are particularly useful in the lumbar region, where sublaminar hook insertion is often difficult because of the presence of the massive lumbar laminae and often hypertrophied facet joints. All hooks can be inserted by using any of a variety of available tools (Figs. 24–6A, B, and C). These instruments allow the sur-

geon to place the implant securely while under full control of the hook during insertion. In the case of the hook holder, the hook can be held away from the neural elements by pulling up on the hook holder. The method of hook attachment to the hook holder is via a tongue-and-groove configuration. This configuration replaces an older two-pin design (Fig. 24–6C).

The lateral eyebolt orientation of the TSRH system often causes moderate difficulty with regard to bolt tightening. The facet joints or laterally retracted muscle tissues can be annoying obstacles. The availability of newer wrench designs and prototype tools for hook/rod attachment has obviated this problem to some degree. The central-post hook configuration has further minimized this problem by providing more room for nut tightening and in situ hook manipulation (Figs. 24–7A, B, and C).

The fundamental hook configurations available with the TSRH system are similar to those available with the CD System. Contours for attachment to superior and inferior laminar surfaces are offered as well as offset hooks to allow combinations of pedicle or transverse process fixation with laminar fixation. There are also low-profile hooks and pediatric sizes available. The bone contact portions of the TSRH hooks are larger than their CD counterparts. The TSRH hooks differ substantially from the configurations of other systems, such as the ISOLA system. The latter offers essentially one hook in varying sizes, whereas the TSRH system offers a wide variety of hook configurations.

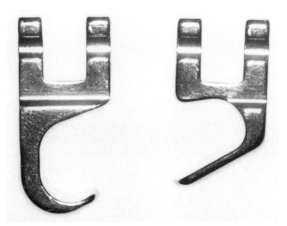

Figure 24–5. The cranial (left) and caudal (right) hooks for sublaminar placement in the lumbar spine.

The Rod

The CD system uses a knurled rod and set-screw configuration. The TSRH system can be considered the equivalent of a racing slick on a dragster that requires significant road-to-tire surface area contact to obtain the desired traction. The CD system can be considered the equivalent of a knobby tire

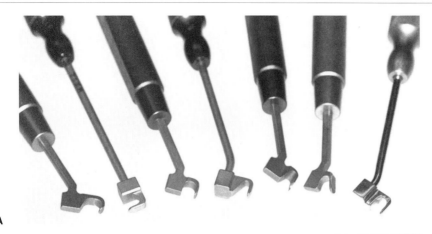

A

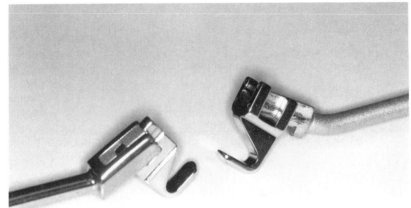

B

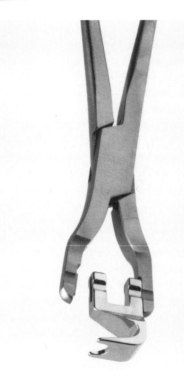

C

Figure 24–6. The variety of TSRH hook insertion tools. (**A**). The trial hooks for each of the available hooks allow the testing of the hook insertion site prior to actual hook insertion. (**B**). Hook inserters (left, central post, and right, full top hook inserters) with or without the hook holder are used for insertion of the hook into its bed. (**C**). Note the tongue-and-groove method of attachment of the hook holder to the hook.

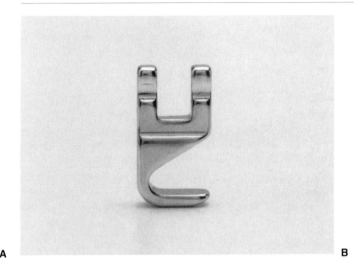

A

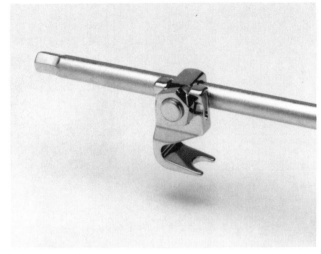

B

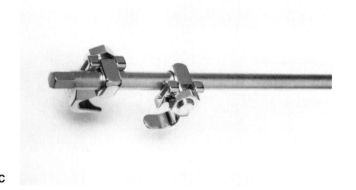

C

Figure 24–7. (**A**). The central-post hook (thoracic laminar hook). (**B**). The method of attachment of a central-post hook to the rod obviously allows for more room for hook manipulation and nut tightening. (**C**). The hooks may be attached on opposite sides of the rod if necessary.

on an off-road vehicle that requires the friction provided by a relative conformation between the tire and the ground surface. Both achieve their desired result effectively. The racing slick, however, would not be effective off road. Similarly, an off-road tire would not be effective on a dragster. If one were to utilize a three-point shear clamp device, such as a TSRH crossmember on a knurled rod, the surface area of contact would be reduced, thereby creating a weaker construct with greater chance for slippage. The TSRH crossmember can, however, be utilized effectively with any rod of the appropriate size without clinically significant sequelae.

The friction-slide intermediate extent of hook/rod tightness is achieved more simply and effectively with the TSRH than the CD system. Excess or unpredictable friction with the CD system can cause distraction, compression, or rotational grabbing, possibly with untoward results.[4] The TSRH system facilitates the achievement of friction-slide tightness with less difficulty.

The TSRH rods are cold-rolled, shot-peened stainless steel. The peening process compresses the outer layer of the rod, thereby adding approximately 10% to its fatigue resistance. The peening process results in a matte finish appearance of the rod (Fig. 24–1). The rods are available in three

sizes: $\frac{3}{16}$ in, $\frac{1}{4}$ in, and 7 mm. The $\frac{1}{4}$-in rod is available with rigid (stiff) or malleable (flex) characteristics. The rods may be bent and cut ex vivo and may also be bent in situ with available equipment (as are the rods of all other commonly and currently utilized USI systems). The TSRH rods are less malleable than CD rods. Thus, they require more force to contour but they also offer greater resistance to bending in vivo.

Crossfixation

A fundamental difference between the TSRH system and the variety of currently available USI systems is the type of crossfixation utilized. The TSRH system uses a rigid crossmember that interconnects the two rods (Fig. 24–8A). This crossmember allows for the most rigid quadrilateral construct currently available.[2] It is not a variable-length crossmember in the strictest sense (as are the CD and ISOLA crossmembers), but varying interrod widths can be accommodated by utilizing one of a variety of crossmember sizes available (Fig. 24–8B). The TSRH crossmembers are also available in off-set and end-to-end configurations (Fig. 24–8C). These facilitate the linkage of rods to previously placed implants.

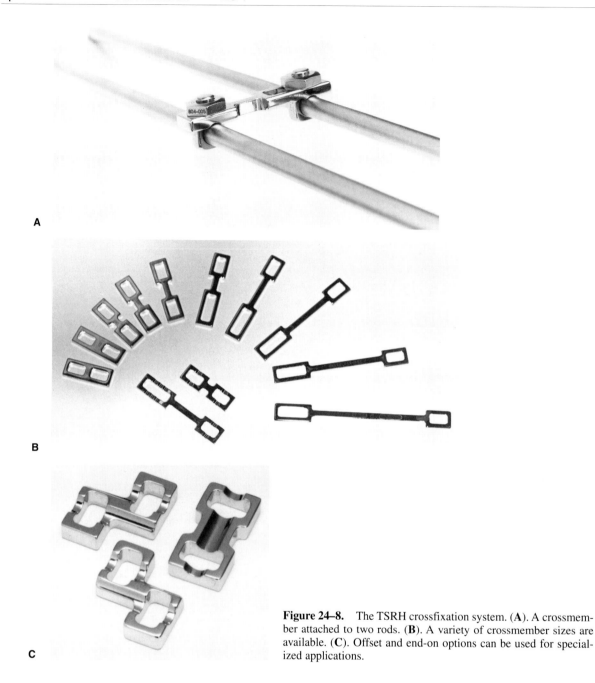

A

B

C

Figure 24–8. The TSRH crossfixation system. (**A**). A crossmember attached to two rods. (**B**). A variety of crossmember sizes are available. (**C**). Offset and end-on options can be used for specialized applications.

The TSRH crossmembers and hooks, as mentioned, utilize a three-point, shear-clamp type of fixation to the rods. The surface characteristics of the crossmember and the rod are similar (both relatively smooth), thus allowing for substantial surface area contact between these metal components. The friction thus created affords a secure attachment.

Versatility

The TSRH hook/rod spinal fixation system is versatile, offering a variety of hook options as described earlier, as well

as the option of utilizing either variable-angle or fixed-angle screws. The former are available with several sizes of spacers that allow for lateral or medial variability of rod placement (Fig. 24–9).

INSERTION TECHNIQUES

The two insertion techniques for the TSRH hook/rod system are the traditional drop-in technique utilized by all systems and an additional technique that is currently unique to

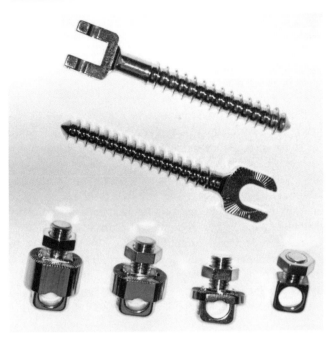

Figure 24–9. The TSRH screws and their attachment mechanisms. The standard fixed-angle screw (upper) and variable-angle screw (middle) are depicted. Attachment eyebolts for the variable-angle screw (left three; lower) allow for varying distances of lateral displacement of the screw from the rod. The bottom right eyebolt is used to affix the fixed-angle screw to the rod. The variable-angle screw can be attached to the rod at any angle.

the TSRH central-post system, the SHI technique. Each is described here. The latter, however, is described in more detail because the relative lack of familiarity with this method.

The Traditional Drop-In Technique

A drop-in technique of insertion of the rod into the hooks, or a variant thereof, is used by most traditional and commonly available USI hook/rod techniques.[3,5,6] What varies is the mechanism of attachment of the hook to the rod.

With the drop-in technique, the hooks are first inserted into their respective bony sites after the site is prepared and "tried" with a trial hook specific for the hook size and type to be inserted. Following placement of the hooks and the protection of all hooks from entering the spinal canal when appropriate (observe in Fig. 24–10 the utilization of hook holders to prevent the latter), the rod is configured by a rod bender to fit the desired contour of the spine. If desired, a large-gauge wire can first be fitted and used as a template for rod contouring. After contouring, the eyebolts for connecting the hooks and crossmembers to the rod are placed on the rod and it is dropped into place. This aspect of the procedure can be fraught with frustration, requiring at least one assistant to facilitate insertion and often another to protect the neural elements by maintaining the hooks in a safe position

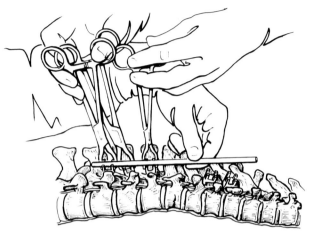

Figure 24–10. The traditional drop-in technique. The hooks are inserted into their respective sites prior to rod attachment. As illustrated, rod attachment often requires substantial assistance to secure the hooks in a safe position.

(Fig. 24–10). Each eyebolt must be fitted into a slot in its respective hook.

After positioning the rod properly, the eyebolts are tightened individually. In situ rod bending can be used if needed to ensure a close fit. However, regardless of the system utilized, the more accurately the rod is contoured to the spine and hook arrangement prior to actual attachment, the less will be the frustration involved with this aspect of the procedure. In situ bending carries with it a risk of neural injury due to instrumentation manipulation. It also stresses the hook/bone interfaces substantially.

Once the hooks are secured to the rod but the eyebolts are not tightened fully (friction-slide tightness), the hooks may

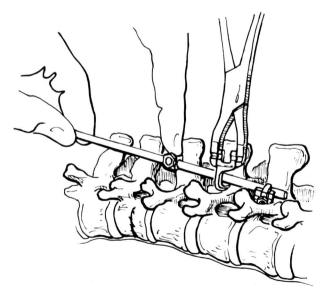

Figure 24–11. A central-post hook positioned lateral to the rod. It is secured at its hook/bone interface position while the second half of the claw (second hook) is inserted.

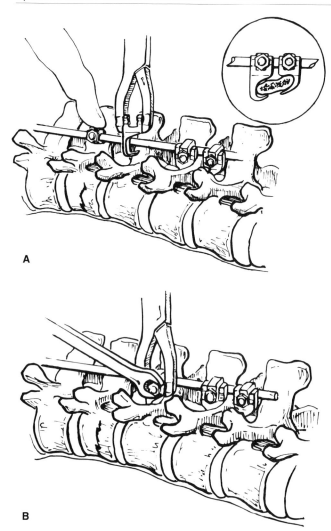

A

B

Figure 24–12. Following the attainment of security of the rod-claw combination (inset), the third hook is inserted (**A**) and secured (**B**). The remaining hooks are sequentially inserted and secured in a similar manner.

be slid up and down the rod (with appropriate compression and distraction instruments) to obtain the desired force application to the spine. Spinal kyphotic deformity reduction is somewhat difficult and potentially dangerous with the drop-in technique if significant force application is required during construct insertion.

The central-post TSRH hook configuration can be used in a similar fashion. However, because of its narrow profile, the central-post hook offers the surgeon more room for manipulation of the relationship of the hook to the rod.

The SHI Technique

The SHI technique of TSRH hook/rod insertion allows the avoidance of many of the problems and complications associated with the traditional drop-in technique.[7] The narrow body facilitates the fixation of the hook to the rod. It also facilitates the possibility of inserting the hook into position while the rod is fixed in situ, as is the case with the tradi-

tional drop-in technique. Hook insertion with the rod already positioned is an integral component of the SHI technique, as discussed later. All of these attributes are unique to the TSRH central-post system. Neither threading a rod through a closed hook or a drop-in to a trough (as is required with all traditional techniques) is required. Finally, the SHI technique facilitates the safe reduction of deformities by allowing an easy method of applying translational forces to the spine via a three-point bending force application.

The method of insertion is similar in some respects to the more traditional techniques. First, hook sites are prepared in the routine manner. These sites are then fashioned for each hook by using the trial hooks if deemed appropriate. Then the most caudal (or rostral) hook is attached to a rod that has been bent to the desired configuration. The hook is positioned lateral to the rod and secured firmly. The next hook is inserted into its site while an assistant prevents neural injury by holding the rod medially (Fig. 24–11). The second hook is then secured firmly after it is placed into its ultimately desired position by a compressor or distractor. The third hook is then placed in a similar manner (Fig. 24–12A) and secured (Fig. 24–12B). The medial location of the rod allows for the attachment of the hook to the rod with the rod in place while not disturbing the relationship of the previously placed hooks. Usually a claw configuration is utilized for the first two hooks (Fig. 24–12A, inset). Therefore, a safe and secure fixation of the rod to the spine is achieved after the insertion of only the first two hooks.

If a reduction of a kyphotic deformity is desired, the SHI technique can be used to apply a lever-arm force to the deformity site in a safe manner with the lower (or upper) half of the construct's hooks affixed firmly to the rod. Crossmember eyebolts should be positioned in sequence as

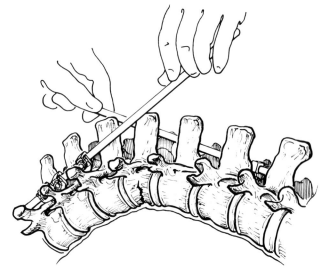

Figure 24–13. The crossed-rod technique of deformity correction. The rostral three hooks were inserted on the left and the caudal three on the right. Ventral force application on both rods then results in deformity correction. The remaining hooks are then secured in a sequential manner.

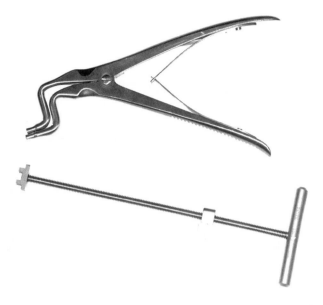

A

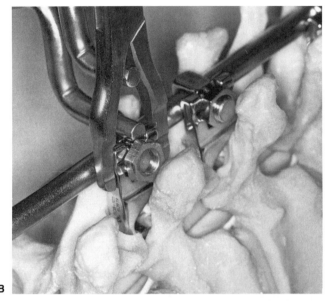

B

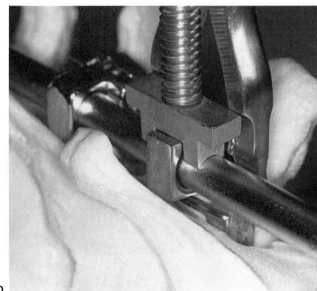

D

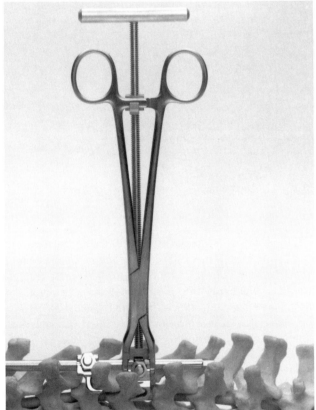

C

Figure 24–14. The rod may be brought down to the hook by using the elephant nose (top) or the mini-corkscrew (bottom) (**A**). The elephant nose (**B**) is used for moderate force application and the mini-corkscrew for more substantial force application (**C** and **D**).

indicated. The eyebolts can be positioned sequentially as well with this technique, thus minimizing the fiddle factor associated with dealing simultaneously with multiple eyebolts positioned on the rod.

The remainder of the hooks are placed in a similar manner, and the rod of the opposite side is positioned similarly. If significant reduction forces are required, the crossed-rod insertion technique can be applied by starting the hook in-

sertion rostrally on one side and caudally on the other. When all of the upper half of the hooks on the rostral component and the lower hooks on the caudal component are attached, the rods can be manipulated to obtain reduction by the application of two simultaneous ventrally directed forces. This results in the application of a three-point bending force complex to the spine; the end result is kyphosis reduction (Fig. 24–13). Two instruments, the elephant nose and the mini-

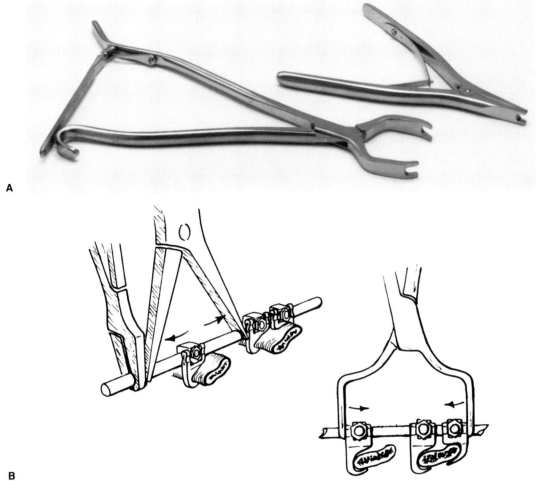

Figure 24–15.   (**A**). Hook compression or distraction is achieved with a compressor (left) and distractor (right). (**B**). An example of distraction (left) and compression (right).

corkscrew, can be used to bring the hook to the rod in difficult circumstances (Figs. 24–14A, B, C, and D). Both (particularly the latter) can apply significant and perhaps excessive force to the construct. Therefore, care must be taken in this regard.

Manipulation of the hook relationships and applied forces can be achieved with the distractor and compressor instruments (Figs. 24–15A and B). Complex force application can, thus, be achieved. The finished product is illustrated in Figure 24–16.

RESULTS AND COMPLICATIONS

The early results of TSRH spinal instrumentation have been published.[3,4] Unfortunately, comparisons with other implant types are not available. Major universal spinal instrumentation manufacturers have been extremely responsive to surgeons and have, therefore, produced products that are, to varying degrees, user friendly and efficacious. The TSRH instrumentation system is a good example of an outgrowth from this responsiveness.

Complications of universal spinal instrumentation are usually not manufacturer dependent. The misapplication of spinal implants is much more likely to cause complications than the actual implant itself. In the authors' experience, the most common complications associated with the TSRH system are related to the time required for insertion, the frustations associated with the technical aspects of application, and the use of an insufficiently long construct when distraction is the mode of application used.

The frustations associated with implant application are predominantly related to the mechanism of connection of the hooks to the rod via eyebolts. This aspect of the procedure is often challenging because of the lateral location and confining nature of nut tightening. The central-post SHI technique has, for the most part, eliminated this problem. This, in turn, has decreased operative time significantly.

The use of an insufficiently long construct can lead to postoperative deformity progression. When instrumentation-related distraction is planned, the authors usually extend the construct to at least three spinal levels above and two below the spinal level of the pathology. A longer lever arm (particularly above the spinal level of the pathology) de-

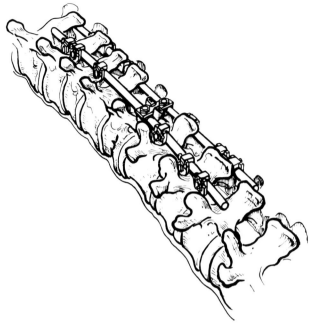

Figure 24–16. The finished product. A single crossmember has been applied in the center of the construct. Torsional stability may be increased by using two crossmembers, thereby creating a quadrilateral frame construct.

creases the chance for failure.

CONCLUSION

The TSRH system of spinal fixation is versatile. The variety of TSRH components provides for significant flexibility. In-

The TSRH system is well suited to congenital, traumatic, and degenerative applications. The SHI technique, using TSRH instrumentation, allows reduction of traumatic or nontraumatic deformities with greater ease and less operative risk. The hook/rod aspect of the system can be combined with a pedicle screw fixation mode of construct/bone interface. Therefore, it fulfills the requirements for a universal spinal instrumentation system in the truest sense.

Acknowledgment. The authors recognize and appreciate the expert assistance of Michael F. Norviel, medical illustrator.

REFERENCES

1. Cotrel Y, Dubousset J, Guillaumat M. New universal instrumentation in spinal surgery. *Clin Orthop.* 1988;227:110–123.
2. Johnston CE, Ashman RB, Corin JD. Mechanical effects of cross-linking rods in Cotrel-Dubousset instrumentation. Presented at the Scoliosis Research Society combined with the British Scoliosis Society; 21st annual meeting; September 21–25, 1986; Hamilton, Bermuda.
3. Benzel EC, Kesterson L, Marchand EP. Texas Scottish Rite Hospital rod instrumentation for thoracic and lumbar spine trauma. *J Neurosurg.* 1991;75:382–387.
4. Ashman RB, Herring JA, Johnston CE II. Texas Scottish Rite Hospital (TSRH) instrumentation system. In: Bridwell KH, De Wald RL, eds. *The Textbook of Spinal Surgery.* Vol 1. Philadelphia, Pa: JB Lippincott; 1991:219–248.
5. Engler GL. Cotrel-Dubousset instrumentation for reduction of fracture dislocations of the spine. *J Spinal Disord.* 1990; 3:62–66.
6. Gurr KR, McAfee PC. Cotrel-Dubousset instrumentation in adults: a preliminary report. *Spine.* 1988;13:510–520.
7. Benzel EC, Ball PA, Baldwin NG, Marchand EP. The sequential hook insertion technique for universal spinal instrumentation application. *J Neurosurg.* 1993;79:608–611.

25 Transpedicular Screw Fixation of the Thoracic and Lumbar Spine

Patrick W. Hitchon, M.D., Kenneth A. Follett, M.D., Ph.D.

INTRODUCTION

The vertebral pedicle constitutes the junction of five vertebral body components. These are the superior and inferior facets, the lamina and the transverse process posteriorly, and the vertebral body anteriorly. If we look on the vertebral body as being composed of two columns, an anterior one made of the vertebral body and a posterior one consisting of the neural arch, the pedicle is therefore the fulcrum or point of convergence of the two vertebral columns.[1] Due to these anatomic features of the pedicle with a fairly large cortex-to-cancellous ratio, the pedicle was recognized early on as a potential site for spinal fixation. Fixation of the spine by means of pedicular screws incorporates both anterior and posterior columns.[2,3] The biomechanics of pedicular screw and plate fixation have been studied in cadaveric spines.[3] When the lumbar spine is destabilized to simulate burst fractures, pedicular screws with plates have been shown to increase stiffness compared to the injured spine without instrumentation.[3] Fixation with pedicular screws and plates was still unable, however, to achieve the stiffness of the normal spine. In isolated cadaveric lumbar spines destabilized with bilateral laminectomy, facetectomy, and diskectomy, comparative studies have been undertaken with pedicle screws and plates (Steffee) and Luque rectangles.[4] These studies have shown a greater degree of stiffness with the Steffee system as compared to the Luque loop in flexion, extension, lateral bending, as well as axial rotation.

In the isolated calf lumbar spine, several anterior and posterior devices were tested following corpectomy of L3.[2] Transpedicular screws (Cottrell-Dubousset [CD] and Steffee) and the Kaneda devices were significantly more rigid than Harrington rods, Luque rectangles, or anterior iliac crest grafting. Similar studies in the in vitro calf spine have shown that transpedicular screws (Arbeitsgemeinschaft für Osteosynthesefragen/Association for the Study of Internal Fixation [AO–ASIF] fixateur interne, Steffee plates, and the Kluger fixateur interne) allow significantly more strain across the unstable site (L3) than posteriorly placed devices (Harrington and Luque).[5] Isolated calf spines have also been utilized to simulate isthmic spondylolisthesis.[6] Here again, pedicular screws (CD and Steffee) provided the most rgidity under flexural, extensile, and torsional forces compared to the destabilized spine, posterior lumbar interbody fusion (PLIF), and Harrington instrumentation.

Clinical studies have favored pedicular screw and plate fixation (Steffee or variable screw placement, VSP) in immobilizing fewer segments and maintaining lumbar lordosis vis-à-vis Luque rectangles and Harrington rods.[7–9] These results have been overwhelming in their support for the utilization of pedicular screws in the treatment of thoracic and

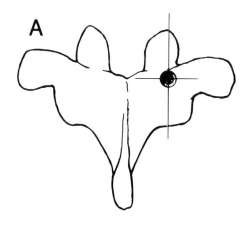

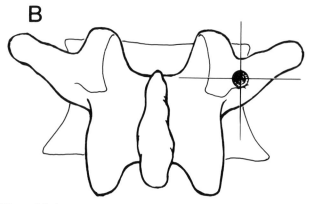

Figure 25–1. Entry point to the thoracic (**A**) and lumbar (**B**) pedicle is identified by the intersection of two lines. The first bisects the transverse process, and the second is longitudinal and lies lateral to the superior facet. In the lumbar spine, the entry point corresponds to the accessory process at the base of the transverse process.

lumbar fractures. Additionally, pedicular screws have the advantage of providing for stability in the absence of laminae. Screw fixation has also been acclaimed for improvement in lumbar fusion rates performed regardless of etiology.[8,10–13]

In spite of the many attributes of pedicular screws, their limitations should also be recognized. Pedicular screws are limited in the absence of anterior load sharing.[3,10,12,14] In the isolated lumbar spine with an L3 corpectomy, pedicular screws and plates fail in axial loading and perform poorly when compared to other devices incorporating an anterior strut.[14] Clinically, such occurrences are present in disease processes involving the vertebral body secondary to infection, neoplasm, or severe burst fractures. The limitations inherent in the use of pedicular screws and plates or rods need to be recognized to prevent progressive angulation postoperatively.

TECHNIQUE

The author prefers to perform these procedures on padded laminectomy rolls, suspending the abdomen and allowing for free respiratory excursions. Pneumatic compression stockings are applied over full-length leg hoses with the knees flexed at least 30°. The potential blood loss during these procedures necessitates an arterial line. Cell savers are not routinely used. In general, patients being operated on for cord compression with or without partial neurological deficit undergo monitoring of somatosensory evoked potentials. Baseline studies are usually obtained the day prior to surgery. Following incision, an intraoperative lateral roentgenogram or radiograph is obtained to identify the level of surgery and the orientation of the vertebral bodies and disk spaces. The incision is carried at least one level ros-

tral and caudal to those being instrumented. The dissection is extended laterally to the tips of the transverse process using a combination of electrocautery and large Cobb elevators. Retraction is achieved with a combination of D'Errico, Miskimon, and Adson-Beckman retractors. The lumbar transverse processes are significantly smaller than those of the thoracic spine and can be fractured easily. Every effort should be made to maintain the integrity of the interspinous ligament if it has not been ruptured by the trauma. Unilateral or bilateral laminotomy is performed to assess adequately the spinal canal and the neural foramina. The laminotomy must be sufficiently large to allow intraoperative ultrasonic visualization of the canal and anterior compression (in this case by retropulsed bone from a burst fracture). The laminotomy may have to be extended laterally, incorporating the medial aspect of the facets and pedicle for proper decompression. A 3-mm drill can be utilized to undermine the retropulsed bone fragment unilaterally or bilaterally. Thereafter, reduction of the bone can be accomplished with ease using a bone tamp (Redmond Surgical Instruments, Lake Zurich, Ill). Restoration of the canal can sometimes be accomplished without sacrificing the integrity of the posterior longitudinal ligament if it has not already been lacerated by the trauma. It is important not to disrupt the normal spine anatomy until the pedicular entry points have been selected. Dural rents encountered can be repaired with 6-0 proline following intradural reduction of any herniated nerve rootlets.

The selection of entry points for pedicular screws is based on published anatomic criteria.[1,15–17] The entry point is usually the intersection of two lines, one bisecting the transverse process and one longitudinal coinciding with the lateral margin of the superior facet. A bony prominence is usually encountered at this point in the lumbar spine, the accessory process.[18] These landmarks are not as pronounced

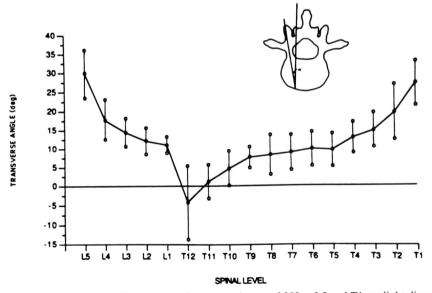

Figure 25–2. Pedicular angle gradually decreases from a maximum of 30° at L5 and T1 to slight divergence at T12. (Reproduced from Zindrick MR, et al. *Spine.* 1987;12:160–166, with permission from JB Lippincott.)

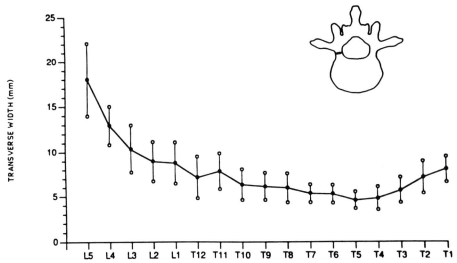

Figure 25–3. Transverse diameter of the pedicle increases caudally from 5 mm at T4 to 15 mm at L5. (Reproduced from Zindrick MR, et al. *Spine.* 1987;12:160–166, with permission from JB Lippincott.)

in the thoracic spine and require close inspection of the exposed spine and the computed tomographic (CT) scan being viewed in the operating room (Figs. 25–1A and B). The proposed entry point is now eburnated with either an air drill or a rongeur and the proposed transpedicular trajectory is made utilizing a probe or gear shift (ACROMED Corporation, Cleveland, Ohio). The trajectory is nearly perpendicular at

T12 and increases in a lateral-to-medial direction rostrally and caudally with a maximum of 30° at L5 and T1 (Fig. 25–2).[19–21] The convergence of pedicular screws is an important feature that contributes to resistance of screw pullout as well as the prevention of lateral translation.[20,22] The more parallel the screw trajectories are, the less stable is the structure. Once the channel has been made through the cancel-

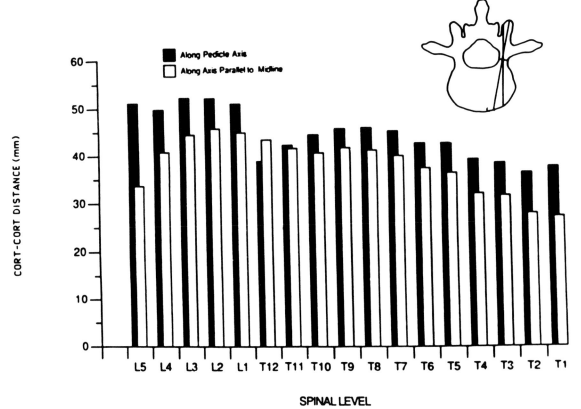

Figure 25–4. Length of pedicular trajectory to the anterior vertebral body cortex increases gradually from 40 mm at T1 to 50 mm at L5. (Reproduced from Zindrick MR, et al. *Spine.* 1987;12:160–166, with permission from JB Lippincott.)

lous bone within the confines of the pedicle, it is then tapped with one of three taps: 5.5 mm, 6.25 mm, or 7.0 mm. The size of the tap used is based on published anatomic data[19–21] and intraoperative examination of the patient's CT scan (Figs. 25–3 and 25–4). The transverse diameter of the L5 pedicles is 15 mm, and this dimension decreases gradually to a minimum of 5 mm at T4.[21] In case of uncertainty regarding the trajectory made, this can be confirmed through the laminotomy. The length of the channel created by the tap is generally 35 mm.

Following withdrawal of the tap, the trajectory is examined with a number 4 Penfield or sound. This is to confirm the intraosseous course, avoiding the disk space as well as a possible paravertebral course. Bleeding from the entry point is usually controlled with a small amount of bone wax, and markers such as Steinmann pins are inserted in each hole. An intraoperative roentgenogram may now be obtained to confirm the proper trajectory. On occasion, a second route may have to be made if the first route traverses a disk space. Thereafter, a screw of appropriate size and length is advanced into the hole. Generally, screws 40 mm long are used in the lumbar spine and 35 mm in the thoracic. Here again, the selection is individualized and based in part on studies from osteological collections[19,21] as well as patient CT scans.[20] In cadaveric studies, larger screws were found to have greater pull-out strength than smaller screws.[23] Hence, it is important to select the largest screw (5.5, 6.25, or 7.0 mm) that engages the pedicular cortex. In addition, in cyclic loading (both cephalocaudal and mediolateral), longer screws were more resistant to loosening than shorter screws.[23] Therefore, longer screws are preferable to shorter ones. With the exception of sacral fixation, it is not necessary or recommended to engage the anterior cortex of the vertebral body. Due to the large size of sacral pedicles at S1 and S2, engagement of the anterior body cortex enhances screw pullout strength. Occasionally in osteoporotic bone of poor density, the screw may strip the threads in the bone. Fixation under such circumstances can be augmented by forcefully injecting methyl methacrylate into the bony channels.[23]

If the intent of the procedure is to perform a posterior lumbar interbody fusion (PLIF), distraction of the appropriate screws and the use of a temporary plate may be indicated. The use of a laminar distractor allows the screws to be separated, opening up the interspace. The distraction is maintained by utilizing temporary nesting nuts and spacers, holding the screws of the two adjacent vertebral bodies apart. Following disk excision and eburnation of the disk space, bone is packed into the disk cavity from both sides and countersunk. In case of spondylolysis, the neural arch can be used for bone grafting. Additional banked or preferably autologous iliac crest bone may be required. Having completed the PLIF, the temporary plate is removed and one or more flat or tapered washers are spaced between the final plate and the integrated screw nut. These spacers allow for the packing of bone beneath the plate.

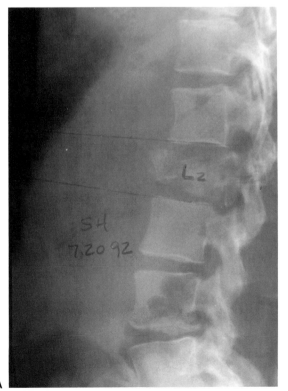
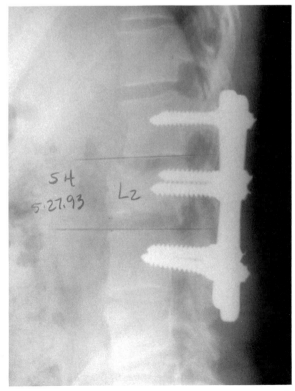

A   B

Figure 25–5.   A burst fracture of L2 in a 24-year-old male. (**A**). Loss in height and an angulation of 4° at L2. (**B**). Postoperative film 10 months later shows improved alignment with partial reconstitution of the body of L2.

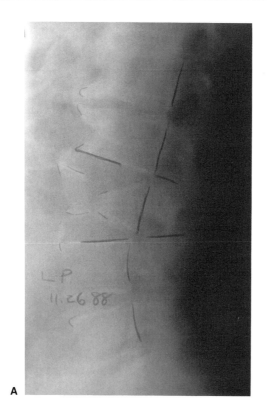

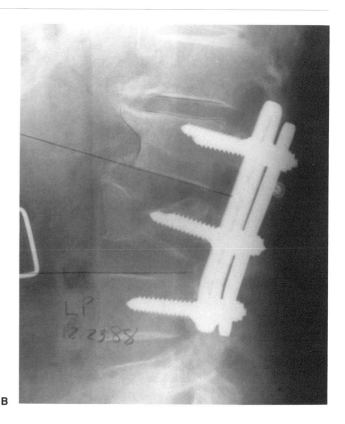

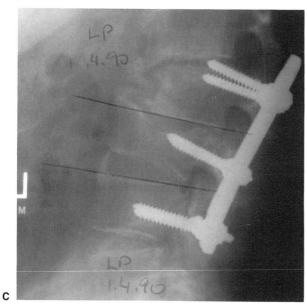

Figure 25–6. A burst fracture of L3 in a 67-year-old farmer. (**A**). Upon admission, normal lordosis is maintained in the supine position. (**B**). Lordosis is unchanged immediately following surgery with VSP screw and plate fixation and a posterolateral bony fusion. (**C**). Progressive angulation occurs in the absence of anterior load sharing. Rostral migration of the screws within the body of L2 occurs, facilitated by poor bone density. Stability is finally achieved with bone healing, but with some loss of lumbar lordosis.

The bone for the posterior lateral fusion can be harvested through a second incision over the posterior iliac crest. Matchsticks of cortical and cancellous bone are placed over the eburnated facets and transverse processes of the involved adjacent bodies. The final plate should allow for restoration of the normal spinal curvature, usually lordosis in the lumbar spine, as well as compression of the bone graft, in the case of a PLIF. If instrumentation spans five to seven levels, it may be impossible to engage the screws in the slots of the

plate. Under such circumstances, an ISOLA rod may be used (ACROMED Corporation). Rods may be secured to pedicular screws using straight or angled slotted connectors (catalog number 5000-55 or 5000-55AN). With appropriate contouring of the rods and due to the slots in the connectors, final fixation of the device is achieved. Perfect apposition between the integral nut and washers and the plates or connectors is mandatory to enhance the strength of the final implant. This is necessary to eliminate the claw-hammer pullout effect of a loose junction between the screw and longitudinal component of the fixature, be it plate or rod. At least one transverse rod connector (catalog number 2030-00, ACROMED Corporation) is necessary for every three levels of instrumentation. This connector can also be utilized in plates and stabilizes the construct particularly against torsional forces and lateral displacement.[22,24] A final intraoperative roentgenogram is obtained to confirm spinal alignment. Once the nesting nuts are tightened securely, the excess portion of the machine-threaded screw is removed with a pin cutter.

The dura is then covered with Gelfoam and residual bone is packed ventral and lateral to the plates or rods. A suction drain is brought out through a lateral stab wound so that it can be removed on the second postoperative day with facility. The fascia is then approximated with 0 vicryl (Ethicon, Summerville, NJ) in the cases of degenerative disease or trauma. Where preoperative radiation has been delivered or postoperative radiation anticipated, nonabsorbable 0 suture is recommended. The subcutaneous tissue is brought together with absorbable 3-0 or 2-0 suture and the skin is closed with staples or nylon. A thin dressing is applied to avoid discomfort when in the supine position. Postoperatively, patient-controlled analgesia is often necessary and hence a pulse oximeter is recommended. The drain is removed on the second postoperative day or earlier if a cerebrospinal fluid (CSF) leak is suspected based on the volume and clarity of fluid in the vacuum suction. The patient is usually mobilized in a thoracolumbar clam-shell orthosis 7 to 10 days following surgery, depending on the availability of the orthosis. Mobilization is performed with careful monitoring of neu-

rological function and sequential x-rays at 45 and 90 degrees. The shells are worn whenever out of bed for a period of 3 months after surgery. Careful monitoring of the patient's blood count is performed every 6 hours for the first 2 days. Transfusion may often be necessary as late as the second or third postoperative day. Because most of these cases are not elective or planned, autologous transfusions have not been utilized. In general, the blood loss has been on the order of 1000 cc, and a transfusion is often rendered unnecessary.

RESULTS

The advantages of pedicular screws for spinal fixation in trauma have been accepted universally. The authors have recently adopted pedicular screws with rods or plates in the treatment of 17 patients with thoracic and lumbar fractures. Pedicular screws alone were utilized in 13 patients, and in combination with ISOLA hooks and rods in four other patients. A combination of hooks and screws were used for fractures involving the thoracolumbar junction (T11, T12, and L1). These patients were scored using the Frankel scale, with 1 the score for total paralysis and 5 for normal neurological function. The mean score on admission ± standard deviation was 2.75 ± 1.5. Thus the majority of patients had neurological deficit; in others surgery was performed to expedite mobility. Mean angulation on admission was 5.4° and that at discharge 2.6°, with an improvement in angulation of 2.75°. Decompression of the canal was performed in all cases using a unilateral or bilateral extradural approach. Where the pedicle was not compromised, a screw was also

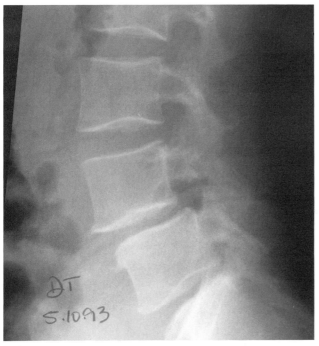

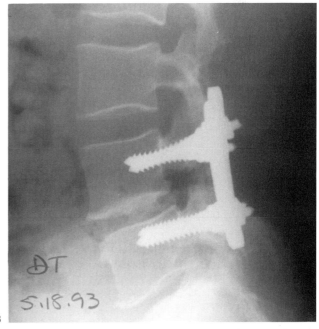

A   B

Figure 25–7.   Intractable postural pain in a 50-year-old man secondary to spondylolysis and listhesis of L4. (**A**). Lysis of the pars-interarticularis of L4 is noted with a grade I listhesis. (**B**). Reduction and stabilization is achieved with VSP screws and plates. Stabilization is augmented with PLIF utilizing the neural arch for grafting.

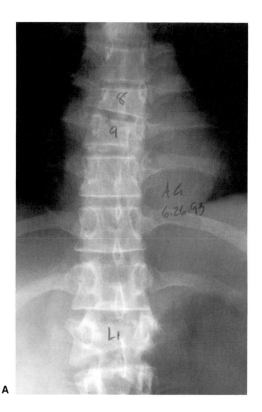

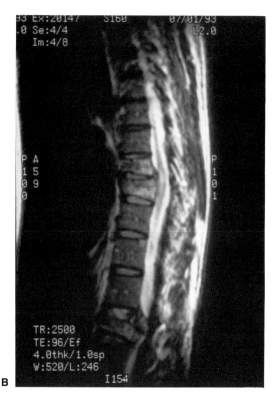

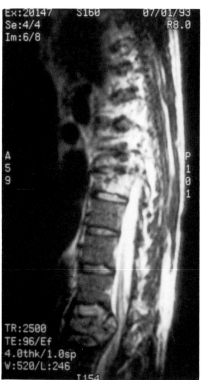

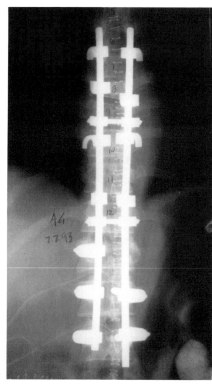

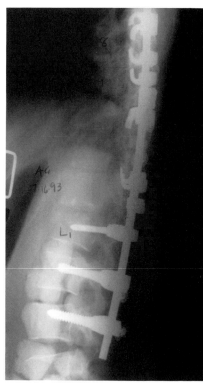

Figure 25–8. Burst fracture of L1 and flexion-compression fractures of T8 and T9 in a 46-year-old man with paraplegia. (**A**). Collapse of the bodies of T8, T9, and L1 with widening of the interpedicular distance is noted on this AP projection. (**B**). T2-weighted sagittal MRI shows compromise of the canal and increased signal within the cord at T8 to T9. (**C**). T2-weighted sagittal MRI shows the burst fracture at L1 with retropulsion of bone into the canal associated with conus contusion manifested with increased signal within the cord. (**D**). Postoperative AP projection shows the transpedicular screws in L1, L2, L3 with ISOLA hooks in the thoracic spine. Two transverse rod connectors stabilize the construct against torsional forces. (**E**). Pedicular screws are used in the lumbar spine and ISOLA hooks in the thoracic. A claw configuration of the hooks is necessary to stabilize the spine in axial, sagittal, and lateral planes.

placed into the fractured body on one or both sides. Figure 25–5 shows the preoperative and postoperative images of an L2 burst fracture in a patient with sphincter disturbance. Angular deformity was improved from +4° on admission to −5° at latest follow-up. Vertebral body height as well as lumbar lordosis have been restored. These results were achieved with one level of instrumentation above and below the fractured body in a 24-year-old man. A similar burst fracture of L3 is presented in Figure 25–6 in a 67-year-old man who was intact. Screws and plates spanned L2 to L4. At latest follow-up, angular deformity had progressed from −14° on admission to 2° at latest follow-up. This progression occurred due to excessive anterior load bearing in the presence of a severely fractured vertebral body compounded by osteoporosis.

Pedicular screws have proven effective in the restoration of normal spinal alignment in patients with iatrogenic, degenerative, or isthmic spondylolisthesis. Figure 25–7 shows a 50-year-old man with an L4 to L5 isthmic spondylolysis with grade I listhesis. His alignment was restored, and his pain was alleviated subsequent to an L4 to L5 PLIF with VSP stabilization.

CONCLUSIONS

Pedicular screws with rods or plates constitute an effective method of spinal stabilization regardless of cause. The construct created utilizing pedicular screws is not always sufficient to withstand anterior-column load bearing in the presence of a diseased or fractured vertebral body.[3,10,12,14] Such failure can be averted by resorting to either a ventral struct graft or possibly by extending stabilization two levels rostral and two levels caudal to the site of fracture. Where pedicles are too small for pedicular screws, ISOLA hooks in the thoracic spine can be used in conjunction with pedicular screws in the lumbar spine (Fig. 25–8). Pedicular screws are ideal in the lumbar spine in achieving normal lumbar lordosis with short segments of fixation. The latter have not been achieved using older distractive devices.

Acknowledgment. The authors recognize the help of Judy Rehbehn in the preparation of this manuscript.

REFERENCES

1. Steffee AD. The variable screw placement system with posterior lumbar interbody fusion. In: Lin PM, Gill K, eds. *Lumbar Interbody Fusion: Principles and Techniques in Spine Surgery.* Aspen Publishers, Inc.; 1989:81–93.
2. Gurr KR, McAfee PC, Shih CM. Biomechanical analysis of anterior and posterior instrumentation systems after corpectomy. *J Bone Joint Surg.* 1988;70A:1182–1191.
3. Yoganandan N, Larson SJ, Pintar F, et al. Biomechanics of lumbar pedicle screw/plate fixation in trauma. *Neurosurgery.* 1990;27:873–811.
4. Goel VK, Lim T, Gwon J, et al. Biomechanics of fusion. In: Andersson BDJ, McNeil PW, eds. *Spinal Stenosis.* St Louis, Mo: CV Mosby; 1992:403–414.
5. Wittenberg RH, Shea M, Edwards WT, et al. A biomechanical study of the fatigue characteristics of thoracolumbar fixation implants in a calf spine model. *Spine.* 1992;17:S121–S128.
6. Shirado O, Zdeblick TA, McAffee PC, et al. Biomechanical evaluation of methods of posterior stabilization of the spine and posterior lumbar interbody arthrodesis for lumbosacral isthmic spondylolisthesis. *J Bone Joint Surg.* 1991;73A:518–526.
7. An HS, Vaccaro A, Colter JM, et al. Low lumbar burst fractures: Comparison among body cast, Harrington rod, Luque rod and Steffee plate. *Spine.* 1991;16:S440–S444.
8. Davne SH, Myers DL. Complications of lumbar spinal fusion with transpedicular instrumentation. *Spine.* 1992;17:S184–S189.
9. Sasso RC, Cotler HB. Posterior instrumentation and fusion for unstable fractures and fracture-dislocations of the thoracic and lumbar spine. *Spine.* 1993;18:450–460.
10. Brantigan JW, Steffee AD, Keppler L, et al. Posterior lumbar interbody fusion technique using the variable screw placement spinal fixation system. *Spine.* 1992;6:175–200.
11. Lorenz M, Zindrick M, Schwaegler P, et al. A comparison of single-level fusions with and without hardware. *Spine.* 1991;16:S455–S458.
12. Steffee AD, Brantigam JW. The variable screw placement spinal fixation system. *Spine.* 1993;18:1160–1172.
13. West JL, Ogilvie JW, Bradford DS. Complications of the variable screw plate pedicle screw fixation. *Spine.* 1991;16:576–579.
14. Gurwitz GS, Dawson JM, McNamara MJ, et al. Biomechanical analysis of three surgical approaches for lumbar burst fractures using short-segment instrumentation. *Spine.* 1993;18:977–982.
15. Steffee AD, Keppler L. *VSP Plating System Technique Manual.* ACROMED Corporation, 3303 Carnegie Avenue, Cleveland, Ohio 44115.
16. Henstorf JE, Gaines RW, Steffee AD. Transpedicular fixation of spinal disorders with Steffee plates. *Surg Rounds Orthop.* March 1987; pp. 35–43.
17. Weinstein JN, Spratt KF, Spengler D, et al. Spinal pedicle fixation: reliability and validity of roentgenogram-based assessment and surgical factors on successful screw placement. *Spine.* 1988;13:1012–1018.
18. Gray H, Goss CM, ed. *Gray's Anatomy: Anatomy of the Human Body.* 29th ed. Philadelphia, Pa: Lea and Febiger; 1973:95–285.
19. Berry JL, Moran JM, Berg WS, et al. A morphometric study of human lumbar and selected thoracic vertebrae. *Spine.* 1987;12:362–367.
20. Krag MH, Weaver DL, Beynnon BD, et al. Morphometry of the thoracic and lumbar spine related to transpedicular screw placement for surgical spinal fixation. *Spine.* 1988;13:27–32.
21. Zindrick MR, Wiltse LL, Doornik A, et al. Analysis of the morphometric characteristics of the thoracic and lumbar pedicles. *Spine.* 1987;12:160–166.
22. Carson WL, Duffield RC, Arendt M, et al. Internal forces and moments in transpedicular spine instrumentation: the effect of pedicle screw angle and transfixation—the 4R-4Bar linkage concept. *Spine.* 1990;15:893–901.
23. Zindrick MR, Wiltse LL, Widell EH, et al. A biomechanical study of intrapeduncular screw fixation in the lumbosacral spine. *Clin Orthop.* 1986;203:99–112.
24. Asher M, Carson W, Heinig C, et al. A modular spinal rod linkage system to provide rotational stability. *Spine.* 1988;13:272–277.

26 The Fixatuer Interne (AO Modular Spine System)

Kenneth J. Easton, M.D., Emad A. El-Mehy, M.D., Hansen A. Yuan, M.D.

HISTORIC PERSPECTIVE

In 1977, Freidrich Magerl of Switzerland began using an external spinal skeletal fixation device (ESSF) for the stabilization of the lower thoracic and lumbar spine. This device was developed in an attempt to approach the stability observed with plate-pedicle screw systems[1] and to decrease the number of motion segments immobilized compared with the conventional rod-hook systems available at that time.[2,3] In 1984, Magerl published his data on 52 patients, including 42 acute fractures. His clinical results were encouraging, and the stability of the ESSF construct was shown to be superior compared with dorsal plating, Harrington distraction, and Jacobs distraction systems.[4]

The fixatuer interne (FI) was developed by Walter Dick at the Basle University Orthopedic Department in an attempt to decrease the bulkiness noted with the ESSF but retain the aforementioned advantages. These goals were accomplished and reported in 1987.[5] The clinical data consisted of 183 patients (111 fractures, 20 posttraumatic deformities, 16 degenerative, 16 spondylolistheses, 11 tumors, and 9 salvage procedures) with a minimum follow-up of 6 months. The results were excellent and gave good reason to be optimistic about the potential versatility of rod-pedicle screw fixation devices in treating a variety of orthopedic spine problems.

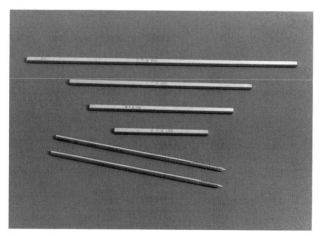

Figure 26–1. The 7-mm threaded rods come in lengths of 70 mm, 100 mm, 200 mm, and 300 mm. The 5-mm Schanz screws are available in 25-mm and 35-mm thread lengths. The 6-mm Schanz screws have a 35-mm thread length.

THE CURRENT DEVICE

The newest design of the fixatuer interne preserves the structural advantages of the original ESSF but adds even more user friendliness. The implant consists of Schanz screws (5 mm or 6 mm), a 7-mm threaded rod with flat sides (four different lengths), and clamps that rotate in the transverse plane (to allow ease of application of the clamps to the pedicle screws) and rotate and lock (via posterior nuts) in the sagittal plane (to correct any kyphotic deformity). These clamps can also translate and lock (via collared nuts) in a cephalad-caudad direction (to distract or compress). Figures 26–1 and 26–2 show the components of the system.

INDICATIONS FOR USE

Although used primarily for reduction and stabilization of thoracolumbar and lumbar burst fractures, the versatility of this device makes it useful in fracture dislocations (device used in a buttress mode) and Chance fractures (compression mode). The fixatuer interne has also been used in adult degenerative conditions, spondylolisthesis, tumor surgery, and for stabilization after correction of posttraumatic deformities.[5]

SURGICAL TECHNIQUE

Sequential compression devices and somatosensory evoked potential monitoring are used routinely during the operative procedure. The patient is positioned in the prone position on rolled blankets (or on any frame that permits postural reduction).

Pedicle Screw Insertion

The technique for insertion of the Schanz screws should be a method the surgeon finds comfortable and reproducible in his or her own hands. Many authors have noted the difficulty of inserting pedicle screws within the confines of the pedicle even under biplanar fluoroscopy. We describe a technique that has worked well for many years under the supervision of the senior author.

After midline exposure of the spine, the posterior landmarks for the pedicles are identified (Fig. 26–3), and a 3-mm burr is used to create a small entry site. Next, a 2-mm

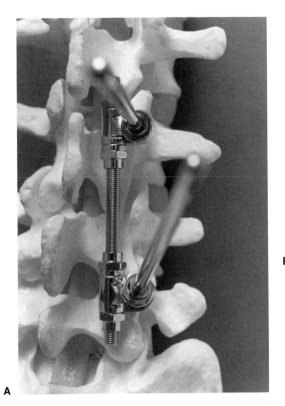

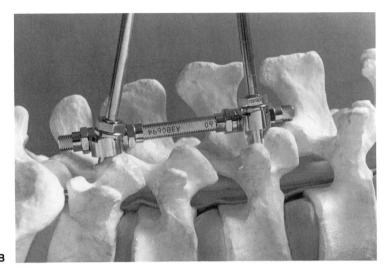

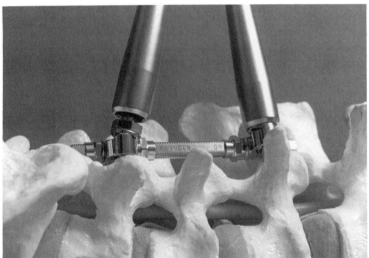

Figure 26–2. (**A**). The assembled fixatuer interne. (**B**). The fixator allows rotation and locking (via posterior nuts) in the sagittal plane. (**C**). The cannulated socket wrenches allow you to use the long-lever arm to restore the normal sagittal plane contour.

Kirschner wire is inserted. After all four wires are inserted, their position is checked on an anteroposterior (AP) projection (Fig. 26–4). The wires should converge slightly but not cross. A fluoroscopic lateral projection of the vertebrae is obtained to verify that the Kirschner wires are parallel to, or slightly angling toward, the superior endplate of the superior vertebrae and the inferior endplate of the inferior vertebrae. If the position of the Kirschner wires is optimal, they are sequentially removed and replaced with Schanz screws. The lateral soft tissue tends to push the surgeon's hand too medial and push the tip of the screw out laterally. A controlled

insertion of the screw following the exact path of the Kirschner wire is essential. Do not allow the screw to define its own path, or it will cut out of the pedicle a fair percentage of the time. In addition, do not penetrate the anterior cortex because the risk of injuring the vascular structures far outweighs the greater bone purchase obtained.

Assembling the Fixator

The flat sides of the threaded rods are placed in the sagittal plane to increase the flexion stability of the construct and to facilitate final crimping of the nut collars. The threaded rods

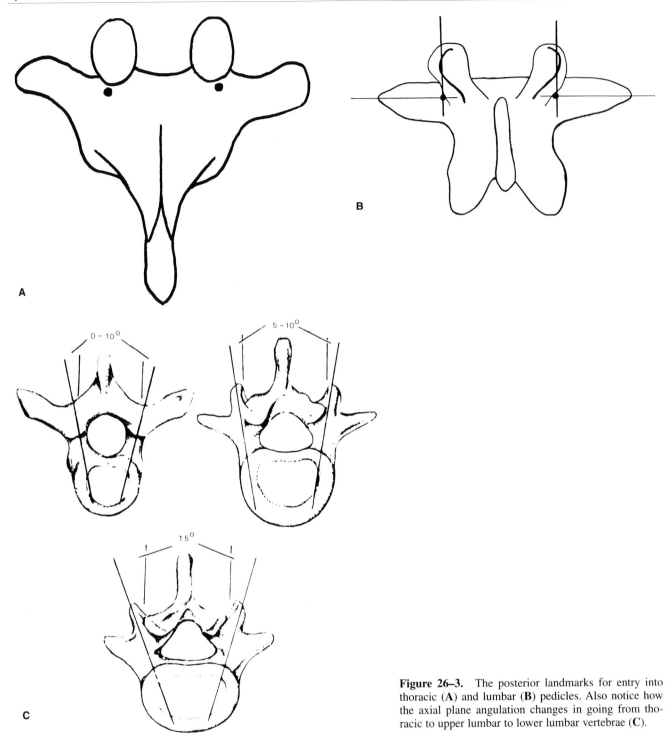

Figure 26–3. The posterior landmarks for entry into thoracic (**A**) and lumbar (**B**) pedicles. Also notice how the axial plane angulation changes in going from thoracic to upper lumbar to lower lumbar vertebrae (**C**).

of desired length are selected and the clamps and nuts are preassembled. The collared nuts are then loosened to allow free movement of the clamps, and the preassembled apparatus is slipped on the Schanz screws.

Fracture Reduction

The reduction sequence varies depending on the type of fracture one is reducing. The advantage of this system is that

one can rotate the screws (via clamps) in the sagittal plane, lock them in this position, and then distract or compress via the collared nuts.

BURST FRACTURES

The long-lever arm of the cannulated socket wrench on the Schanz screw makes correction of the kyphotic deformity simple. It is important that some distraction be ob-

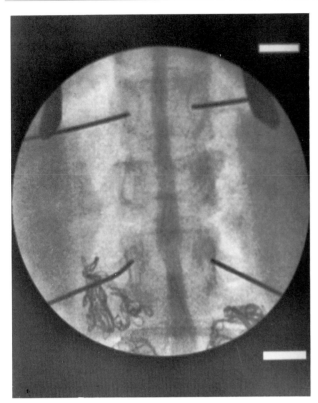

Figure 26–4. The Kirschner wires are shown optimally placed within the center of each pedicle.

tained prior to correction of kyphosis. Our technique is to distract until approximately 90% of the posterior vertebral height is restored and then loosen ("back off") both of the distraction nuts by 4 mm. The linkage now provides a safe fulcrum for lordosis restoration. To regain lordosis, place the socket wrenches on the posterior nuts, bring the handles together manually (in line with the rods), and then lock these nuts by turning the socket wrench handles clockwise. The inner distraction nuts are used to push the clamps away from one another and regain vertebral height. Finally, retighten all of the posterior nuts and crimp the distraction nut collars. Because the rod has two flat sides, crimping will prevent the nuts from loosening. Figures 26–5 and 26–6 shows the aforementioned reduction sequence.

FRACTURE DISLOCATIONS

Because these are extremely unstable injuries, they should be realigned carefully and stabilized with the fixator in a buttress mode. Crosslinking with 16-gauge wires is essential (Fig. 26–7).

CHANCE FRACTURES

The fixator should be placed in a compression mode (used as a tension band) to stabilize these fractures.

CLINICAL STUDY

Materials and Methods

From January 1987 to March 1991, we treated 32 unstable thoracolumbar fractures with posterior short-segment fusion and stabilization using the fixatuer interne. There were 22 males and 10 females whose average age at the time of fracture was 31 years (range 16 to 60 years). There was one fracture at T11, four at T12, nine at L1, eight at L2, six at L3, and four at L4. Among these were 23 burst fractures, six fracture dislocations, two seatbelt-type fractures, and one severe compression fracture. The average delay before operative intervention was 3 days (range 1 to 19 days). More than half of the patients were stabilized on the day of injury, and 90% were operated on within the first week. All patients were followed up a minimum of 6 months postoperative, with an average follow-up of 2 years.

The four radiographic measurements we obtained preoperatively, postoperatively, and at latest follow-up included kyphosis (degrees), anterior vertebral height loss (percentage of normal), anterior translation (percentage), and spinal canal compromise (percentage). A complete clinical assessment of each patient in the study was also done.

Results

RADIOGRAPHIC ASSESSMENT

The average preoperative kyphosis was 15 degrees (range of 6 degrees of lordosis to 36 degrees of kyphosis). The postoperative correction was to an average of 5 degrees lordosis, and at final follow-up the deformity averaged 8 degrees kyphosis (ie, 13 degrees loss of correction). The average peroperative anterior vertebral height loss was 60% (range 30% to 92%). The postoperative height was restored to 90%, and this was maintained at latest follow-up. The average preoperative anterior translation was 16% (range 3% to 50%). The postoperative translation measured 7% and worsened to 10% at final follow-up. The preoperative canal compromise averaged 60% (range 25% to 90%). This was corrected postoperatively to an average of 30%, and at final follow-up it measured only 20%. Ninety-four percent of our patients had a solid fusion radiographically.

CLINICAL ASSESSMENT

Twenty-five patients (78%) had complete relief of pain. Six patients (19%) had mild pain with activity that necessitated infrequent analgesics, and one patient required regular analgesics for moderate pain. The overall results were good in 23 patients (72%), fair in seven (22%), and poor in two (6%).

COMPLICATIONS

One dural tear occurred due to accidental slippage of the rongeur. This was repaired primarily, and there were no sub-

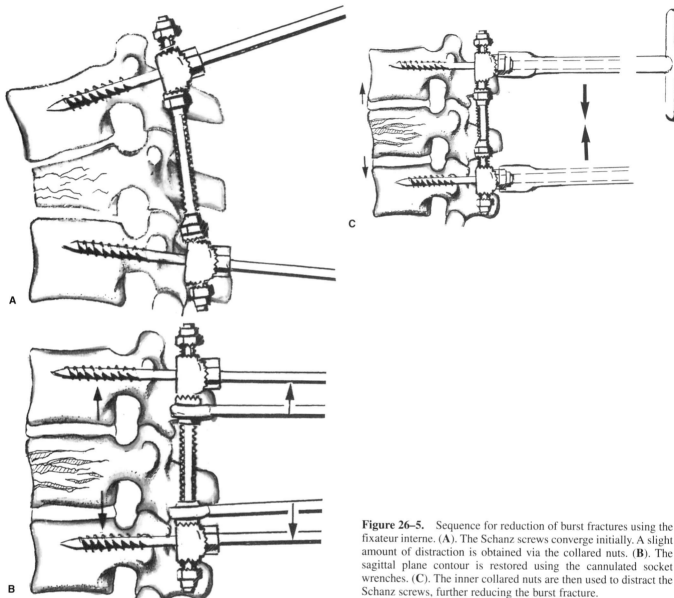

Figure 26–5. Sequence for reduction of burst fractures using the fixateur interne. (**A**). The Schanz screws converge initially. A slight amount of distraction is obtained via the collared nuts. (**B**). The sagittal plane contour is restored using the cannulated socket wrenches. (**C**). The inner collared nuts are then used to distract the Schanz screws, further reducing the burst fracture.

sequent neurological sequelae. In two cases there was penetration of the pedicle screw through the lateral cortex of the vertebral body, and in three cases there was late screw breakage. Two thin patients requested removal of the hardware because of irritation of the skin.

Discussion

KYPHOSIS CORRECTION

Other authors have reported the ability of the fixatuer interne to correct 10 to 15 degrees of sagittal plane deformity, but then lose 3 or 4 degrees correction at 1-year follow-up.[6–8] Our results were more dismal with regard to maintenance of this sagittal plane contour (we showed a loss of 13 degrees of correction). Because the anterior vertebral height

was initially well restored and stayed that way at latest follow-up, we feel that the recurrence of kyphotic deformity was most likely related to disk space collapse. This can be anticipated by evaluating the disk disruption noted (by magnetic resonance imaging, MRI) on initial films.

ANTERIOR VERTEBRAL HEIGHT

Aebi[6] noted initial anterior vertebral height of 57%, which was restored to 92% postoperatively and maintained at 88% at follow-up. These results are comparable with our results (ie, maintenance of 90% vertebral height).

ANTERIOR TRANSLATION

There are no other reports in the literature that address the correction of anterior translation with the fixatuer interne.

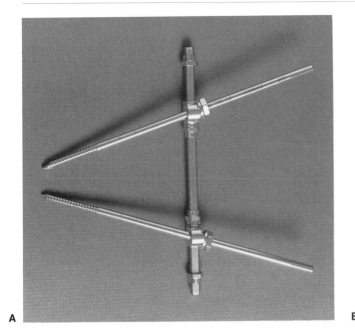

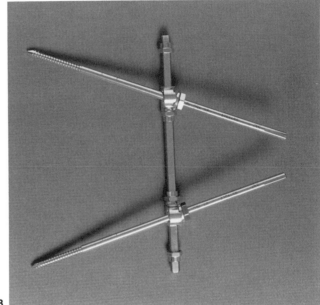

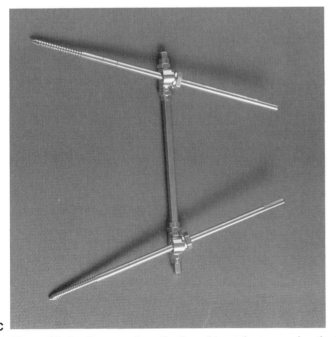

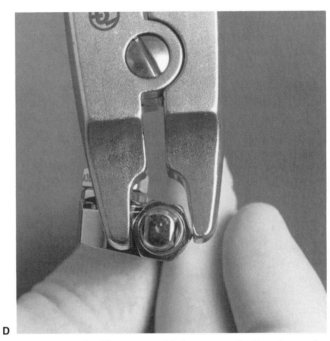

Figure 26–6.   Sequence for reduction of burst fractures using the fixatuer interne. (**A**). The preassembled apparatus is slipped over the Schanz screws. The Schanz screws are in a significant amount of kyphosis (ie, they converge) initially. A slight amount of distraction (as described in the text) is obtained via the collared nuts; then the sagittal plane contour is restored using the cannulated socket wrenches. (**B**). The lordosis is locked into place by tightening the posterior nuts. (**C**). Finally, the inner collared nuts are used to distract the Schanz screws. This is the most important step in reduction of the burst fracture. (**D**). The collared nuts are then crimped.

CANAL COMPROMISE

Esses[7] reported 60% canal compromise corrected to 30% postoperatively, and Gertzbein[8] noted canal compromise improvement from 54% to 40%. Oure results are slightly better than those and verify that remodeling can result in even more of a decrease in canal compromise with later follow-up. We feel, as do other authors, that the most important step in the reduction of a burst fracture is distraction.[9] Recent

studies have shown that it is the annulus fibrosis, and not the posterior longitudinal ligament, that is the important structure in the reduction of these difficult fractures.[10]

REFERENCES

1. Roy-Camille R, Saillant G, Berteaux D, Salgado V. Osteosynthesis of thoracolumbar spine fractures with metal plates

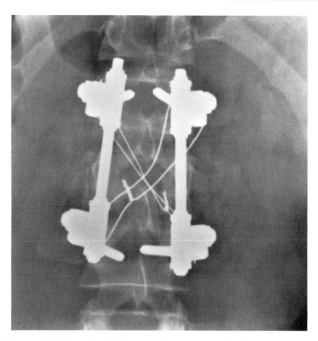

Figure 26–7. Crosslinking with 16-gauge wire is an effective means of adding more stability to the construct when a three-column injury exists.

screwed through the vertebral pedicles. *Reconstr Surg Traumatol.* 1976;15:2–16.

2. Dickson JH, Harrington PR, Erwin WD. Results of reduction and stabilization of the severely fractured thoracic and lumbar spine. *J Bone Joint Surg.* 1978;60A:799–805.

3. Flesch JR, Leider LL, Erickson DL, Chou SN, Bradford DS. Harrington instrumentation and spine fusion for unstable fractures and fracture-dislocations of the thoracic and lumbar spine. *J Bone Joint Surg.* 1977;59A:143–153.

4. Magerl FP. Stabilization of the lower thoracic and lumbar spine with external skeletal fixation. *Clin Orthop.* 1984;189:125–141.

5. Dick W. The "Fixatuer Interne" as a versatile implant for spine surgery. *Spine.* 1987;12:882–900.

6. Aebi M, Etter C, Kehl T, Thalgot J. Stabilization of the lower thoracic and lumbar spine with the internal spinal skeletal fixation system. *Spine.* 1987;12:544–551.

7. Esses SI, Botsford DJ, Wright T. Operative treatment of spinal fractures with the AO internal fixator. *Spine.* 1992;16:558–560.

8. Gertzbein SD, Crowe PJ, Fazl M, Schwartz M, Rowed D. Canal clearance in burst fractures using the AO internal fixator. *Spine.* 1992;17:558–560.

9. Fredrickson BE, Mann KA, Yuan HA, Lubicky JP. Reduction of the intracanal fragment in experimental burst fractures. *Spine.* 1988;13:267–271.

10. Fredrickson BE, Edwards WT, Rausching W, Bayley JC, Yuan HA. Vertebral burst fractures: an experimental, morphologic, and radiographic study. *Spine.* 1992;17:1012–1021.

27 Reduction–Fixation System for the Thoracic and Lumbar Spine

Robert Jacobson, M.D.

SYSTEM EVOLUTION

The reduction-fixation (RF) system was developed following a 5-year comprehensive study of the clinical problems confronted routinely by the practicing spine surgeon. The complexities faced in the treatment of spinal fractures and spondylolisthesis, coupled with the limitations of the instrumentation systems available to treat such conditions, pose significant challenges to the practicing spine surgeon.[1-4]

Although the use of Harrington rods has been considered the gold standard in the treatment of scoliosis and thoracolumbar fractures, the system lacked the versatility needed to correct most lumbar deformities without anterior or transpinal releases and forced manipulation.[4-6] More recently developed instrumentation systems (CD, TSRH, and ISOLA), though clearly answering some the technical problems encountered with the Harrington rod system, continue to encounter problems of hook dislodgement and laminar edge resorption, resulting in loosening of the construct. These systems lacked the capability to apply corrective forces gradually and maintain stable fixation in all dimensions or the ability to translate individual vertebrae in any direction.

FRACTURE CONSTRUCT DESIGN GOAL

Because most thoracolumbar fractures are caused by compression, flexion, and rotational forces, a system was needed that could generate controlled distraction, restore lordosis, and provide rotational control.[4-6] The system should provide the capability of controlling the position of individual vertebrae in all planes of motion, thereby allowing all necessary corrective forces to be applied by the implants. The system must also provide for the use of the shortest construct needed to reduce and fix the fracture to avoid the inclusion of noninvolved motion segments.

SPONDYLOLISTHESIS CONSTRUCT DESIGN GOAL

In situ posterior lateral fusion, with or without decompression, has been the standard treatment for spondylolisthesis. Many surgeons have encountered an unacceptable rate of pseudarthrosis, progression of the slip, loss of motion in normal segments above the slip, and residual deformity.[7,8] Because the spondylolisthesis deformity results from anterior slippage, loss of disk space height, and lumbosacral kyphosis, these forces must be counteracted to correct the deformity and provide for solid fusion.[5,9,10] The goal is to achieve full correction of the spondylolisthesis deformity with less surgery and morbidity.

To achieve this goal, a system that provides for simultaneous application of distraction, posterior translation, and double fixation at the sacrum is needed to correct the forces causing the spondylolisthesis. Additionally, the system should maintain the normal lordosis of the spine to allow for normal spine mechanics and prevent the cosmetic deformity.

The RF system was designed to counteract the forces of deformation and the resulting planes of instability that are secondary to vertebral body fracture or spondylolisthesis. By applying corrective forces to achieve both mechanical stabilization and restoration of normal anatomic alignment at each motion segment, reconstruction of the injured spine can be achieved.[3,7,9]

RF SYSTEM COMPONENTS

The RF system has five basic components, which are used to develop the constructs required to provide distraction, reduction, compression, translational stability, and rigid fixation.

RF Screws

The RF screws are offered in three designs (angled, threaded transpedicular, and self-locking) to accommodate the anatomic and biomechanical requirements encountered routinely in the reduction and stable fixation of spinal abnormalities.

The angled pedicle screws (Fig. 27–1) are designed to permit controlled application of corrective forces to produce kyphosis, lordosis, distraction, and compression. The screws are offered in four angles: 0°, 5°, 10°, and 15°. This measurement is the degree of angle between the U-shaped screw head and the shank of the screw. Each angled screw is offered in five diameters from 5.75 mm to 7 mm and four lengths, ranging from 35 mm to 50 mm. Versatility in screw

255

diameter, length, and angle provides for the variances in sizes required to meet a broad patient population. The U-shaped head of the screw, with a flat and concave side, prevents unwanted rotation of the screw within the pedicle yet provides for the application of corrective forces to control the vertebrae in all planes.

The normal thoracic kyphosis is used as a reference and the lumbar lordosis is created equal to, or slightly larger than, this measurement. In general, for T12 and L1 vertebral bodies, RF screws with 0° angulation are used to create a straight thoracolumbar junction. For vertebral bodies below L1 (L2 to L5), screws of 5° or 10° angulation are used to create lumbar lordosis, gradually increasing the degree of angulation at each level caudally. RF screws of 15° angulation are used for sacral fixation.

The RF transpedicular screw (Fig. 27–2) is offered in three lengths, ranging from 40 mm to 50 mm and provided in 6.25-mm and 6.50-mm diameters. An integrated hexagonal nut is located at the proximal end of the cancellous threaded section of the screw, which is used to insert the screw into the pedicle canal. There is also a hexagonal drive end at the proximal end of the machine-threaded section of the screw, which can be used to reduce a spondylolisthesis once the construct has been established.

The RF 6-mm self-locking screws (Fig. 27–3) are offered in five lengths, ranging from 25 mm to 45 mm. Self-locking screws are designed with two sets of threads. The distal cancellous threads provide secure fixation in the vertebral body,

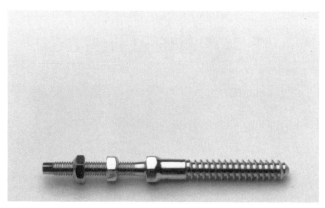

Figure 27–2. Transpedicular screws are used to reduce and stabilize in the AP plane, thereby avoiding the need to contour rods.

whereas the proximal threads lock the screw into the sacral block at the desired angle. The application of the self-locking screw/sacral block component provides double sacral fixation when L5 to S1 deformities are being treated.

RF Threaded Rods

The RF threaded longitudinal rods (Fig. 27–4) are 8 mm in diameter and are offered in 10 lengths, ranging from 35 mm to 150 mm. One side of the rod is flat; the other side of the rod is slotted to accommodate a set screw. When applied to the U-shaped screw heads, the rods prevent the screws from rotating within the pedicles, and the U-shaped head of the screws prevents the rod from rotating about the screws. The fully threaded rod permits controlled movement in both directions for segmental compression, distraction, or neutralization. Although not required in the majority of cases, the rods can be contoured in axial and sagittal planes up to 26° without destruction of the threads.

Two RF traction nuts (Fig. 27–5) are used to secure the U-shaped head screws to the threaded rods. A convex-sided traction nut is threaded onto the rod to engage the concave side of the U-shaped head screw. The flat-sided traction nut is threaded onto the rod to abut the flat side of the U-shaped head screw. Each traction nut is designed to accept 3-mm set screws, which prevent loosening of the traction nuts along the rod.

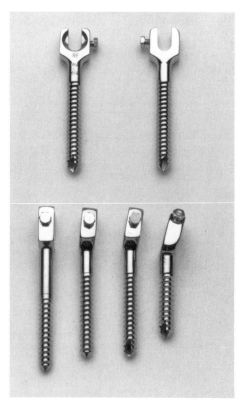

Figure 27–1. Four angled screw heads are used to develop and maintain lordosis.

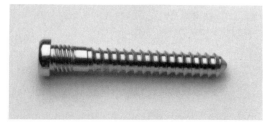

Figure 27–3. Self-locking screws are used primarily to provide additional fixation in the sacrum.

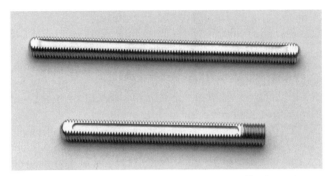

Figure 27–4. Threaded rods allow for the application of controlled compression or distraction.

RF Spondylolisthesis Block

The RF spondy block (Fig. 27–6) is used in conjunction with the threaded transpedicular screw gradually to reduce kyphosis, lateral, retro, or spondylolisthesis. The spondy block is designed to slide onto the threaded rod and be secured in place by a set screw. This block allows for the secure connection of the threaded transpedicular screw to the rod when lateral or medial insertion of the screw within the pedicle is required due to anatomic anomalies.

RF Sacral Block

The RF sacral block (Fig. 27–7) is used when double sacral fixation is desired. The block is threaded onto the end of the rod to abut the flat side to the 15° screw used in the S1 pedicle. It can be rotated to the desired angle to provide medial

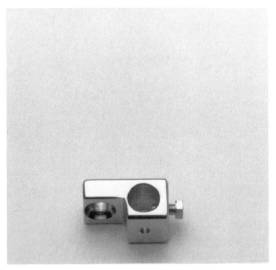

Figure 27–6. The spondy block is placed onto the threaded rod and can be positioned at the desired position to accept a screw placement that is more lateral or medial than superior or inferior screws.

or lateral placement of the self-locking screw. The sacral block is used primarily in the reduction and stabilization of L5 spondys when only the L5 to S1 disk space is being bridged by the construct.

RF Pullback Block

The RF pullback block (Fig. 27–8) is used for short-segment reduction and stabilization when one disk space is being bridged. Used in conjunction with the threaded transpedicular screw, the pullback block is threaded onto the end of the appropriate length rod (35, 40, or 50 mm). The pullback block is then placed over the threaded transpedicular screw and secured in place by tightening the hexagonal nuts on the threaded transpedicular screw. The rod is inserted into the U-shaped screw at the lower level and secured by use of the traction nuts. The use of this construct configuration provides the capability to stabilize and reduce a low-grade spondy yet minimize the number of levels included in the fusion.

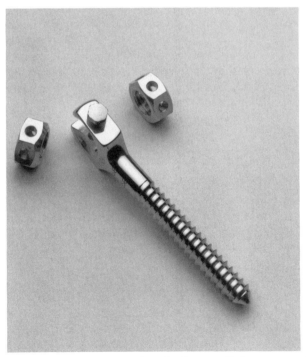

Figure 27–5. Traction nuts allow for the controlled movement of the R screws and blocks along the threaded rod and firm attachment of the screws to the rod.

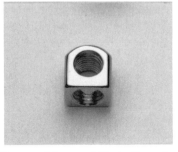

Figure 27–7. The use of the sacral block allows for the application of double sacral fixation when additional points of fixation are desired.

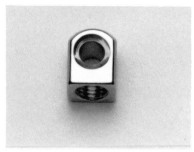

Figure 27–8. A pullback can be used when a single level reduction of grade I or II spondy is to be completed. The use of the pullback block allows for application of the construct even at the lowest lumbar level.

RF Transverse Fixation Assembly

The RF transverse fixation assembly (Fig. 27–9) is applied to the threaded rods to add strength to the total construct and to resist translational forces. Two transverse fixation assemblies are used in all fracture cases above L3, and one assembly is commonly used in nonfracture cases that span three levels above S1. They serve to improve the reduction of coronal plane deformity and to enhance construct stability.

CONSTRUCT DEVELOPMENT

The initial step in planning spinal reconstruction, following review of the radiographs, is selection of the construct. The RF components are assembled in various constructs depending on the biomechanical needs of the case. The application of compression or distraction forces is available with all RF constructs yet is not required for a stable construct.

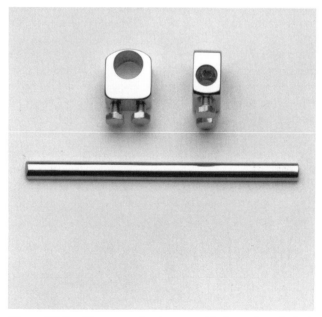

Figure 27–9. Transverse fixation assembly is used routinely in the treatment of unstable burst fracture or when three levels are to be fused.

Preoperative Planning

Careful review and analysis of standing and bending films—as well as contrast studies to determine the direction of forces causing the deformity, sites of neural compression, and the presence of bony obstacles that could prevent reduction and–or anatomic alignment—should be noted and planned for resection prior to instrumentation.

The selection of the most proximal and distal vertebrae that will be instrumented to maintain stable fixation without excessive construct length or incorporation of noninvolved motion segments is an important step in the planning process and will assist in the reduction of the overall operative time.

Selection of the implants and the order of their insertion is another important step in the planning process that allows for reduced operating room time and reduction of intraoperative blood loss.

SURGICAL TECHNIQUE

Posterior exposure with localization of the appropriate pedicle and placement of a 3-mm guide pin in each of the pedicles to be included in the reconstruction is done according to the description of Yuan.[7] The position of the guide pin should be centered within the pedicle canal and parallel to the endplate. Confirmation of pin placement is obtained by anteroposterior (AP) and lateral radiographs using an image intensifier.

Once the guide pins are in the correct position, the holes are tapped with a bone tap for insertion of the pedicle screw. The depth of the tapping is monitored in the lateral view by image intensifier, and screws of the appropriate length are determined. Appropriate angled screws are chosen before surgery for creating normal lumbar lordosis. For patients who have preinjury lateral plain films, the lordosis is gauged based on these films. For patients without preinjury lateral lumbar plain films, the thoracic kyphosis is used as a reference and the lumbar lordosis is created equal to or slightly larger than this measurement.

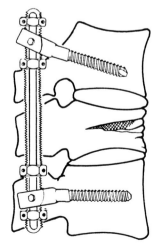

Figure 27–10. Initial location of RF screws within the pedicle canal prior to tightening of the traction nuts.

Treatment of Vertebral Body Fractures

The predetermined angled screws are only implanted into the vertebrae above and below the fractured vertebra. The threaded rods with paired traction nuts are inserted into the U-shaped screw heads and locked onto the screw head by tightening the set screws (Fig. 27–10).

Reduction of the burst fracture is completed as follows:

1. The traction nuts are tightened to the U-shaped head screw to create the lordosis necessary, as determined before surgery. Creating lordosis will not only reduce kyphotic deformity but also force the posterior longitudinal ligament, with its attaching bony fragments, anteriorly away from the neural tissue to enhance the effect of indirect neurological decompression (Fig. 27–11).

2. The angled screws are moved in opposite directions from each other by rotating the traction nuts. Such movement provides symmetric lordotic distraction for further reduction of vertebral height and intracanal fragments (Fig. 27–12).

3. After satisfactory reduction has been achieved, all nuts are locked to the rods by tightening the set screws. Two transverse fixation assemblies are applied routinely to provide additional stability. After secure reduction and fixation has been completed, a short fusion of the length of the instrumentation is completed using bone grafts (Fig. 27–13).

This construct configuration provides for the restoration of the disk space height, indirect decompression of the neural elements, alignment of the vertebral bodies to their normal anatomic position, and stable fixation of the fracture. Clinical and biomechanical reports[7,9,11] indicate that the RF fracture construct maintains the desired correction during

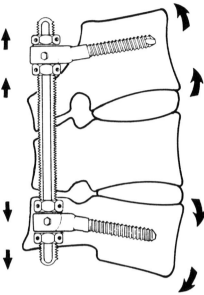

Figure 27–12. Compression or distraction of the vertebral bodies is achieved by moving the traction nuts towards or away from the end of the rod.

the bone consolidation period, thereby reducing the incidence of pseudarthrosis.[12,13]

Treatment of Degenerative Spondylolisthesis

The reduction and fixation of spondylolisthesis provides many advantages that are worthy of consideration. It (1) stops progression of the deformity, (2) limits fusion length, (3) permits decompression of the nerve root, (4) restores normal spine mechanics and alignment, (5) promotes union, and (6) reduces postoperative pain.

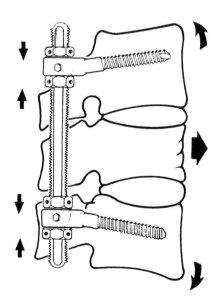

Figure 27–11. Tightening of the traction nuts against the angled heads of the screws places the vertebral body in the desired lordosis.

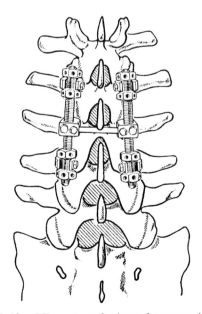

Figure 27–13. RF construct for burst fractures with transverse fixation assembly in place. Screws are not applied to the fractured vertebral body.

When necessary, decompressive laminectomies to correct stenosis in the central canal, lateral recess, and neural foramina are performed.[14,15] After decompression, reduction of the preexisting deformities and rigid fixation can be accomplished with the RF system.

With cases that present with a 50% slip or greater, three levels are included in the instrumentation. The U-shaped head screws of the appropriate length and angle are inserted into the level above and below the abnormal vertebra. The threaded transpedicular screws are inserted into the abnormal vertebra. A spondy block is attached to the threaded rod and secured in place with the flat traction nuts. The corresponding pairs of traction nuts are applied to the rod for securing the U-shaped head screws to the rod (Fig. 27–14). The rod, with the spondy block and traction nuts, is placed into the U-shaped head screw and over the threaded transpedicular screw.

The set screws on each U-shaped head screw are secured to the rod. Correction of the preexisting deformity is completed by distraction for longitudinal reduction of height and kyphotic reduction by tightening the traction nuts to the U-shaped screw head. Correction of the spondylolisthetic deformity in the sagittal plane is achieved by the posterior tightening of the threaded transpedicular screws (Fig. 27–15). Confirmation of alignment and vertebral body height is confirmed via image intensifier. Bone graft material is applied to a well-prepared fusion bed spanned by the instrumentation. A free fat graft obtained from subcutaneous tissue can be placed over exposed dura and nerve roots.

When the patients presents with less than a 50% slip and the bone stock is viable, a two-level construct can be used to reduce the spondy and provide anatomic alignment.

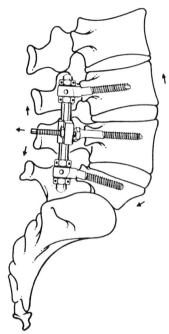

Figure 27–15. When the traction nut of the threaded transpedicular screw is tightened to the block, the deformity is reduced uniformly.

Threaded transpedicular screws are inserted into the abnormal vertebra in the method described previously. The pullback block is attached to the proximal end of a 35- or 40-mm threaded rod, and traction nuts are applied to the rod to secure the U-shaped screw at the lower level. The rod, with pullback block, is positioned over the the threaded transpedicular screw and seated within the U-shaped head of the distal screw. A locking nut is placed on the transpedicular screw and seated on the pullback block. Distraction is applied to the traction nuts on the distal screw, and posterior translation of the abnormal vertebra is achieved by seating the locking nut on the transpedicular screw (Fig. 27–16).

Until recently, the morbidity associated with the multistaged procedures needed for the reduction of major spondylolisthetic deformities severly restricted the indications for reduction. With the availability of an instrumentation system that provides for immediate anatomic alignment, controlled translational reduction, and two-level fixation, the indications for reduction have been expanded.

CLINICAL STUDIES

Treatment of Unstable Thoracolumbar Burst Fractures

Chang's[7,11] recently published study included 33 patients with thoracolumbar burst fractures treated by open reduction and internal fixation with the RF system, with a minimum postoperative follow-up period of 2 years. The mean follow-up was 32.7 months (range, 24 to 36 months). The average age of the patients was 33.5 years (range, 19 to 59 years). The vertebral level of injury was T12 in seven pa-

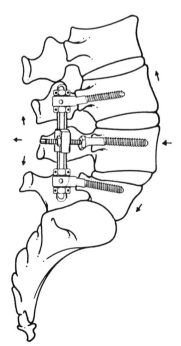

Figure 27–14. RF construct for treatment of spondylolisthesis where block and threaded transpedicular screw is used to reduce deformity to anatomic alignment.

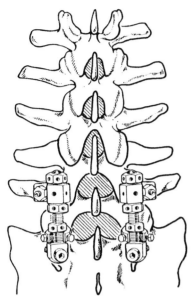

Figure 27–16. Application of the pullback block to treat an L5 spondy with only a construct that incorporates the L5 and S1 level.

tients, L1 in eight, L2 in five, L3 in seven, both L2 and L3 in one, and L4 in five. Twenty-seven patients had been injured in traffic accidents or in falling from heights and five in suicide attempts. Denis's classification of burst fractures[8] was used in the evaluation of all patients in this series: type A (9 patients), type B (15 patients), type C (5 patients), and type E (4 patients).

Plain roentgenography was performed before and after surgery and at follow-up. Computed tomography (CT) was performed before and after surgery for all patients. Spinal alignment, restoration of vertebral body height, and reduction of intracanal fragments were evaluated radiographically.

Alignment
Average preoperative vertebral body plus disk space height was 52% of normal (range, 39% to 77%). Average postoperative restoration of vertebral body plus disk space height for all constructs was 98% (range, 95% to 100%). The mean correction obtained at surgery was 48%. Maximum preoperative anteroposterior or lateral displacement was 11 mm

(range, 3 to 17 mm). Maximum postoperative anteroposterior or lateral displacement averaged 0.07 mm (range, 0 to 2 mm). For the majority of patients in this series, kyphosis was corrected completely. Average angulation was –1° of of kyphosis or 1° relative lordosis and 0° scoliosis (Table 27–1).

Neurological Decompression
Every patient presenting with incomplete neurological deficit showed significant neurological improvement. Of the five Frankel B patients, two improved to Frankel C, one improved to Frankel D, and two improved to Frankel E. Of the nine patients who were Frankel C, three improved to Frankel D and six improved to Frankel E. All seven patients who were Frankel D before surgery recovered normal strength and sensation after RF instrumentation (Table 27–2).

Maintenance of Correction
The effectiveness of any fixation device lies in its ability to provide maintenance of correction. The average loss of height for the disrupted disk space and fractured vertebral body was limited to 1%. The resulting average vertebral height plus disk space height at 24-month follow-up remained approximately 97% of normal. Maximum anteroposterior or lateral angulation (kyphosis or scoliosis) and correction of horizontal displacement (translation) were maintained with no significant loss in position. Overall, at 24-month follow-up, the RF system maintained average correction to within 97% of normal vertebral body plus disk space height, 0° angulation, and 0.7 mm of translation (Table 27–1).

All patients had a pain level evaluation at their 24-month follow-up. Twenty-three patients were in group 1 and reported themselves to be completely free of pain; 10 patients were in group 2 and had only occasional pain not requiring analgesics. No patients were in groups 3 or 4.

All patients had a minimum number of segments fixated (the fractured vertebra, one above and one below). Mean operating time was 2.0 hours (range, 1.7 to 2.4 hours). The average blood loss was 2 units. The rigidity of this system appeared to minimize postoperative pain and facilitate mobilization; all patients could begin rehabilitation in a

Table 27–1. Radiographic Evaluation in 33 Patients with Thoracolumbar Fractures.

	VERTEBRAL HEIGHT (%)		TRANSLATION (MM)		ANGULATION COBB METHOD (DEGREES)	
	Range	*Mean*	*Range*	*Mean*	*Range*	*Mean*
Preoperative	39–77	52	3–17	11	15–30	21
Postoperative	95–100	98	0–2	0.7	–1–+1	0
Correction	23–59	48	3–15	9.5	15–26	21
Follow-up (24 mo)	94–100	97	0–2	0.7	–1–+1	0
Loss of correction	0–1	1	None	None	None	None

Table 27–2. Preoperative and Postoperative Functional Neurological Levels.

| | | POSTOPERATIVE | | | | | |
| | FRANKEL FUNCTIONAL NEUROLOGICAL LEVEL | | | | | | |
Preoperative		A	B	C	D	E	Total
A	0	0	0	0	0	0	0
B	5	0	0	2	1	2	5
C	9	0	0	0	3	6	9
D	7	0	0	0	0	7	7
E	0	0	0	0	0	0	0
Total	21	0	0	2	4	15	21

light, external orthosis within 1 week. The mean hospitalization time was 15 days (range, 12 to 21 days).

Complications

There were no wound infections and no iatrogenic neurological deficits. Two cases had screw breakage occurring at 9 and 11 months because of nonunion of the fusion. Both cases were treated by repair of the nonunion and replacement of the broken screws, and results in both cases were satisfactory.

Medical complications were also relatively minor and all were resolved. The most common problem was catheter-related urinary tract infection in four cases.

Treatment of Degenerative Spondylolisthesis

In a 1989 study, Chang[12] reported a series of 16 consecutive patients with low-back pain presenting with degenerative spondylolisthesis, lumbar radiculopathy, and intermittent claudication who were treated with decompressive laminectomy and posterior lateral fusion, with reduction of deformities and rigid fixation using the RF system.

No patients had undergone prior lumbar surgery. Twelve patients were women and four were men. The average age at operation was 57.2 years (range, 48 to 75 years). Follow-up time averaged 27.5 months, with a minimum of 24 months and a maximum of 30 months.

All patients exhibited with grade II degenerative spondylolisthesis, as confirmed by radiographic films, and with an intact neural arch at the L4 to L5 level. Myelography demonstrated high-grade blockage at the L4 to L5 level with an hourglass-type constriction or complete blockage of radiographic contrast material. Decompressive laminectomy was performed at the L4 to L5 level in all 16 patients; decompression was also performed at L3 to L4 in three patients because of spinal stenosis at this level. A satisfactory outcome occurred in 14 patients (87%) and an unsatisfactory outcome in two (13%).

The average operating time was 167 minutes (range, 140 to 220 minutes), with an estimated blood loss averaging 950 mL (range, 350 to 1450 mL). The patients were generally ambulatory on the fourth or fifth postoperative day (average, 4.3; range, 2 to 7 days) and hospitalized for an average of 10.2 days (range, 8 to 19 days) after surgery. There were no intraoperative complications and no wound infections. No patients were neurologically worse postoperatively. The average blood loss averaged 950 mL (range, 350 to 1450 mL).

Maintenance of Correction

The spines of all patients in this series showed evidence of distraction with an increase in the height of the intervertebral disk space and neural foramena. All patients exhibited a decrease in their preoperative spondylolisthesis after surgery. Stress lateral flexion-extension radiographs at 1-year follow-up examination were obtained in all patients and showed no motion at fused sites. The degree of lumbar lordosis was determined by measuring the angle formed by a line drawn on the upper surface of the L1 vertebral body and a line drawn at the upper surface of the sacrum. This demonstrates that there were no cases of iatrogenic flat-back syndrome as the patient's lumbar lordosis was preserved in the presence of RF instrumentation.

SUMMARY

The RF system provided symmetric three-column lordotic distraction and rigid fixation, achieving near-anatomic reduction and maintenance of fixation in both series. The average vertebral body height was restored to 98% of normal, maximal translation was reduced to 0.7 mm, near complete correction of angulation was obtained, and 33% of additional canal cross-sectional area was restored. The rigidity of this system allowed rapid mobilization in a light, external orthosis within 1 week. The minimum follow-up in both series was 24 months. The RF system achieved the surgical goals of posterior instrumentation for treatment of thoracolumbar burst fractures and degenerative spondylolisthesis and thereby offers an effective tool in the spinal surgeon's reduction and fixation armamentarium.

REFERENCES

1. Aebi M, Etter C, Kehl T, Thalgott J. Stabilization of the lower thoracic and lumbar spine with the internal spinal skeletal fixation system. Indications, techniques and first results of treatment. *Spine.* 1987;12:544–551.

2. Akbarnia B, Fogarty J, Tayob A. Contoured Harrington instrumentation in the treatment of unstable spinal fractures. *Clin Orthop.* 1984;189:186–194.

3. Dove J. Internal fixation of the lumbar spine. *Clin Orthop.* 1986;203:134–140.

4. McAfee PC, Yuan HA, Glisson RR. A biomechanical analysis of spinal instrumentation systems in thoracolumbar fracture. *Spine.* 1985;10:204–217.

5. Edwards CC. Reduction of spondylolisthesis. In: DeWald RF, Bridwell K, eds. *Spinal Disorders.* Philadelphia, Pa: JB Lippincott; 1991.

6. Edwards CC, York JJ, Levine AM, et al. Determinants of spinal hook dislodgement. (Abstract). *Orthop Trans.* 1986;10:8.

7. Chang Kao-Wha, Zou DW, Donna MD, Fredrickson BE, Yuan HA. Mechanics of reduction of intracanal fragments thoracolumbar burst fractures. Presented at the International Conference on Spinal Surgery; November 1990; Taipei, Taiwan.

8. Denis F. The three column spine and its significance in the classification of acute thoracolumbar spinal injuries. *Spine.* 1983;8:817–831.

9. Chang KW, Zou DW, McAfee PC, et al. A comparative biomechanical study of spinal fixation using the combination spinal rod-plate and transpedicular screw fixation system. *J Spinal Disord.* 1989;1:257–266.

10. Kaneda K, Kazama H, Satoh S, Fujiya M. Follow-up study of medial facetectomies and posterolateral fusion with instrumentation in unstable degenerative spondylolisthesis. *Clin Orthop.* 1986;203:159–167.

11. Chang Kao-Wha. *A Reduction-Fixation Instrumentation System for Unstable Thoracolumbar and Lumbar Fractures. Spine.* 1992;17:879–886.

12. Chang Kao-Wha. Degenerative spondylolisthesis treated with reduction fixation system. *J Surg Assoc.* 1990;23:120–127.

13. Burton CV, Kirdaldy-Wills WH, Yong Hing K, Heithoff KB. Causes of failure of surgery on the lumbar spine. *Clin Orthop.* 1981;157:191–199.

14. Burton CV. Diagnosis and treatment of lateral spinal stenosis: Implications regarding the "failed back surgery syndrome." In Genant HK ed. *Spine.* San Francisco: University of California Press; 1984.

15. Ray CD. New methods for decompression in spinal stenosis. Audiocassettes CU-09, CU-10, from Symposium on Spinal Stenosis. American Association of Neurological Surgeons. Annual Meeting. April, 1983.

28 Kaneda Anterior Spinal Instrumentation

Mitchell G. Cohen, M.D., Paul C. McAfee, M.D.

INDICATIONS

Anterior procedures to the thoracolumbar spine have increased in prevalence among spine surgeons. The primary indication cited is to achieve anterior spinal canal decompression. Other indications are (1) the need to stabilize anteriorly in the presence of deficient bone secondary to trauma, tumor, infection, congenital causes, or deformity; (2) deficient bone posteriorly; (3) late kyphosis status postlaminectomy; and (4) late posttraumatic kyphosis. The evolution of anterior spinal instrumentation has made anterior spinal stabilization more desirable. The goals and benefits of internal fixation with a spinal fusion are to correct deformity, maintain rigidity and anatomic alignment, decrease pseudarthrosis rate, enhance postoperative management, and obviate the need for a second-stage posterior instrumentation procedure.

HISTORY

Anterior decompression and instrumentation of the thoracolumbar spine have become more common over the last 10 years. The spinal cord or cauda equina can become compromised secondary to tumor, fracture, degenerative disease, or other type of deformity. These pathologic conditions compromise the anterior spinal canal more than the posterior spinal canal. Therefore, it is only logical that an anterior spinal canal decompression would be the method of choice when there is anterior spinal canal compromise. In addition, anterior spinal reconstruction is frequently necessary after the decompression. To help stabilize and correct spinal alignment, anterior instrumentation has been developed and improved over the years.

Dwyer et al first used anterior spinal instrumentation in 1964 for correction of scoliosis using a cable and screw system.[1–3] A screw-staple assembly was drilled into each vertebral body on the convex side of the curvature. A braided titanium wire was passed through the screw heads and tension was applied (Fig. 28–1). Excellent results have been reported with its use.[1,4] However, the flexible cable resists only the tension force, and the elastic connection of the implants may lead to cable or screw failure with subsequent pseudarthrosis.[5,6] In addition, serious vascular and urologic complications have been documented.[7,8]

Zielke modified the Dwyer system in 1975 by substituting a compression rod with nuts for the cable and introducing a derotator to correct rotation and prevent kyphosis.[9] The system was made of stainless steel rather than titanium and appeared to have better pullout characteristics. It was designed for correction and stabilization of scoliosis and not designed to withstand the compressive forces in the anterior vertebral column following hemicorpectomy or total corpectomy or correction of kyphosis.

Slot[10] reported a distraction system using a heavy single rod device fixed to Zielke screws for the anterior correction of kyphotic deformities. The design is poor because it uses only one rod that does not control rotational forces well.

Kostuik developed an anterior modification of the classic posterior Harrington instrumentation (Fig. 28–2). Spinal screws are placed into the vertebral bodies and a Harrington distraction rod is placed through the screw heads and distracted. C washers lock the rod into place. A second, heavier Harrington compression rod is then placed posteriorly to the first rod. Complications have included screw breakage, rod breakage, and vertebral body fractures.[11,12] Although this is a two-rod system, it does not afford rotational stability because there are no crosslinks between the paravertebral rods. This was shown by Zdeblick et al[13] using a calf spine corpectomy model.

Dunn introduced his original device (Fig. 28–3) for use anteriorly in fractures of the anterior and middle column primarily for burst fractures.[14,15] Use of the Dunn device has been complicated by aortic rupture due to erosion of the device into the aorta.[16]

In 1984, Kaneda first reported the use of his own anterior spinal fixation device for stabilization after anterior decompression in the treatment of thoracolumbar burst fracture with neurological deficit.[17] The most recent configuration of the Kaneda anterior spinal device was tested biomechanically in comparison with the posterior instrumentation systems after a corpectomy model by Gurr et al in 1988.[18] They found that the Kaneda device compared favorably when compared with the Cotrel-Dubousset and Steffee posterior systems, which require the incorporation of two more motion segments. Another advantage of the Kaneda device is that an additional posterior procedure is not needed. If the Kaneda device does not cause a significant reduction in the stability before a solid fusion is obtained and if it is not as-

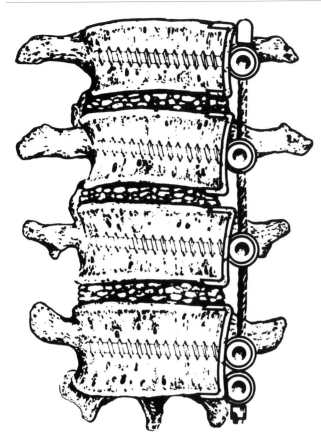

Figure 28–1. Dwyer cable.

sociated with any long-term problems related to its proximity to the abdominal viscera, it may offer specific advantages compared with other systems in stabilizing the spine after corpectomy. We have had favorable experience with the Kaneda device in anterior reconstruction of the thoracolumbar spine in the treatment of thoracolumbar burst fractures, tumors, degenerative disease, and deformity with or without neurological deficit.[19]

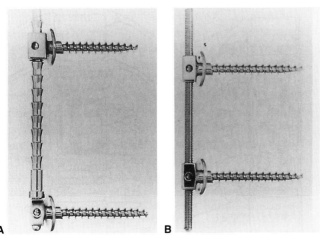

Figure 28–2. Kostuik anterior spinal system. (**A**). Harrington distraction rod and spinal screws with washers. (**B**). Harrington compression rod and spinal screws with washers.

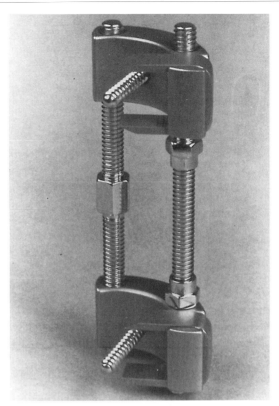

Figure 28–3. Dunn device.

KANEDA INSTRUMENTATION

The Kaneda anterior spinal device (Figs. 28–4A through G) consists of multiple parts: vertebral plate, vertebral body screw, rigid threaded rod, nut, and transverse fixators. The vertebral plate has four spikes that are seated into the lateral vertebral body. The vertebral screw is self-tapping. The rod diameter is 5.2 mm. The nuts are fixed into the screw head hole on the rod from both sides (Fig. 28–5). The final construct is shown in Figure 28–6. Multiple segments can be used for fixation with the Kaneda device. Figure 28–7 shows the scheme of anterior multisegmental fixation using the one-hole vertebral plate and screw. The most superior and inferior vertebral bodies are fixed with two screws, and the vertebral bodies in between are fixed with one screw. The transverse fixators are important biomechanically for elimination of the rotatory and flexion-extension instability. The Kaneda device can support both compressive and distractive forces. By turning the nuts on the rod, compressive or distractive forces can be applied.

ANTERIOR APPROACH TO THE THORACOLUMBAR SPINE

Positioning

The patient is placed on the operating table on two large rolls, left side up. One roll is anterior and one is posterior. Both rolls are parallel with the patient in the lateral decubi-

diaphragm is not necessary and the parietal pleural should be preserved intact; therefore, a chest tube is not necessary. In a series of 185 cases reported by McAfee et al,[23] there was not a single case of entrance into the visceral pleura of the ipsilateral lung. The major pulmonary problem was atelectasis of the contralateral lung from the surgery. Atelectasis and postoperative pneumonia developed on the dependent side. This can be prevented by the anesthesiologist performing vigorous endotracheal suctioning of the dependent lung immediately prior to extubation.

Complications of the Decompression

Prevention of neurological injury and optimizing the environment for neurological recovery is the main priority of anterior spinal surgery. There have been few reports of iatrogenic neurological injury in most series of anterior approaches. For trauma and unstable spinal conditions, there appears to be safety in visualizing directly the anterior aspect of the thecal sac. Anterior direct decompression of the spinal cord is safer than relying on ligamentotaxis and indirect, closed reduction of thoracolumbar fractures using posterior instrumentation.

We recommend thorough anterior disectomies above and below the fractured vertebral body prior to corpectomy. This orients the surgeon to the depth of the spinal canal and posterior longitudinal ligament. For infection cases wherein the fascial planes are disturbed and tissues are edematous, it is helpful to follow an intercostal nerve or the genitofemoral nerve into the thecal sac for orientation.

Dural tears must be closed meticulously, particularly in the thoracic levels, because there is less surrounding muscle to tamponade cerebrospinal fluid (CSF) leakage. Resistant CSF fistulas should be treated by inserting a diverting subarachnoid drain for 3 to 4 days, as was described by Kitchel et al.[24] If the subarachnoid drain cannot be placed in the spine, then a diverting ventriculostomy (temporary) can be considered.

Ipsilateral sympathectomy is an inadvertent result of the anterior decompression and to our knowledge leads to no long-term complications.

The segmental vessels must be transected in the anterior half of the vertebral bodies to allow for anastomotic channels to maintain cord viability. Spinal cord injury thought to be secondary to vascular interruption of segmental vessels has been reported with neuromuscular scoliosis. We prefer to use spinal cord monitoring for all anterior spinal decompressive procedures, but it is debatable if the cases of intraoperative deficit secondary to vascular interruption would be reversible.

Complications of Stabilization

Graft extrusion, penetration of the graft into the vertebral endplates, graft breakage, and pseudarthrosis are all more common in osteoporotic patients. In an effort to decrease these problems, we have been working with Brantigan et al in the development of a carbon fiber composite.[25,26] The car-

bon fiber is machined into a cagelike configuration that gives immediate stability, and the cancellous bone graft inside the cage confers long-term stability after arthrodesis.

The anterior instrumentation (usually consisting of 316 LVM stainless steel) is associated with breakage, loosening, vascular erosion, and metal allergy. The Dunn anterior spinal device had a large profile and was reported to cause six cases of late erosion of the vena cava. There are no known published cases of the Kaneda device eroding into the great vessels.

Infections are more difficult to treat with anterior instrumentation, but the incidence of infections is low even in Zielke and Dwyer's combined large series of over 1000 anterior procedures.[2]

An important concept to remember is that in the event of anterior instrumentation failure, it is rarely necessary to revise through an additional anterior approach. Almost all anterior instrumentation failures can be treated successfully with posterior segmental instrumentation (TSRH or CD) and fusion.

APPLICATIONS

The following are several examples of applications of the Kaneda device after our experience with 35 consecutive cases of the Kaneda device with two or more years follow-up.[21] Two of thirty-five cases of Kaneda instrumentation (5.7%) had breakage of Kaneda screws with pseudarthrosis 1 year postoperatively. This is comparable to the incidence encountered by Kaneda after his first 100 cases (6%). All cases were treated successfully by posterior spinal instrumentation and fusion. It was not necessary to remove the anterior hardware. One case had a deep wound infection 10 months postoperatively. Cultures were negative, and the patient recovered uneventfully (Table 28–1).

Table 28–1.   Baltimore Experience with Kaneda Instrumentation: 35 Cases.

Pseudarthrosis	2 cases
Iatrogenic neurological deficit	0 cases
Deep wound infection	1 case
Vascular complication	0 cases
Pneumothorax	0 cases
Migration of hardware requiring removal	0 cases
Postoperative kyphosis (>20 degrees)	0 cases

The first case presented is that of a 19-year-old male who jumped feet first into a water hole from about 20 feet. He suffered a burst fracture of L1 with retropulsion and canal compromise of at least 50% of the canal (Fig. 28–9). Physical exam was normal, but the patient complained of bilateral posterior thigh dysesthesia. He was treated with L1 corpectomy and iliac crest strut graft fusion with Kaneda instrumentation (Fig. 28–10). Postoperatively he had no complaints and was neurologically intact.

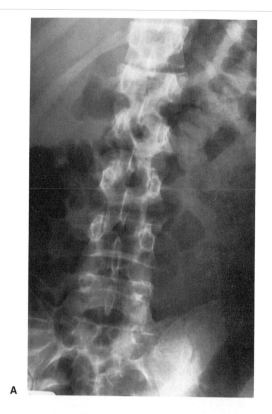

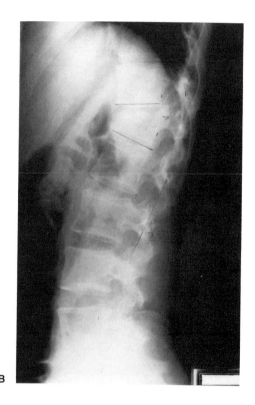

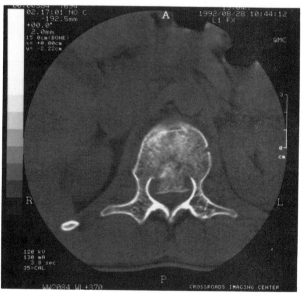

Figure 28–9. Preoperative radiographs of an L1 burst fracture. (**A**). AP view. (**B**). Lateral view with 28 degrees of kyphosis and retropulsed fragment. (**C**). CT scan of retropulsed fragment compromising at least 50% of the canal.

The next case is a 30-year-old male who sustained an L1 burst fracture from a motorcycle accident. He had an incomplete conus medularis injury with weakness in the left leg. He underwent Kaneda anterior instrumentation (Fig. 28–11) and postoperatively had a complete neurological recovery. Figure 28–12 shows ligamentotaxis with anterior instrumentation such as the Kaneda device. The posterior springing open of the neural arch is reduced by the use of distraction with the Kaneda instrumentation.

The next patient is a 34-year-old female who had a fracture dislocation T5 on T6 (Fig. 28–13). When she was log rolled at the referring hospital, she developed a T6 sensory level. This indicated the severe unstable nature of her injury. She underwent initial anterior decompression with insertion of Kaneda instrumentation. She was then stabilized posteriorly the same day with Cotrel-Dubosset instrumentation (Fig. 28–14). The key point this case shows is that anterior instrumentation should never be used alone with fracture dislocations. As it turned out, when we explored the patient posteriorly, she had four levels of lamina fractures and gross instability.

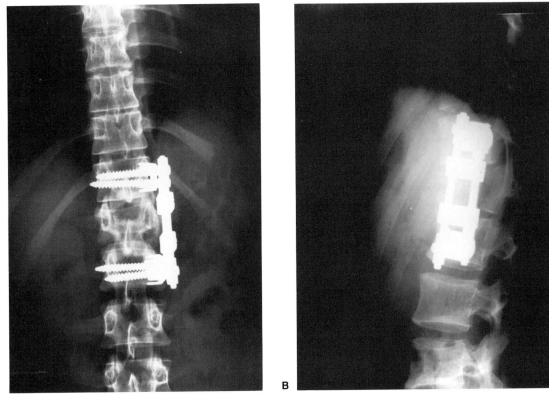

Figure 28–10. Postoperative radiograph. (**A**). AP view. (**B**). Lateral view.

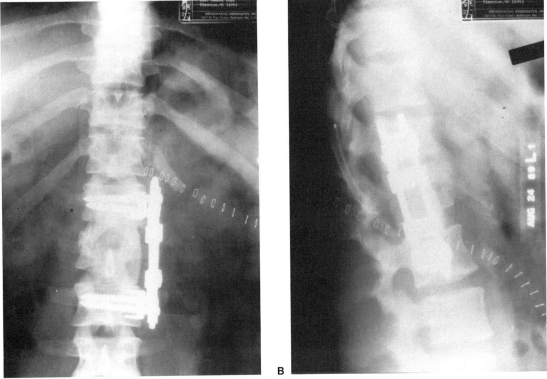

Figure 28–11. Postoperative radiograph. (**A**). AP view. (**B**). Lateral view.

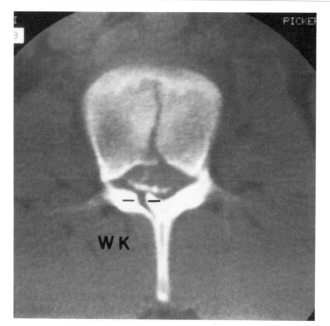

Figure 28–12. (A). CT scan with retropulsed fragment and fracture of posterior neural arch. (B). Postoperative CT scan demonstrating decompression of spinal canal and reduction of posterior neural arch fracture.

AVOIDING COMPLICATIONS

There are a number of techniques that one should remember while approaching the thoracolumbar spine anteriorly and implanting the Kaneda device and that should decrease the incidence of anterior instrumentation failure with the Kaneda device. First, during the approach to the thoracolumbar spine one must identify the genitofemoral nerve. The nerve originates from the spinal segment L1 and L2. It runs obliquely and caudad over the anterior surface of the psoas muscle. The nerve can be injured if retraction posteriorly to the psoas muscle is done too vigorously. The psoas muscle should be stripped adequately enough in a posterior direction to allow lateral placement of the device. This will also help in directing the screws in a coronal direction, staying out of the spinal canal. Additionally, all metal should be 1 cm away from the great vessels to avoid vascular complications.

While doing the anterior decompression of the retropulsed fragments, it is safest to start at the neural foramen level. By using a nerve root retractor, the nerve can be retracted and protected posteriorly at the neural foramen. The posterior longitudinal ligament should be stripped off the posterior aspect of the vertebral body. This will help decrease bleeding from the spinal canal. If there is epidural bleeding that cannot be coagulated directly with bipolar cauterization, Gelfoam packing may be used around the dura.

The vertebral plate should be placed directly into the lateral aspect of the vertebral body. The spikes on the plate must not enter the vertebral disk space. If the vertebral plate is too anterior, the instrumentation may rest on the aorta. Therefore, correct placement of the vertebral plate will allow for correct placement of the vertebral screws.

The screw tips should penetrate the contralateral cortex of the vertebral body. Blunt dissection with one's finger should

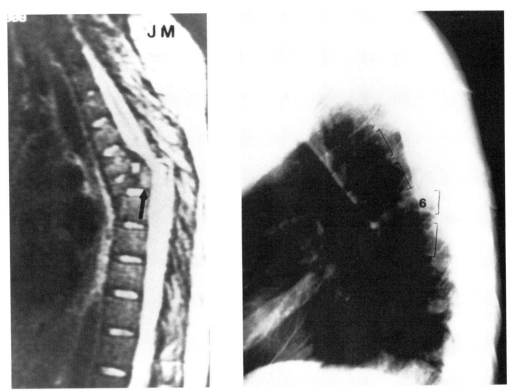

Figure 28–13. (**A**). MRI of thoracic spine showing a fracture/dislocation T5 on T6 with retropulsed fragment (arrow). (**B**). Lateral radiograph T5 on T6 fracture dislocation.

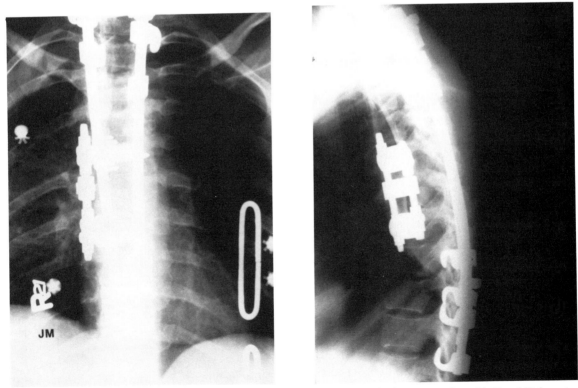

Figure 28–14. Postoperative radiograph. (**A**). AP view showing Kaneda anterior instrumentation with Cotrel-Dubosset instrumentation posteriorly. (**B**). Lateral view showing Kaneda and Cotrel-Dubosset instrumentation.

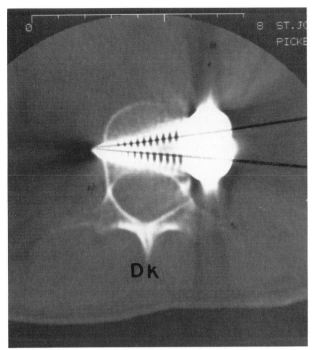

Figure 28–15. CT scan showing triangulation of vertebral body screws.

be done while protecting the great vessels to palpate the screw tips. In addition, the screws should converge within the vertebral bodies in a triangulated fashion to increase vertebral fixation at the metal-bone interface, particularly in osteopenic patients[21] (Fig. 28–15). The transverse approximators should always be applied to the construct because this improves the torsional rigidity of the Kaneda system.

Finally, it is essential to use tricortical iliac crest graft for anterior strut grafting. Bone chips from the resected vertebral body or rib are then packed between the anterior vertebral wall and the tricortical graft. The strut graft must be placed in compression by tightening the outer nuts on the paraverte-

bral rods. If the grafting is done in this fashion, it should allow for a stable anterior pillar that will not collapse.

An additional problem is osteoporosis. One innovative development in reconstructing anterior vertebral column defects is the Brantigan carbon fiber reinforced (CFR) cage.[25–28] The carbon fiber implant is radiolucent and it is machined into a cagelike configuration. It is packed with autogenous bone graft, combining the superior immediate compressive strength of the carbon fiber composite material with the advantages of long-term strength of autogenous bony fusion (Fig. 28–16). In our laboratory, the CFR cage demonstrated 10 times the compressive strength of allograft or autograft bone.[29]

SUMMARY

Anterior approaches to the thoracolumbar spine are often necessary in the treatment of a variety of pathologic conditions, including fractures, tumors, degenerative diseases, or infections. Reconstruction of the anterior spine includes resection of the pathologic lesion, anterior spinal canal decompression, correction of the deformity, and restoration of spinal stability. Over the last few years, anterior spinal instrumentation has evolved to become an accepted and safe technique for stabilizing the spine. Anterior spinal canal decompression can be performed safely and effectively because of advances in surgical instrumentation and techniques. As the clinical experience increases, anterior spinal decompression and instrumentation will become an even safer and more effective approach to the thoracolumbar spine.

REFERENCES

1. Dwyer AF, Newton NC, Sherwood AA. An anterior approach to scoliosis—a preliminary report. *Clin Orthop.* 1969;62:192–202.
2. Dwyer AF. Experience of anterior correction of scoliosis. *Clin Orthop.* 1973;93:191–214.

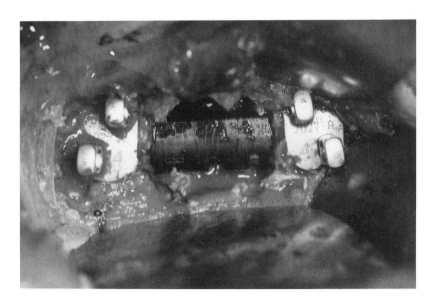

Figure 28–16. Carbon fiber cage in place.

3. Hall JE. Dwyer instrumentation in anterior fusion of the spine. *J Bone Joint Surg Am.* 1981;63:1188–1190.

4. Dwyer AF. Anterior instrumentation in scoliosis. *J Bone Joint Surg Br.* 1970;52:782–783.

5. Hall JE. The anterior approach to spinal deformities. *Orthop Clin Am.* 1972;3:81–98.

6. Hall JE, Gray J, Allen M. Dwyer instrumentation and spinal fusion. *J Bone Joint Surg.* 1977;59B:117.

7. Dwyer AP, O'Brien JP, Seal PP, et al. The late complications after the Dwyer anterior spinal instrumentation for scoliosis. *J Bone Joint Surg Br.* 1977;59:117.

8. McMaster WC, Silber I. An urological complication of Dwyer instrumentation. *J Bone Joint Surg Am.* 1975;57:710–711.

9. Chan DP. Zielke instrumentation. *AAOS Instructional Course Lectures.* 1983;32:208–209.

10. Slot GH. A new distraction system for the correction of kyphosis using the anterior approach. Presented at the Scoliosis Research Society, 1981, Montreal.

11. Kostuik JP. Anterior spinal cord decompression for lesions of the thoracic and lumbar spine, techniques, new methods of internal fixation results. *Spine.* 1983;8:512–531.

12. Kostuik JP. Anterior fixation for fractures of the thoracic and lumbar spine with or without neurologic involvement. *Clin Orthop.* 1984;189:103–115.

13. Zdeblick TA, Warden KE, Zou D, McAfee PC, Abitbol JJ. Anterior spinal fixators: a biomechanical in-vitro study. *Spine.* Vol 18:4,513–517.

14. Dunn HK. Anterior stabilization and decompression for thoracolumbar injuries. *Orthop Clin Am.* 1986;17:113–119.

15. Dunn HK. Spinal instrumentation. Part 1. Principles of posterior and anterior instrumentation. *AAOS Instructional Course Lectures.* 1983;32:192–202.

16. Jendrisak MD. Spontaneous abdominal aortic rupture from erosion by a lumbar spine fixation device. A case report. *Surgery.* 1986;99:631–633.

17. Kaneda A, Abumi K, Fujiya K. Burst fractures with neurologic deficits of the thoracolumbar spine, results of anterior decompression and stabilization with anterior instrumentation. *Spine.* 1984;9:788–795.

18. Gurr KR, McAfee PC, Shih CM. Biomechanical analysis of anterior and posterior instrumentation system after corpectomy: a calf spine model. *J Bone Joint Surg.* 1988;70A:1182–1191.

19. Kaneda K. Anterior approach and Kaneda instrumentation for lesions of the thoracic and lumbar spine. In: *The Textbook of Spinal Surgery.* Vol 2. Philadelphia, Pa: JP Lippincott; 1991:959–990.

20. Kostuik JP. Surgical approaches to the thoracic spine. In: *The Adult Spine Principles and Practice.* Vol 2. New York, NY: Raven Press; 1991:1243–1266.

21. Ruland CM, McAfee PC, Warden KE, Cunningham BW. Triangulation of pedicular instrumentation. A biomechanical analysis. *Spine.* 1991;6:5270–5276.

22. McAfee PC. Complications of anterior approaches to the thoracolumbar spine: emphasis on Kaneda instrumentation. *Clin Orthop.* In press.

23. McAfee PC, Bohlman HH, Yuan HA. Anterior decompression of traumatic thoracolumbar fractures with incomplete neural deficit using a retroperitoneal approach. *J Bone Joint Surg.* 1985;67A:89–104.

24. Kitchel S, Eismont F. Closed subarachnoid drainage for management of cerebro-spinal fluid leakage after an operation on the spine. *J Bone Joint Surg.* 1989;71A:984–987.

25. Brantigan JW, McAfee PC, Wang H, Orbegoso CM, Cunningham BC, Warden KE. The use of a carbon fiber implant in reconstructing anterior spinal column defects. *Orthop Trans.* 1992;16:139–140.

26. Brantigan JW, McAfee PC, Wang H, et al. Interbody lumbar fusion using a carbon fiber cage implant vs. allograft bone—an investigational study in the spanish goat. *Spine.* In press.

27. Shono Y, McAfee, PC, Cunningham BW, Brantigan JW. A biomechanical analysis of decompression and reconstruction methods in the cervical spine—emphasis on a carbon fiber composite cage. *J Bone Joint Surg.* In press.

28. Cunningham BW, Brantigan J, McAfee PC, Shono Y, Steffee AD. Reconstruction of the anterior spinal column defects utilizing a carbon fiber reinforced composite. In: *Transactions of the Thirty-Eighth Annual Meeting of the Orthopaedic Research Society, 1992.* Chicago, Ill: Ricter, Dickenson; 1992:168.

29. Brantigan JW, Steffee AD, Geiger JM. A carbon fiber implant to aid interbody fusion: mechanical testing. *Spine.* 1991;16:S277–S282.

29   Z-Plate Anterior Thoracolumbar Instrumentation

Thomas A. Zdeblick, M.D.

INTRODUCTION

The treatment of thoracolumbar burst fractures is evolving rapidly. Although fractures of the spine have been recognized for centuries, treatment of burst fractures is a relatively modern development. Historically, burst fractures with paralysis were treated with prolonged bed rest, which led to a 90% mortality rate.[1] Lorenz Boehler was the first physician to advocate postural reduction of the kyphotic spine using hyperextension and a body cast.[2] He then encouraged early ambulation and trunk-strengthening exercises to ensure patient rehabilitation. This treatment was echoed by Holdsworth in 1970, when he first classified spinal injuries and formally described the burst fracture.[3] His recommended treatment was postural reduction followed by bed rest and, eventually, a molded plaster body cast.

The adaptation of the Harrington distraction rods for the treatment of displaced burst fractures was a great step forward.[4–9] Distraction allowed some restoration of the height of the injured vertebrae, and fixation led to a higher percentage of fusions and to earlier patient mobilization. With modifications such as rod contouring and the use of sleeves, some reduction of the kyphosis and spinal canal clearance was possible. However, posterior distraction instrumentation has some drawbacks, such as the need for fixation two levels caudad and three levels cephalad to the fracture. Also, only semirigid fixation is achieved and supplemental external support is often necessary. Most importantly, posterior distraction utilizing ligamentotaxis may not lead to adequate clearance of the spinal canal and hence residual neurological compression.[10] Direct spinal canal decompression could only be achieved through an anterior or anterolateral decompression.

The anterolateral approach to the thoracolumbar spine was first described by Hodgson and Stock.[11] This approach was a retroperitoneal muscle-splitting approach. Their procedures were developed primarily for the drainage of tuberculous abscesses. In the 1950s, the anterior approach had begun to be utilized for the anterior fusion of scoliosis. Capener advocated anterior disk space fusion of the scoliotic curve.[12] Dwyer,[13] Hall,[14] and Zielke[15] all developed anterior instrumentation devices for the correction of scoliosis. In general, these fixation devices included a single vertebral body screw placed laterally, connected by a flexible cable or threaded rod that could then be compressed to help reduce the convexity of the scoliotic curve. This fixation was not rigid but was primarily a device used for reduction.

The retroperitoneal approach to the thoracolumbar spine for the decompression of late, malunited burst fractures was developed by Bohman.[16,17] These fractures were primarily treated late, after healing with a kyphotic malunion. McAfee et al noted substantial neurological recovery with late anterior decompression.[18] Anterior strut grafting alone, however, cannot stabilize an acutely fractured spine that has disruption of the posterior column. The nonunion rate when anterior fusion is performed without instrumentation ranges from 18% to 100% and averages 10% to 20%.[19–24] Because of this, several surgeons began recommending a two-stage operative procedure.[25–29] Typically, this entailed posterior instrumentation with distraction followed by the performance of intraoperative studies such as myelography or ultrasonography to assess canal clearance.[28,29] If compression of the canal persisted, an anterior or posterolateral decompression would then be carried out.

To reduce morbidity of a two-stage operation, anterior instrumentation after anterior decompression has been advocated as a single-stage procedure.[6,20,30–33] An anterior fixation device designed by Dunn had initial excellent results in both the reduction and fixation of thoracolumbar burst fractures.[20,21] This device was applied in the anterior/anterolateral spine with a screw and staple used for fixation. Although this device was eventually withdrawn because of late vascular injuries, other surgeons were more successful with the use of anterior thoracolumbar devices. Kostuik et al reported on 80 sequential patients treated with single-stage anterior decompression, bone grafting, and stabilization using the Kostuik-Harrington device.[31,32] He noted excellent neurological recovery in those patients with incomplete deficit. Kostuik found a nonunion rate of only 4%, although 16% had some type of hardware failure. Bradford and McBride compared 20 patients treated by anterior decompression and stabilization with 39 patients treated by posterior decompression and stabilization.[25] The neurological recovery rate was greater for those with anterior surgery (88% versus 64%), and inferior results correlated with residual

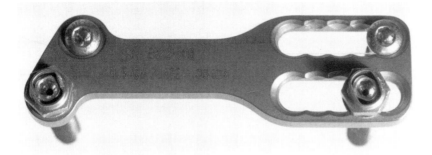

Figure 29–1. The Z-Plate (Danek Medical, Memphis, Tenn) is a titanium plate designed for use in the anterior thoracolumbar spine. It consists of two slots and two holes through which bolts and screws are placed.

bony canal stenosis identified on postoperative computed tomography (CT) scans.

Kaneda and coworkers have developed an anterior fixation device that employs vertebral body staples and screws connected by two threaded longitudinal rods that are crosslinked.[30] In the first 100 cases in the United States, 96% of patients have had some neurological recovery and the nonunion rate was 6%. More importantly, no vascular or neurological complications have occurred with this device. Static devices, such as the Armstrong plate or the Yuan I Plate, have also been effective in performing anterolateral fixation following decompression for fracture and–or tumor resection.[34] Most recently, Heller et al and Lowery have reported their early results using the Texas Scottish Rite Hospital (TSRH) screw and rod system as an anterior fixation device following corpectomy.[35,36] Both studies have shown low rates of hardware failure, high fusion rates, and excellent neurological recovery.

Few animal studies have been performed on the efficacy of anterior fixation followed by corpectomy. Zdeblick et al created a model of burst fracture treated by anterior corpectomy in the dog.[37] They performed anterior corpectomy and spacer application in seven dogs, anterior corpectomy followed by anterior arthrodesis with an ulnar strut in seven dogs, and an ulnar strut plus an anterior Kaneda-type instrumentation in seven dogs. They analyzed their results in terms of the rate of fusion, biomechanical rigidity, neuropathologic findings, and histomorphometric data. They found that the rate of fusion was significantly higher in the group using anterior instrumentation. In addition, the spines were stiffer in torsion than those that were uninstrumented. Minimal device-related osteopenia occurred in those spines treated with the anterior fixation device. Their conclusion was that, in the unstable spine, anterior bone grafting alone led to a high rate of nonunion and less mechanical rigidity than anterior grafting plus instrumentation.

Bench-top testing of anterior thoracolumbar fixation devices has led to a determination of the initial stability provided by these devices.[8,38–44] Jacobs et al tested the biomechanical stiffness of spinal constructs with simulated spine injuries.[8] Although he tested anterior vertebral body plates, he failed to report on their effectiveness. Gurr et al compared the mechanical stiffness of the Kaneda device construct with traditional posterior spinal constructs in a calf spine model.[38,39] They found that posterior pedicle screw

systems spanning five levels were equivalent to the Kaneda device spanning three levels. Ashman et al tested four anterior fixation systems: the Zielke-Slot, the Kostuik-Harrington device, the ASIF T plate, and a broad compression plate.[45,46] They found that the broad dynamic compression plate was stiffer in axial load and torsion than the other systems tested; in particular, they found the Kostuik-Harrington system to be less stiff in torsion.

Abumi et al compared an anterior Kaneda-type device with posterior Harrington compression rods and a transpedicular external fixator.[47] They found that the external fixator was superior in returning spinal stability in flexion extension and rotation. They felt that the Kaneda device, although it performed well in flexion and extension, was not as stable in rotation. However, this device did not include crosslink bars. Zdeblick et al, in a calf spine model, compared the biomechanical stiffness of the Kaneda device, the Kostuik-Harrington device, the TSRH vertebral body screw construct, and the Armstrong CASP plate.[44] Their tests were performed under torsion, flexion extension, and axial compression. They found that in torsion the Kostuik-Harrington device was unstable, whereas the Kaneda device was most rigid. In axial loading and flexion, the Kaneda device and the TSRH construct proved to be the most stiff. They concluded that the TSRH anterior vertebral body screw construct or the Kaneda device were most effective in restoring acute stability to the lumbar spine after corpectomy.

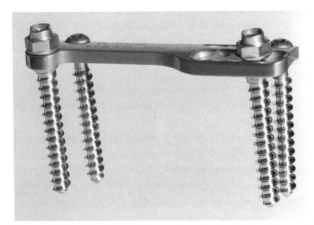

Figure 29–2. The rigid bolts are placed posteriorly and have a titanium nut that is crimped at the end of the procedure. The bolts are 7 mm in diameter. Titanium 6.5-mm screws are placed in the anterior hole and slot and engage the opposite cortex.

CLINICAL INDICATIONS

It appears clear that anterior decompression and stabilization plays a significant role in the treatment of thoracolumbar burst fractures. For those fractures without neurological deficit and with mild deformity, postural reduction followed by bed rest and casting is still indicated.[33,48,49] In general, those patients with less than 20 degrees of local kyphosis and less than 50% canal compromise can be treated adequately in this manner. With greater degrees of deformity but without neurological deficit, posterior reduction and stabilization with fusion is the treatment of choice. Fractures in the proximal thoracolumbar spine are best treated with either rod-hook devices or pedicle screw-rod devices.[50–56] In the mid to lower lumbar spine, pedicle screw fixation of one level above and below the fracture is indicated.[54,55]

In those patients with neurological deficit from a thoracolumbar burst fracture, I prefer to perform both anterior decompression and stabilization. This is based on the higher degree of neurological recovery following anterior decompression, the restoration of the height of the anterior and middle columns possible with the anterior approach, and the lower incidence of late collapse and settling with restoration of the anterior and middle columns.

If one is to treat with a single-stage anterior decompression and stabilization, the most rigid system should be chosen. However, there are numerous perceived difficulties of the current anterolateral fixation devices. Although the Kaneda device and the anterior TSRH system were rigid under biomechanical testing, both are high-profile systems with difficult insertion of the rods and crosslink. In addition, both devices are stainless steel, which makes postoperative imaging difficult. In cases of fracture, imaging for postoperative syringomyelia is best achieved with a magnetic resonance imaging (MRI) scan, which is precluded by the use of a stainless steel fixation device. For patients with tumor decompressions, following the tumor with either computed tomography (CT) scan or MRI scan is difficult with these stainless steel devices. Although plate devices such as the CASP or the Yuan plate are low-profile and easier to insert, they have shortcomings as well. With either plate device, one is not able to utilize the device in reduction of the kyphotic deformity (ie, distraction). In addition, once the device is placed, placing compression across the bone graft further increases the stability that can be achieved. Neither of these plate devices allows bone graft compression.

Z-PLATE DESIGN CRITERIA

The impetus for the design of a new anterior thoracolumbar fixation system was to remedy some of the difficulties with existing systems. The results of animal studies have shown that the increased rigidity of a fixation system will lead to an increased fusion rate and more rigid fusion mass. Therefore, we felt that the system should be as rigid as possible in the connections of the screws to the longitudinal member. In ad-

dition, it should have high pulloff strength (ie, the construct should not fail by pulling off of the vertebral body). This system should be low profile to prevent late vascular complications and to allow easy repair of the diaphragm. In addition, we felt that a system that was top loading versus using threaded rods or closed screws would be much easier for surgeon insertion, with a low "fiddle factor." Due to success using the Kaneda device as a dynamic device, we felt that the ability to distract (to help in the reduction of kyphosis) as well as the ability to compress after bone grafting were useful criteria. Finally, the materials that were used should be both MRI and CT compatible to allow postoperative imaging of the fracture and–or tumor site.

Implant design should incorporate a design for failure and removal. It was felt that this system should fail by loosening rather than screw or plate fracture. This would help reduce the incidence of loose implants in an inaccessible body cavity. It was felt that in-line loosening (ie, loosening of the bolt-plate interface without the loss of alignment) would be the preferred failure mode. We feel that we have met all of these criteria in the design of the Z-Plate anterior thoracolumbar system.

The plate is a titanium system with titanium bolts and screws. There are slots at the superior end and fixed holes at the inferior end of the plate (Fig. 29–1). The plate has a radius of curvature so that it is more closely applied to the curvature of the vertebral body (Fig. 29–2). The longer plates and the thoracic plates also have a curvature over their length to adapt to the normal kyphosis of the thoracic spine. There is both a thoracolumbar size and a thoracic size. It is recommended that the thoracic plates be used from T3 to T9 and the thoracolumbar plates be used from T9 to L4.

The system is utilized by placing a bolt into the vertebral body above and below, as well as a screw into the vertebral body above and below. The bolt-plate interface is rigid and the screw-plate interface is semirigid. However, this combination of a bolt and screw in each vertebra allows the system to be top loading and allows convergence of the bolt and screw for greater pulloff strength. The bolts, once placed, can be used to provide distraction to help reduce a kyphotic deformity. The plate is then applied and the bolts tightened partially. The slot allows compression to be placed across the bolts, compressing the bone graft before final tightening. The screws are placed convergent with the bolts to provide fixation into the vertebrae above and below. Finally, the nuts on the bolts are crimped, which provides additional stability. If the nuts loosen, the crimp will prevent them from disengaging from the bolt and becoming free in the thoracic or retroperitoneal space.

SURGICAL TECHNIQUE

The Z-Plate anterior thoracolumbar system (Danek Medical, Memphis, Tenn) is indicated for anterior spine stabilization following corpectomy for fracture, tumor, or following diskectomy and anterior bone grafting. The thoracolumbar

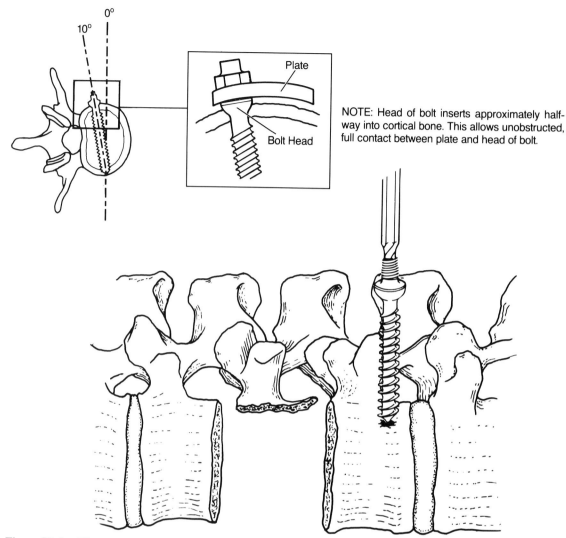

NOTE: Head of bolt inserts approximately half-way into cortical bone. This allows unobstructed, full contact between plate and head of bolt.

Figure 29–5.   The 7.0-mm bolt is inserted using the screwdriver. Tapping is not necessary. Care should be taken to remain parallel to the vertebral endplate and to angle slightly away from the spinal canal.

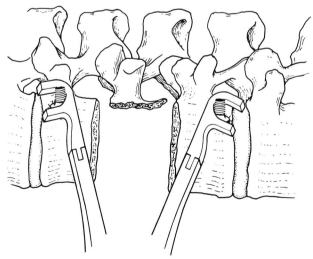

Figure 29–6.   Once both bolts are placed, if fracture reduction is required, reduction maneuvers can be performed at this point. This includes manual pressure on the patient's back, distraction using a laminar spreader within the corpectomy defect, and distraction against the bolts using the Z-Plate distractor.

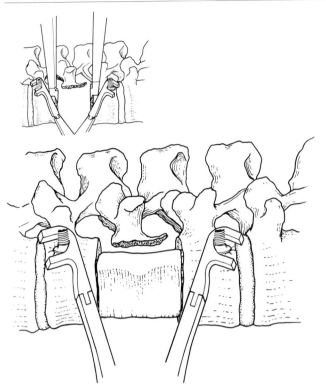

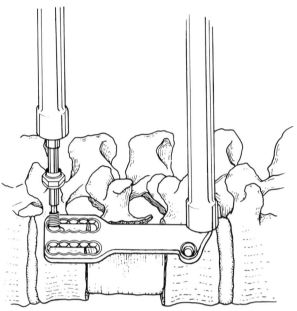

Figure 29–9. The starter shaft is left on the inferior nut as the superior nut is seated. Prior to final tightening, compression across the bone graft can be obtained.

Figure 29–7. Once distraction is complete, the length of bone graft is measured and an appropriate sized bone graft inserted. This maintains the reduced position of the spine.

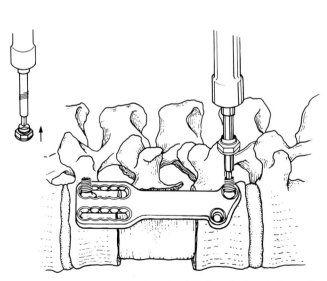

Figure 29–8. The appropriate sized Z-Plate is inserted over the bolts. The nuts are started using the nut starter shafts, the inferior nut first.

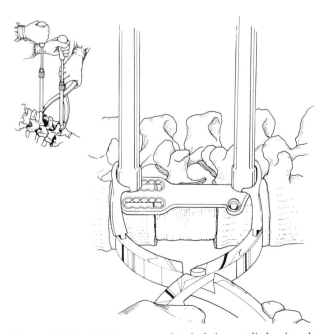

Figure 29–10. While compression is being applied using the Z-Plate compressor, final tightening of the nuts is completed. Care should be taken to maintain the starter shafts in a parallel fashion while compression is being applied.

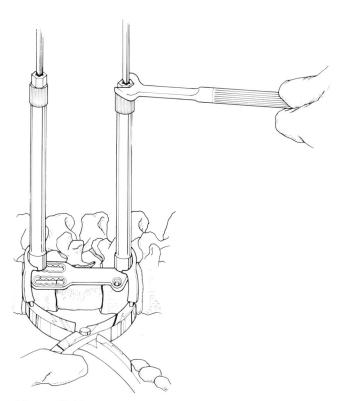

Figure 29–11. Final tightening is performed using the speed wrench and torque wrench while holding counter-torque on the screwdriver shaft.

The Z-Plate compressor is then used to compress the bone graft prior to final nut tightening (Fig. 29–10). The surgical assistant holds the nut starter shafts in a parallel fashion while the surgeon applies the Z-Plate compressor to the base of the nut starter shaft sockets. Compression is then applied and the nuts are then tightened fully while maintaining the parallel plane of the nut starter shafts.

Using the nut starter wrench, the inferior spiral lock nut is tightened while holding countertorque on the shaft handle (Fig. 29–11). Once the inferior nut has been tightened, the superior nut can then also be tightened, again maintaining countertorque on the shaft handle. Compression should be maintained using the compressor during the final tightening of both nuts. The compressor can then be removed. Final tightening of the spiral lock nuts is done using the crow's foot torque wrench. Final tightening should be to a minimum of 80 in-lb.

The two anterior screws are then implanted (Fig. 29–12). Screw placement sites are prepared using the awl. The anterior screws should be placed directly across the vertebral body perpendicular to the proximal cortex. Again, tapping is not necessary, and the screws should engage the opposite cortex. In general, they will need to be 5 mm longer than the bolt implanted in the same vertebral body. When placing the screw in the slot, one should make sure that the starting guide is used with the awl to ensure that the screw head set-

tles firmly into the base of one of the slots. An x-ray can then be obtained to ensure adequate placement of all spinal hardware. The Z-Plate crimper is used to crimp the nut collars onto the flat portion of the bolt. This will prevent postoperative disengagement of the nut from the bolt (Fig. 29–13).

Standard postoperative care should be followed. Typically, a TLSO molded brace is applied on the third postoperative day and ambulation allowed. Bracing is continued for 10 to 12 weeks or until solid fusion is noted on x-ray.

RESULTS

The Z-Plate was approved for use by the FDA in May 1993. Since then, 68 cases have been performed in the United States and 14 by the author. The longest follow-up is 1 year. To date, none of the author's implants have loosened, broken, or required revision, and none of the patients have developed neurological or vascular complications. Posterior instrumentation has not been required, even in the six unstable burst fractures that have been stabilized with the Z-Plate. Of course, longer follow-up is needed, but early clinical results have been encouraging. The system's low profile and ease of insertion have facilitated anterior instrumentation. Sufficient rigidity is present to provide an excellent biomechanical environment for early anterior fusion. Postoperative maintenance of reduction has been excellent. In addition, the use of the postoperative MRI scan has allowed us to visualize the neurological elements to assess the presence of syringomyelia, tumor recurrence, and adequacy of decompression postoperatively.

REFERENCES

1. Bedbrook GM. Treatment of thoracolumbar dislocation and fractures with paraplegia. *Clin Orthop.* 1975;112:27–43.
2. Boehler L. *The Treatment of Fractures.* Philadelphia, Pa: Grune & Stratton; 1956:323–340.
3. Holdsworth F. Fractures, dislocations, and fracture-dislocations of the spine. *J Bone Joint Surg.* 1970;52A:1534–1551.
4. Cotler JM, Vernace JV, Michalski JA. The use of Harrington rods in thoracolumbar fractures. *Orthop Clin Am.* 1986;17:87–103.
5. Dewald RL. Burst fractures of the thoracic and lumbar spine. *Clin Orthop.* 1984;189:150–161.
6. Dickson JH, Harrington PR, Erwin WD. Results of reduction and stabilization of the severely fractured thoracic and lumbar spine. *J Bone Joint Surg.* 1978;60A:799–805.
7. Flesch JR, Leider LL, Erickson DL, Chou SN, Bradford DS. Harrington instrumentation and spine fusion for unstable fractures and fracture-dislocations of the thoracic and lumbar spine. *J Bone Joint Surg.* 1977;59A:143–153.
8. Jacobs RR, Nordwall A, Nachemson A. Reduction, stability, and strength provided by internal fixation systems for thoracolumbar spinal injuries. *Clin Orthop.* 1982;171:300–308.
9. Keene JS, Wackwitz DL, Drummond DS, Breed AL. Compression-distraction instrumentation of unstable thoracolumbar fractures: anatomic results obtained with each type of injury and method of instrumentation. *Spine.* 1986;11:895–902.

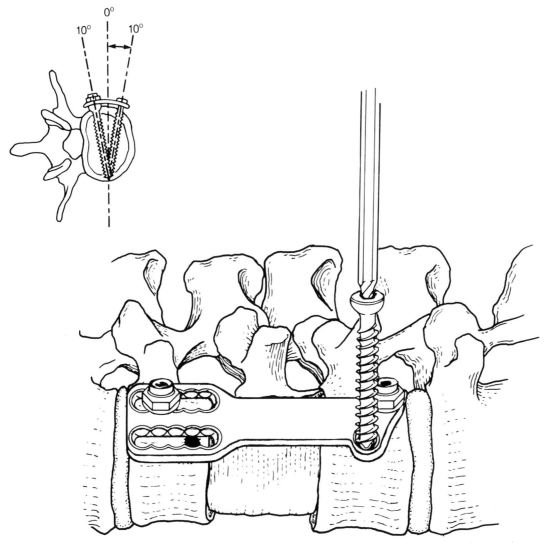

Figure 29–12.   The two anterior 6.5 mm screws are inserted in starting points as shown. These should engage the opposite cortex and angle slightly toward the spinal canal.

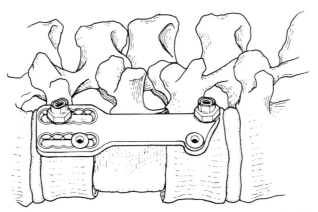

Figure 29–13.   The final step is to crimp the nut collars using the crimp device prior to wound closure.

10. Gertzbein SD, MacMichael D, Tile M. Harrington instrumentation as a method of fixation in fractures of the spine. A critical analysis of deficiencies. *J Bone Joint Surg.* 1982;64B: 526–529.

11. Hodgson AR, Stock FE. Anterior spinal fusion. A preliminary communication on radical treatment of Pott's disease and Pott's paraplegia. *Br J Surg.* 1956;44:266–275.

12. Capener N. The evolution of lateral rachitomy. *J Bone Joint Surg.* 1954;36B:173–179.

13. Dwyer AF, Newton NC. An anterior approach to scoliosis—a preliminary report. *Clin Orthop.* 1969;62:192–202.

14. Hall JE. The anterior approach to spinal deformities. *Orthop Clin N Am.* 1972;3:81–98.

15. Zielke K. Ventral derotation spondylodese: behandlungsergebnisse bei idiopathischen lumbarskoliosen. *Z Orthop.* 1982;120: 320–329.

16. Bohlman HH. Current concepts review. Treatment of fractures and dislocations of the thoracic and lumbar spine. *J Bone Joint Surg.* 1985;67A:165–169.

17. Bohlman HH, Freehafer A, DeJak J. Free anterior decompression of spinal cord injuries. *J Bone Joint Surg.* 1975;57A:1025.

18. McAfee PC, Bohlman HH, Yuan HA. Anterior decompression of traumatic thoracolumbar fractures with incomplete neurological deficit using a retroperitoneal approach. *J Bone Joint Surg.* 1985;67A:89–104.

19. Benzel EC, Larson SJ. Functional recovery after decompressive operation for thoracic and lumbar spine fractures. *Neurosurgery.* 1986;19:772–778.

20. Dunn HK. Anterior stabilization of thoracolumbar injuries. *Clin Orthop.* 1984;189:116–125.

21. Dunn HK, Goble EM, McBride GG, Daniels AU. An implant system for anterior spine stabilization. *Orthop Trans.* 1981; 5:433–434.

22. Flynn JC, Hoque MA. Anterior fusion of the lumbar spine. End-result study with long-term follow-up. *J Bone Joint Surg.* 1979;61A:1143–1150.

23. Freebody D, Bendall R, Taylor RD. Anterior transperitoneal lumbar fusion. *J Bone Joint Surg.* 1971;53B:617–627.

24. Riska EB, Myllynen P, Bostman O. Anterolateral decompression for neural involvement in thoracolumbar fractures. A review of 78 cases. *J Bone Joint Surg.* 1987;69B:704–708.

25. Bradford DS, McBride GG. Surgical management of thoracolumbar spine fractures with incomplete neurologic deficits. *Clin Orthop.* 1987;218:201–216.

26. Dall BE, Stauffer ES. Neurologic injury and recovery patterns in burst fractures at the T12 or L1 motion segment. *Clin Orthop.* 1988;233:171–176.

27. Dennis F, Armstrong GWD, Searls K, Matta L. Acute thoracolumbar burst fractures in the absence of neurologic deficit. A comparison between operative and nonoperative treatment. *Clin Orthop.* 1984;189:142–149.

28. Eismont FJ, Green BA, Berkowitz BM, Montalvo BM, Quencer RM, Brown MJ. The role of intraoperative ultrasonography in the treatment of thoracic and lumbar spine fractures. *Spine.* 1984;9:782–787.

29. Garfin SR, Mowery CA, Guerra J Jr, Marshall LF. Confirmation of the posterolateral technique to decompress and fuse thoracolumbar spine burst fractures. *Spine.* 1985;10:218–223.

30. Kaneda K, Abumi K, Fujiya M. Burst fractures with neurologic deficits of the thoracolumbar spine. Results of anterior decompression and stabilization with anterior instrumentation. *Spine.* 1984;9:788–795.

31. Kostuik JP. Anterior spinal cord decompression for lesions of the thoracic and lumbar spine, techniques, new methods of internal fixation results. *Spine.* 1983;8:512–531.

32. Kostuik JP. Anterior fixation for fractures of the thoracic and lumbar spine with or without neurologic involvement. *Clin Orthop.* 1984;189:103–115.

33. Schmidek HH, Gomes FB, Seligson D, McSherry JW. Management of acute unstable thoracolumbar (T11–L1) fractures with and without neurological deficit. *Neurosurgery.* 1980;7:30–35.

34. Yuan HA, Mann KA, Found EM, et al. Early clinical experience with the Syracuse I-Plate: an anterior spinal fixation device. *Spine.* 1988;13:278–285.

35. Heller JH, Zdeblick TA, Kunz DN, McCabe RP, Cooke ME. Stability of spinal constructs for metastatic disease. Presented at the North American Spine Society Annual Meeting; August 1, 1991; Keystone, Colo.

36. Lowery G. Unpublished data.

37. Zdeblick TA, Shirado O, McAfee PC, deGroot H, Warden KE. Anterior spinal fixation after corpectomy: a study in dogs. *J Bone Joint Surg.* 1991;73A:527–534.

38. Gurr KR, McAfee PC, Shih CM. Biomechanical analysis of anterior and posterior instrumentation systems after corpectomy. A calf spine model. *J Bone Joint Surg.* 1988;70A:1182–1191.

39. Gurr KR, McAfee PC, Warden KE, Shih CM. Roentgenographic and biomechanical analysis of lumbar fusions: a canine model. *J Orthop Res.* 1989;7:838–848.

40. Johnston C. Spinal rigidity following instrumentation. Read at the Combined Meeting of the Scoliosis Research Society and the European Spinal Deformities Society; September 18, 1989; Amsterdam, The Netherlands.

41. McAfee PC. Biomechanical approach to instrumentation of the thoracolumbar spine. A review article. *Adv Orthop Surg.* 1985;8:313–327.

42. McAfee PC, Regan JJ, Farey ID, Gurr KR, Warden KE. The biomechanical and histomorphometric properties of anterior lumbar fusions. A canine model. *J Spinal Dis.* 1988;1:101–110.

43. McAfee PC, Farey ID, Sutterlin CE, Gurr KR, Warden KE, Cunningham BW. Device-related osteoporosis with spinal instrumentation. *Spine.* 1989;14:919–926.

44. Zdeblick TA, Warden KE, Zou D, McAfee PC, Abitbol JJ. Anterior spinal fixators: a biomechanical in-vitro study. *Spine.* 1993;18:513–517.

45. Ashman RB, Bechtold JE, Edwards WT. In-vitro spinal arthrodesis implant mechanical testing protocols. *J Spinal Dis.* 1989;2:274–481.

46. Ashman RB, Birch JG, Bone LB. Mechanical testing of spinal instrumentation. *Clin Orthop.* 1988;227:113–125.

47. Abumi K, Panjabi MM, Duranceau J. Biomechanical evaluation of spinal fixation devices. Part III: stability provided by six spinal fixation devices and interbody bone graft. *Spine.* 1989;14:1249–1255.

48. Reid DC, Hu R, Davis LA, Saboe LA. The nonoperative treatment of burst fractures of the thoracolumbar junction. *J Trauma.* 1988;28:1188–1194.

49. Weinstein JN, Collalto P, Lehmann TR. Thoracolumbar burst fractures treated conservatively: a long-term follow-up. *Spine.* 1988;13:33–38.

50. Aebi M, Etter C, Kehl T, Thalgott J. Stabilization of the lower thoracic and lumbar spine with the internal spinal skeletal fixation system. Indications, techniques, and first results of treatment. *Spine.* 1987;12:544–551.

51. Cotrel Y, Dubousset J, Guillamat M. New universal instrumentation in spinal surgery. *Clin Orthop.* 1988;227:10–23.

52. Dick W. "The fixateur interne" as a versatile implant for spine surgery. *Spine.* 1987;12:882–900.

53. Jelsma RK, Kirsch PT, Jelsma LF, Ramsey WC, Rive JF. Surgical treatment of thoracolumbar fractures. *Surg Neurol.* 1982;18:156–166.

54. Krag MH, Beynnon BD, Pope MH, Frymoyer JW, Haugh LD, Weaver DL. An internal fixator for posterior application to short segments of the thoracic, lumbar, or lumbosacral spine. Design and testing. *Clin Orthop.* 1986;203:75–98.

55. Levine AM, Edwards CC. Low lumbar burst fractures. Reduction and stabilization using the modular spine fixation system. *Orthopedics.* 1988;11:1427–1432.

56. Magerl FP. Stabilization of the lower thoracic and lumbar spine with external skeletal fixation. *Clin Orthop.* 1984;189: 125–141.

30 Anterior Locking Plate System for Anterior Spine Fixation

Jen-Yuh Chen, M.D., Ronald C. Allen, Ph.D.

INTRODUCTION

The standard treatment for incapacitating spinal conditions secondary to congenital deformity, trauma, neoplasia, or degeneration has been the stabilization of the spine in the involved area. The most common method of spinal stabilization has been posterior rod instrumentation using sublaminar hooks. Posterior instrumentation has continued to be used successfully in the treatment of scoliosis, multiple-segment instability, fracture, and spondylolisthesis.[1-3] By applying distraction and ligamentotaxis, the deformity can often be reduced, thereby providing indirect decompression of the neural elements and early ambulation of the patient.[4]

When posterior stabilization failed to decompress the neural elements or control progressive kyphosis, the patient would normally be restudied for an anterior procedure when direct decompression and anterior stabilization would be completed.[4-7] The cost and morbidity associated with multiple procedures has driven the demand for more effective techniques that provide direct neural decompression and spine stabilization[8] without the morbidity associated with earlier anterior techniques.

With the introduction of anterior spinal fixation systems, anterior decompression has been used successfully in treating cord compression caused by a variety of different lesions.[9-12] In a study of 25 patients by Johnson et al,[13] improvement in neurological functions was obtained in all groups treated for fracture, neoplasm, infection, and congenital deformity. The results of the Johnson study have been reinforced by similar experiences of others.[1,5,14,15]

Ideally, neural decompression should be performed in a single anterior operation when the cause of impingement to the neural elements is located in the anterior column. There are several devices available[6,9,10-12] for use in anterior spinal stabilization procedures that assist the spine surgeon in achieving this goal. Of the various devices available, the anterior locking plate system (ALPS) provides effective stabilization and fixation in the treatment of burst fractures, tumor, and progressive kyphosis.

DESIGN GOALS

The ALPS device was designed for use on the dorsolateral aspect of the vertebral bodies. The primary indication for use of the ALPS device is to treat unstable vertebral bodies secondary to fracture, tumor, and kyphotic deformity. It has been well established that fixation devices applied to the anterior vertebral bodies of the lower thoracic and lumbar spine are subjected to axial, torsional, and bending (flexion and extension) forces.[16,17]

Axial loading of the spine occurs repeatedly as an individual stands, sits, or walks. Such loads have been reported[6] to range from 1.5 to 2.5 times the individual's weight above the waist. Early plate and screw constructs, in which the plate and screws do not lock together, often loosen after repeated loading and unloading of the construct due to what we define as progressive loading of the construct. As axial load is applied, it is transmitted to the superior screw, which causes the screw to move inferiorly and disengage from the plate. This progressive form of loading and unloading is believed to be the primary cause of screw loosening and late loss of correction. The ALPS plate and screws have been designed to lock together, to accept axial loading, and to share the load uniformly with the total construct and bone.

Normal torsional forces applied to the vertebral column are limited by the facet joint, ligaments, and muscles. However, the torsional forces encountered when a fracture occurs at a vertebral body can be as high as 7.25 Nm for a complete three-column fracture. Case reports[1,10] indicate that multicomponent rod devices have encountered difficulty in resisting the torsional loads, with secondary loss of correction and late loss of disc space height. To counteract the torsional loads, these devices have incorporated a cross-bracing component. Although they are effective in resisting the torsional loads, the cross braces increase the overall height of the device, thereby presenting a concern for the overlying soft tissues and vessels.

Anterior devices must provide firm stabilization of the involved bodies to allow for bone consolidation during the fusion process. As experienced with many of the rod/screw devices, the capability to resist flexion and extension forces is often difficult due to the method used to secure the components together. Many of the rod/screw devices require the use of large, multicomponent connectors to provide adequate resistance to the flexion and extension forces normally encountered.

The ALPS plate has been designed to match the convex surface of the vertebral body, thereby providing a low profile and effective bone-to-implant interface. The position of the screw holes in the plate provides a built-in resistance to screw pullout due to flexion and extension forces (Fig. 30–1).

ALPS COMPONENTS

The current ALPS plates and screws are made from 316 LVM stainless steel and consist of a combination of straight, contoured, and narrow plates; 7-mm double-locking screws; and 6-mm self-locking screws. Titanium implants are currently being studied and will soon be available.

The straight vertebral locking plates have been designed to fit the dorsolateral aspect of the vertebral bodies from T11 to L5. The contoured vertebral locking plates are designed to provide secure fixation and stabilization when the vertebral bodies are misaligned up to 5° and can be applied to the thoracic-lumbar and lumbar spine. The narrow plates are designed to be used in the thoracic spine from T5 to L2; however, the plate can be used successfully in the midlumbar spine when anatomic restrictions require the use of the lowest-profile construct (Fig. 30–2).

The double-locking screws (with nut and reverse locking set screw) have a diameter of 7 mm and are used posterolaterally on the plate (Fig. 30–3). The design of the double-locking screw prevents the screw from rotating in the plate, thereby providing a secure plate-screw interface.

The self-locking screws have a diameter of 6 mm and are used medially on the plate (Fig. 30–4). To reduce the profile of the overall device in the thoracic spine, self-locking

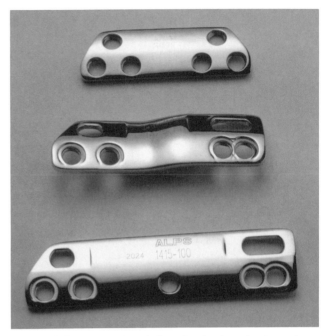

Figure 30–2. ALPS plate designs for the thoracic, thoracolumbar, and lumbar spine.

screws are used both medially and laterally on the narrow plate. Each of the round holes in all ALPS plates is threaded to accept the self-locking screw. This unique design prevents screw pullout and assists in the transfer of the applied forces to the host bone (Fig. 30–5).

PREOPERATIVE PLANNING

Prior to surgery, preoperative x-rays can be used in conjunction with the ALPS templates to determine proper plate length and screw length. The ALPS templates are 15% oversized to allow for x-ray magnification. Using lateral radiographs, measurements are taken from the superior endplate of the highest vertebral body to be fused to the inferior endplate of the lowest vertebral body to be fused (Fig. 30–6). Axial computed tomography (CT) slices of the involved vertebral bodies can then be used to determine proper screw length[18] for both the 7-mm-diameter double-locking screws and the 6-mm-diameter self-locking screws (Fig. 30–7).

PATIENT POSITIONING AND APPROACH

The patient is positioned on the operating table in the lateral decubitus position with the left side up (Fig. 30–8). The transpleural approach (Fig. 30–9) for the thoracolumbar region, or the standard retroperitoneal approach for the lower lumbar region, is used. In the transpleural approach, the skin incision is made two ribs above the affected segment. After thoracotomy, the parietal pleura overlying the vertebral bodies is incised and the exposing segmental vessels are ligated. In the lower lumbar region, the ascending lumbar vein is ligated to allow displacement of vessels. The psoas muscle

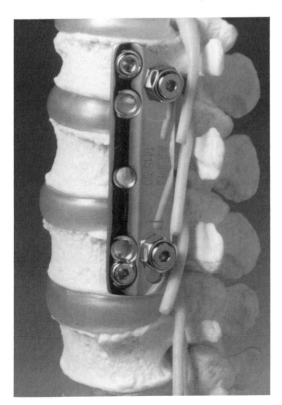

Figure 30–1. Anterior locking plate positioned at L2 to L4.

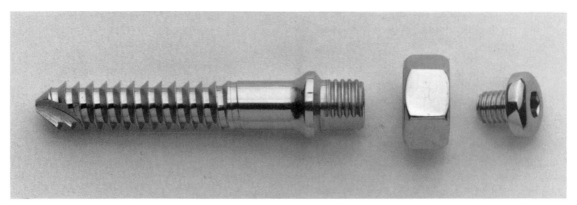

Figure 30–3. ALPS double-locking screw with locking nut and set screw.

must be dissected carefully from the spinal segments that will be instrumented and retracted to avoid nerve root compression.

SURGICAL PROCEDURE

To allow proper alignment of the vertebral locking plate along the posterior lateral aspect of the vertebral body, osteophytes along the endplate should be removed using a curved osteotome or rongeur. Such resection should provide a smooth and flat bone bed for securing the plate.

The adjacent discs above and below the injured vertebral body should be excised extensively. Anterior decompression via vertebrectomy, when necessary, is completed. When the posterior aspect of the vertebral body is excised, Gelfoam (Upjohn, Kalamazoo, MI) is placed on the anterior surface of the spinal canal as a protective barrier following neural decompression. Kyphotic deformity at the concerned level can be corrected with a vertebral body spreader via manual adjustment. The defect is measured, and properly sized tricortical bone grafts are inserted into the defect. The entire bony defect created by the discectomy and vertebrectomy should be filled with bone grafts and tamped into place.

Trial Plate Positioning

The appropriate-length trial plate with drill sleeves is positioned on the involved vertebral bodies. The trial plate should be placed as far lateral as possible on the vertebral body with its longitudinal axis parallel to the sagittal curvature of the spine (Fig. 30–10). When using the contoured plate, the contoured plate spacer is placed on the inferior end of the trial plate. When used at the thoracolumbar levels, the

head of the rib can be excised partially to attain good bone contact between the plate and the vertebral body.

The 4-mm drill bit is used to drill into the superior vertebral body through the appropriate drill sleeve on the trial plate (Fig. 30–11). The depth drilled should correspond with the length of the screws to be used (preoperatively determined with CT). A standard depth gauge can be used intraoperatively to reconfirm the proper screw length.

The screws are not required to penetrate the contralateral cortex but should be just short of the contralateral wall. The angle of the screws when seated in the plate forms a delta. Such screw positioning reduces the need for bicortical fixation of the screws, except when the bone stock quality is below standard. A minimum of 2 cm clearance should be maintained between the implant and the major vessels.

The tap is left in place while drilling and tapping the inferior hole to ensure proper alignment to the superior hole. Then the drill sleeve is removed and the second hole is tapped (Fig. 30–12). The trial plate is then removed.

Double-Locking Screw Insertion

The double-locking screws are first inserted into the superiorly drilled hole and then into the inferiorly drilled hole. Care should be taken during screw insertion to maintain the screws within the predrilled holes. Misalignment of the screws may cause the plate not to set evenly against the vertebral body (Fig. 30–13).

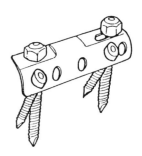

Figure 30–5. ALPS construct that indicates the delta created by the angulation of the screws. The crossing pattern of the screws prevents the screws from pulling out.

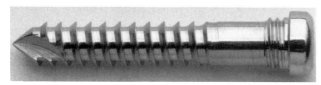

Figure 30–4. ALPS self-locking screw with self-tapping flute and machined locking thread to secure the screw to the ALPS plate.

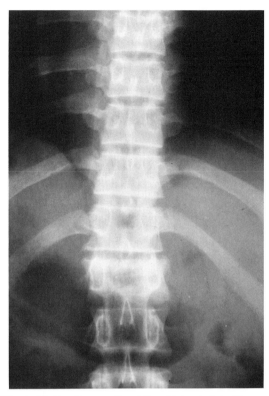
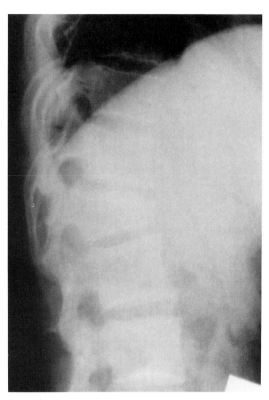

Figure 30–6.   Preoperative AP and lateral plain films are used to plan the procedure.

Vertebral Locking Plate Positioning

Using the plate holder, the plate is placed over the head of the implanted double-locking screws. The larger slotted hole is placed over the screw in the inferior vertebral body (Fig. 30–14). The screws should then be checked in relationship to the plate to determine if the screw heads are at the proper

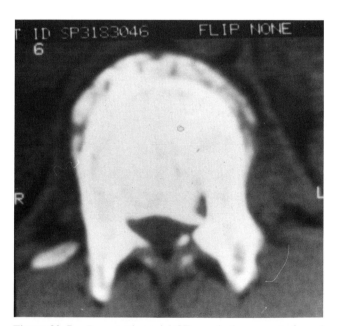

Figure 30–7.   Preoperative axial CT reveals the amount of canal compromise and provides for an accurate screw length measurement.

height above the plate to facilitate the locking nut placement and allow for flush placement of the plate on the vertebral body. A locking nut is placed over each screw, and the nut socket wrench is used to secure them in place (Fig. 30–15). The set screw is then inserted through the nut and into the screw shaft. The set screw provides a secondary protection against loosening of the locking nut.

Two drill guides are threaded onto the selected round holes on the anterior aspect of the plate (one in the superior screw hole and one in the inferior screw hole). If the inferior double-locking screw is positioned in the inferior section of the plate hole, the self-locking screw must be placed in the superior of the two holes on the caudal end of the plate. The plate holder is removed and a hole is drilled through each of the drill guides (Fig. 30–16). The drill guides are removed using the nut socket wrench, if necessary. The holes are

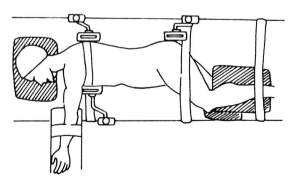

Figure 30–8.   Patient positioned on the OR table that provides for the optimum surgical approach.

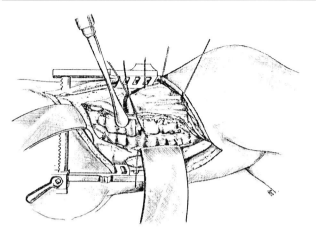

Figure 30–9. Standard retroperitoneal approach.

tapped and the self-locking screws are then inserted with the hex-head screwdriver and seated completely into the plate (Fig. 30–17). When the center vertebral body remains intact, another self-locking screw may be inserted into this vertebra to enhance stabilization, using the same procedure as for inserting the self-locking screws.

Prior to closing, anteroposterior (AP) and lateral x-rays may be obtained to confirm the proper positioning of the screws, reconfirming that the desired vertebral alignment has been achieved and that the neural canal is absent of bone fragments (Fig. 30–18).

In the lower thoracic region, where the vertebral bodies are smaller, a specially designed narrow plate is available, providing for the secure attachment of the plate with the use of four self-locking screws. The narrow plate is inserted in the same manner as the straight lumbar plate, with the exception that only self-locking screws are used in the vertebral body.

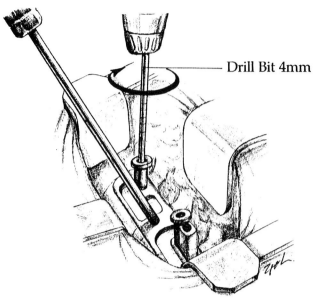

Figure 30–11. With the trial plate in position, a 4-mm drill is used to drill the holes for the double-locking screws.

Wound Closure

If needed, the diaphragm is repaired prior to routine muscle closure. The wound is closed subsequently over Hemovac (Zimmer, Warsaw, Indiana) in the routine manner.

POSTOPERATIVE MANAGEMENT

The patient may be allowed to sit 1 to 3 days after the operation. Wound drains are normally removed 48 hours after the operation. If the patient is able to be ambulated with or

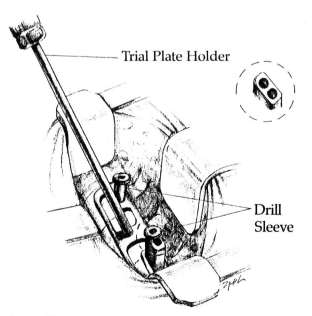

Figure 30–10. Trial plate applied to the involved vertebral bodies.

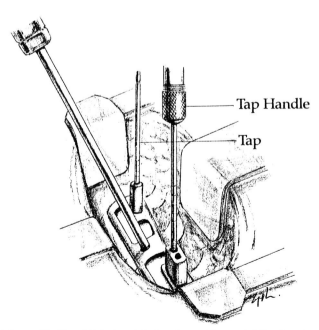

Figure 30–12. With the trial plate in position and following the drilling of the pilot holes, both holes are tapped.

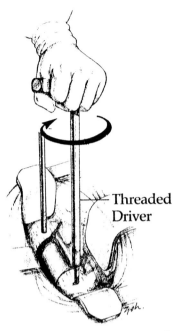

Figure 30–13. The double-locking screws are inserted with the threaded driver.

without crutches, he or she is allowed to do so in 3 to 5 days after the operation. Respiratory therapy, particularly in the first 3 days after the operation, for expansion of the lungs is recommended.

CLINICAL EXPERIENCE

Chen et al[19] report a series of 50 patients who were treated with the ALPS system for burst fracture with incomplete neurological deficit, posttraumatic kyphosis, and metastatic tumor of the spine. All patients in the study have reached a mean follow-up period of 2 years. At last follow-up there had been no screw breakage or loss in correction.

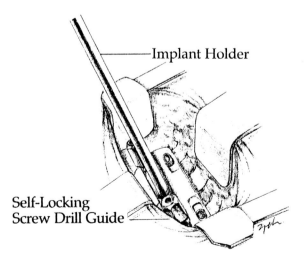

Figure 30–14. The ALPS plate is positioned over the double-locking screws. The larger slot of the plate is placed over the inferior vertebral body to allow for compression of the bone graft.

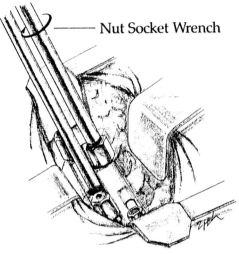

Figure 30–15. The locking nuts are secured to the screws with the ALPS plate in position.

Chen et al have selected three cases to demonstrate the capabilities of the ALPS system in the single-procedure treatment of the patient requiring anterior stabilization.

Case 1

A 28-year-old male sustained a burst fracture of the T12 vertebra with a Frankel C neurological deficit. CT showed a more than 50% of canal encroachment at the T12 level. Anterior decompression by a thoracoabdominal approach was done through the left 10th rib. A tricortical block bone graft was used to bridge the T11 and L1 vertebral bodies. A 90-mm ALPS plate was used for fixation from T11 to L1. The patient was able to sit up on the third postoperative day. A significant neurological improvement to Frankel D was

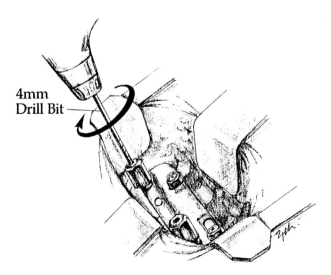

Figure 30–16. With the drill guides in position, the anterior self-locking screw holes are developed.

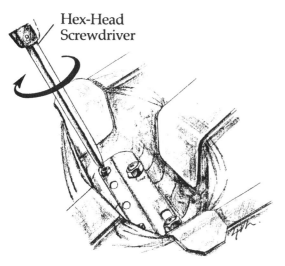

Hex-Head
Screwdriver

Figure 30–17. The self-locking screws are implanted and seated in the ALPS plate. Notice the low profile of the completed construct.

noted at follow-up, 6 months after surgery. The patient was able to ambulate on ankle–foot orthoses (AFO) and was supported with a cane at 2-year follow-up (Fig. 30–19).

Case 2

A 35-year-old female sustained a fall resulting in fracture of the sacrum, calcanei, and burst fracture of L1 with a neuro-

logical status classified as Frankel D. Anterior decompression, fusion with iliac bone graft, and calcaneal fractures were treated by open reduction and internal fixation. Follow-up at 29 months after surgery showed that the instrumentation remained in good position and the patient was able to walk without support (Fig. 30–20).

Case 3

A 31-year-old male sustained a motor vehicle accident resulting in head injury with epidural hematoma and burst fracture of the L4. Emergency craniotomy was done to evacuate the epidural hematoma on the day of the injury. The patient made a good recovery of consciousness on the following day. Subsequent examination revealed a Frankel C neurological status due to a burst fracture of the L4. Anterior decompression, fusion, and a straight ALPS fixation plate were performed 13 days after the injury. The patient has shown a good neurological recovery 2 years after surgery. He has had no significant back pain, although a screw was inadvertently placed in the adjacent disc space at surgery (Fig. 30–21).

SUMMARY

The ALPS device is designed to provide a rigid anterior, short segmental fixation in the lower thoracic, thoracolumbar, and lumbar regions. The device has been effective in the single-stage treatment of fractures, posttraumatic kyphosis, and tumors of the spine. Such treatment has reduced the need for two-

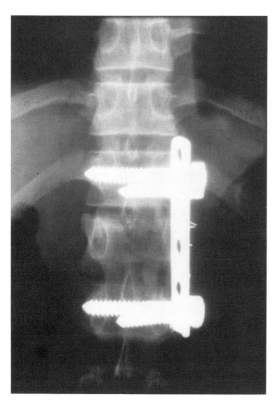
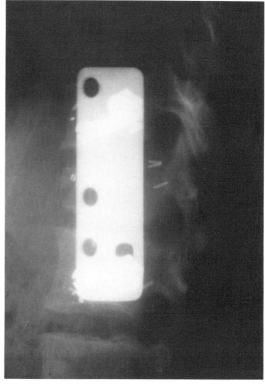

Figure 30–18. AP and lateral films are taken to confirm position of the plate and screws.

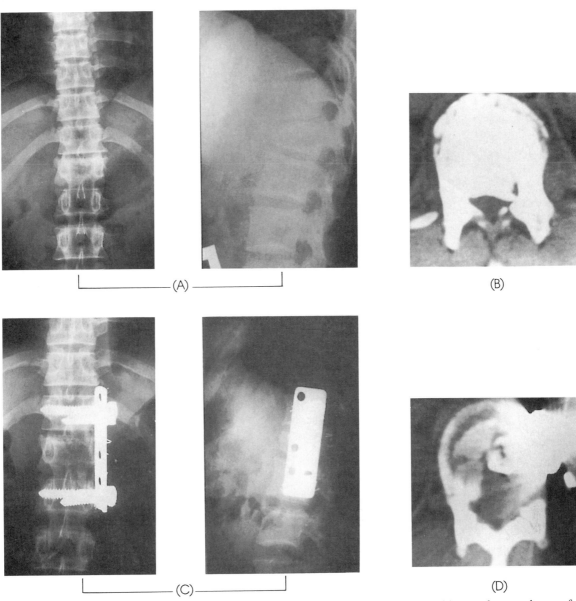

Figure 30–19. Case 1. (**A**) and (**B**). AP, lateral, and CT films of a burst fracture of L1, with a canal encroachment of 50%. (**C**) and (**D**). Postoperative decompression of spinal canal with ALPS from T12 to L2.

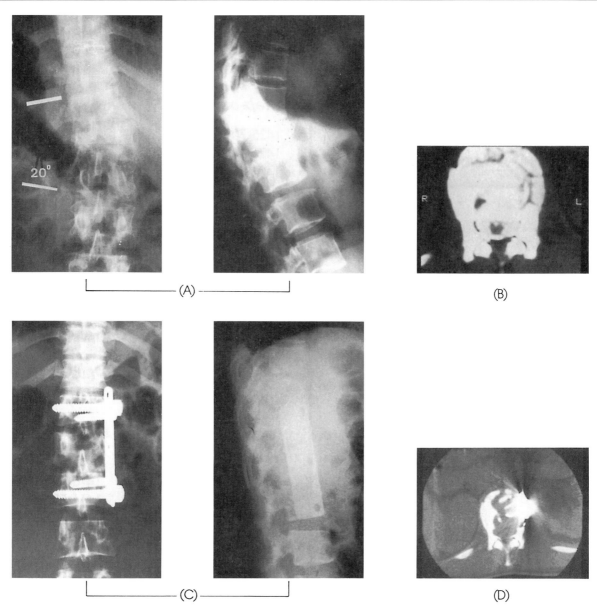

Figure 30–20.   Case 2. (**A**) and (**B**). AP, lateral, and CT films of an L1 burst fracture with kyphoscoliosis. CT scan reveals retropulsion of bone fragments with spinal canal encroachment. (**C**) and (**D**). Postoperative films indicate good correction of kyphoscoliosis and decompression of spinal canal.

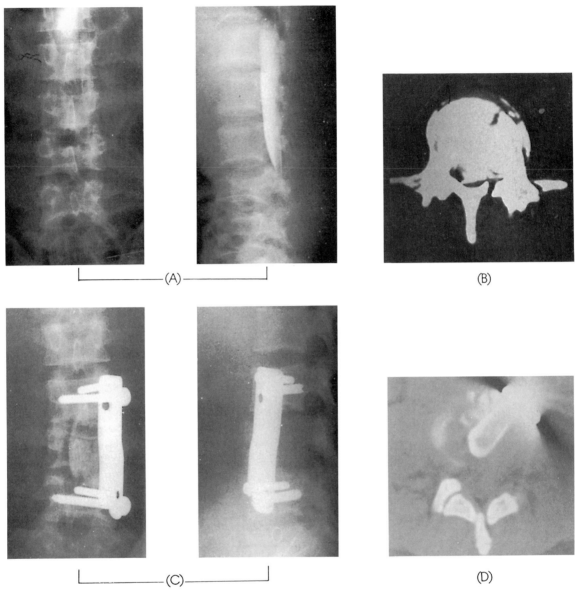

Figure 30–21.   Case 3. (**A**) and (**B**). AP, lateral, and CT films revealing a burst fracture at L4 with Frankel grade C neurological deficit. CT shows severe canal encroachment. (**C**) and (**D**). Postoperative films of decompression, fusion, and rigid fixation with ALPS contoured plate from L3 to L5.

stage procedures for our patient population. Complications have been minor, with no screw breakage or loss of correction.

REFERENCES

1. Dickson JH, Harrington PR, Erwin WE. Results of reduction and stabilization of the severely fractured thoracic and lumbar spine. *J Bone Joint Surg.* 1978;60A:799–805.
2. Holdsworth F. Fractures, dislocations, and fracture-dislocations of the spine. *J Bone Joint Surg.* 1970;52A:1534–1551.
3. Whitesides TE Jr, Shah SGA. On the management of unstable fractures of the thoracolumbar spine. Rationale for use of anterior decompression and posterior stabilization. *Spine.* 1976;1:99–107.
4. McAfee PC, Bohlman HH, Yuan HA. Anterior decompression of traumatic thoracolumbar fractures with incomplete neurological deficit using a retroperitoneal approach. *J Bone Joint Surg.* 1985;67A:89–104.
5. Crock HV. Anterior lumbar interbody fusion—indications of its use and notes on surgical technique. *Clin Orthop.* 1982;165:157–163.
6. Gurr KR, McAfee PC, Shih C-M. Biomechanical analysis of anterior and posterior instrumentation systems following corpectomy. A calf-spine model. *J Bone Joint Surg.* 1988;70A:1182–1191.
7. Streiz W, Brown JC, Bonnett CA. Anterior fibular strut grafting in the treatment of kyphosis. *Clin Orthop.* 1976;128:140–148.
8. Siegal T, Siegal T. Vertebral body resection for epidural compression by malignant tumors. Results of forty-seven consecutive operative procedures. *J Bone Joint Surg.* 1985;67A:375–382.

9. Black RC, Gardner VO, Armstrong GWD, O'Neil J, St. George M. A contoured anterior spinal fixation plate. *Clin Orthop.* 1988;227:135–142.

10. Kaneda K, Abumi K, Fujiya M. The thoracolumbar-lumbar spine: results of anterior decompression and stabilization with anterior instrumentation. *Spine.* 1984;9:788–795.

11. Kostuik JP, Matsusaki H. Anterior stabilization, instrumentation, and decompression for post-traumatic kyphosis. *Spine.* 1989;14:379–386.

12. Ryan MD, Taylor TKF, Sherwood AA. Bolt-plate fixation for anterior spinal fusion. *Clin Orthop.* 1986;203:196–202.

13. Johnson RW, Southwick WO. Surgical approaches to the spine. In: Rothman RH, Simeone FA, eds. *The Spine.* 2nd ed. Vol 1. Philadelphia, Pa: WB Saunders; 1982:171–187.

14. Kostuik JP, Richard R. Single stage anterior decompression and stabilization of thoracolumbar spinal injuries. *Orthop Trans.* 1982;6:9–10.

15. Roberts JB, Curtiss PH. Stability of thoracic and lumbar spine in traumatic paraplegia following fracture or fracture-dislocation. *J Bone Joint Surg.* 1970;52A:1115–1130.

16. Bone LB, Ashman RB, Roach JW, Johnston CE II. Mechanical comparison of anterior spine instrumentation in a burst fracture model. *Orthop Trans.* 1987;11:87–88.

17. Denis F. Spinal instability as defined by the three-column spine concept in acute spinal trauma. *Clin Orthop.* 1984;189:65–76.

18. Handes SF, Lee Y-Y. Computed tomography of spinal fractures. *Radiol Clin N Am.* 1981;19:69–89.

19. Chen JH, Chen WJ, Huang TJ, Shih CH. Anterior locking plate system (ALPS) in burst fractures with incomplete neurologic deficit of the thoracolumbar and lumbar spine. Submitted to ISSLS 1993; Heidelberg, Germany.

31 Posterior Lumbar Interbody Fusion

Paul M. Lin, M.D.

INTRODUCTION

In 1945, Dr Ralph Cloward, a neurosurgeon, first described the concept and technique of posterior lumbar interbody fusion (PLIF).[1] The mechanical advantages of PLIF as compared to the other available techniques of lumbar fusion are indisputable[2]:

1. PLIF has a wider area of bone surface.
2. It has an adequate blood supply through the cancellous portion of the vertebral body, once the subchondral endplate is exposed or removed partially.
3. It is proximate to the center of motion and compression forces.
4. It allows complete visualization of the area of nerve root compression.
5. It allows for complete access for removal of the areas of compression centrally, as well as laterally, at the intervertebral canal.
6. It preserves interbody distance, so there will be no ensuing disk space collapse or possible lateral stenosis as a sequela of disk excision.
7. It annuls the possibility of recurrence of lumbar disk herniation at the fused level.

Unless Cloward's PLIF is performed perfectly as Cloward described it, there will be a high percentage of pseudoarthrodesis or neural damage and graft retropulsion.[3] The purpose of PLIF must be a completion of lumbar arthrodesis or bony fusion. An interbody arthrodesis is a remodeling process whereby the graft is remodeled to that of its host, the vertebral body. The graft must have a cortical rim and a cancellous marrow centrum (Fig. 31–1). A stable nonunion in the form of fibrous osseous union may be clinically satisfactory, but it could not be considered a successful arthrodesis or a fusion. The same can be said about the use of allografts in PLIF. In some allogeneic PLIF, the remodeled arthrodesis may be seen as late as 5 to 10 years after the surgery.

There are three biomechanical principles that must be followed to obtain a high degree of success in PLIF arthrodesis:

1. Adequate osteogenecity of the grafting materials. Until the bone morphogenic protein (BMP) can be synthesized in commercially available quantity, adequate osteogenecity must rely on the cancellous autogeneic graft, where the concentration of the BMP is the highest.[4] Regardless of the types of allograft harvesting and sterilizing techniques, addition of autogeneic cancellous bone mixed with allografts is a good grafting technique. An example is the use of allogeneic femoral ring in anterior interbody fusion, filled tightly with autogeneic cancellous graft. Some surgeons advocate large allografts, with large and strong cortical, bicortical, or even tricortical bone. Not only are large grafts difficult and dangerous to insert, but logic dictates that if we accept that osteosynthesis progresses linearly, then the large graft is slower to be fused. A currently accepted method for fusion of a nonunion fracture is the use of high-density autogenous bone.[5] For a single-level PLIF, an all-autogeneic grafting technique, which will be described in this chapter, is considered the most osteogenic and thus provides a higher success rate for lumbar interbody arthrodesis.

2. Stability of the PLIF construct. Unless the grafts are locked in the disk space in a stable manner, with little or no motion, the fusion will not take place. We can learn from the high success rate of arthrodesis in anterior cervical interbody fusion that the preservation of the posterior portion of the motion segment in the cervical area is responsible for the stable construct of the anterior cervical interbody fusion. The PLIF technique described in this chapter emphasizes the importance of preservation of the posterior motion segment and the mechanical integrity of the facet joint (Fig. 31–2). If one is unable to achieve satisfactory stability of the PLIF construct, either because of technical failure to preserve the posterior segment or because of preexisting instability such as spondylolisthesis, then a mechanical augmentation with an internal fixater must be added (Fig. 31–3). Paraspinal muscles play an important role in the stability of a PLIF construct. Preservation of the posterior motion segment, including the interspinous ligament, affords reattachment of the paraspinal muscles after PLIF by suturing them back to the supraspinous ligament.

3. Sufficient bone grafts. As in all interbody fusion, anterior cervical, or lumbar interbody fusion, to achieve a high fusion rate all the disk space must be packed tightly with bone graft.[6] In PLIF it is not technically possible to remove all disk material and replace it with nothing but bone. However, at least 60% of the disk space must be impacted tightly with bone graft. Although allografts have

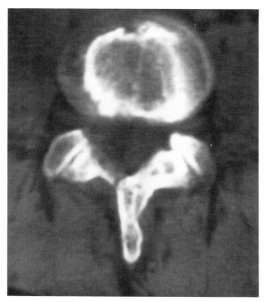

Figure 31–1. Full maturation of an L4 to L5 autograft only 9 months after a posterior lumbar interbody fusion. Note that remodeling has given the graft the osseous characteristics of a vertebral body (ie, a cortical ring and a cancellous centrum).

been found to be successful in achieving arthrodesis in anterior cervical and anterior lumbar interbody fusion, it is the large-size grafts, which fill out nearly the entire disk space, that give the construct its stability. In these situations the relative lack of osteogenicity of the allogeneic interbody fusion is not a hindrance to a successful fusion. The PLIF technique described in this chapter favors the use of smaller autogeneic grafts because of their safety factor to the surrounding neural structures and their higher osteogenecity. We emphasize, however, the impor-

tance of preparing of the largest grafting area and the insertion of the grafts in the most impacted manner.

CLINICAL INDICATIONS

With the advance of internal fixation as an adjunct to spinal fusion, there is a tendency toward overutilization of the mechanical devices in all PLIF. One of the best biomechanical advantages of PLIF is the presence of a compression force on the graft during weight bearing. This facilitates the process of osteosynthesis.[7] Rigid fixation with mechanical devices removes this advantage so that radiologically the speed of osteosynthesis, such as remodeling or evidence of trabeculation, is much delayed (1 to 2 years). Although PLIF alone is inadequate to stabilize a motion segment that is already destabilized, opinions are divided on those that could be done with or without concomitant internal fixation.[8,9]

The following are indications for PLIF without internal fixation:

1. Segmental spinal stenosis and spondylosis This includes lumbar spondylosis with chronic back pain.
2. Recurrent herniated disk with or without spinal stenosis
3. Segmental instability such as postchemonucleolysis pain syndrome or a massive midline disk herniation especially at the L4 to L5 interspace
4. Obesity associated with lateral disk herniation.

The following are indications for PLIF with internal fixation:

1. Moderately severe lytic and degenerative spondylolisthesis
2. Failed back syndrome
3. Iatrogenic destabilization of a motion segment

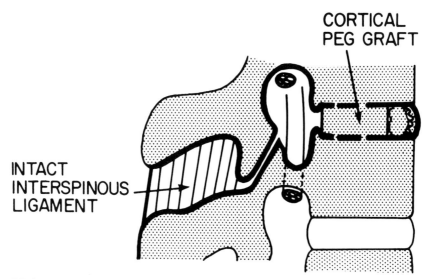

Figure 31–2. Motion segment reconstituted and immobilized by posterior lumbar interbody fusion. If the posterior segment of the motion segment is intact, the distraction of the disk space by bone graft increases the tension of the supraspinous ligament. The keystone locking design of the posterior intervertebral rim helps keep the graft in place and under tension.

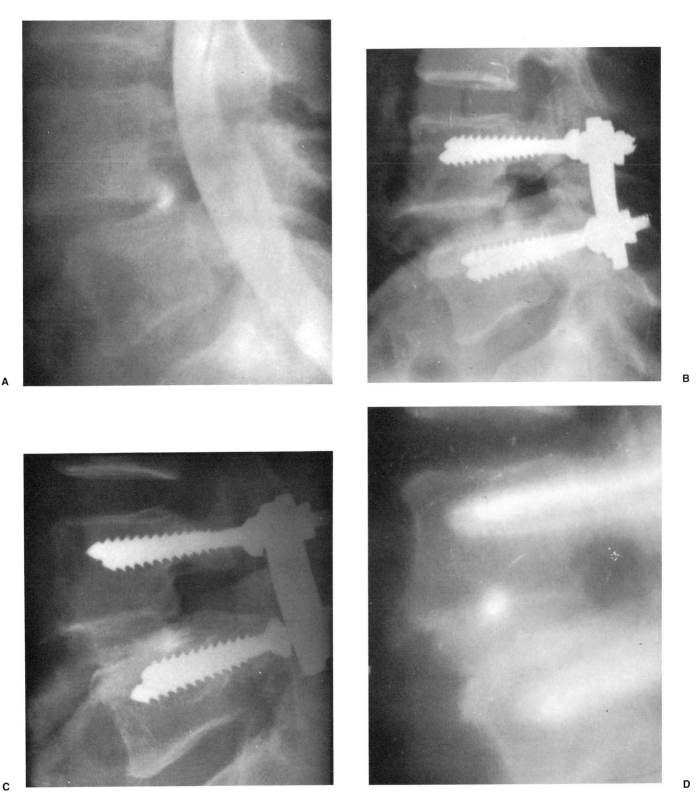

A

B

C

D

Figure 31–3. Posterior lumbar interbody fusion with a transpedicular internal fixation device (VSP) in a 47-year-old man with grade 1 spondylolisthesis and spondylosis at the L4 to L5 level. (**A**). Preoperative lateral myelogram. (**B**). Postoperative lateral radiograph. (**C**). Lateral radiograph done 3 months after surgery. Note the dense, matured bone graft and the sign of early trabeculation. (**D**). Lateral tomogram done 3 months after surgery, demonstrating a similar degree of maturing arthrodesis, with no evidence of disk space collapse or recurrence of listhesis.

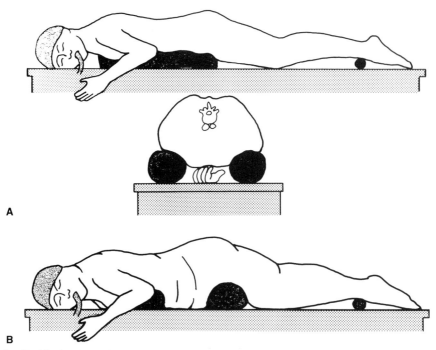

Figure 31–4. Positioning the patient for posterior lumbar interbody fusion. (**A**). Placement of firm rolls for the patient of average size. Rolls are individually tailored to the patient's size. Flexion of the table is not needed. The tension of the anterior abdominal wall should be tested. (**B**). Placement of larger rolls for the obese patient. One is placed horizontally in the middle of the chest, and a larger roll is placed across the upper thigh. The pendulous abdomen is kept in suspension.

4. Other congenitally unstable motion segments, such as an incompetent facet complex.

TECHNIQUE

The use of an operative microscope or fast-speed air drill is optional in doing PLIF. Many experienced PLIF surgeons have used either or both of these options with great success.[8,10,11]

Position of the Patient

The patient is placed in a prone position. The iliac crest, the lateral rib cage, and the clavicles are supported with two firm rolls serving as buttresses to prevent compression of the anterior abdominal wall and the inferior vena cava, thus avoiding excessive epidural bleeding during surgery. Because patients vary in size and height, cotton sheets should be rolled tightly in a customized manner just prior to surgery. After the patient is positioned properly, the surgeon should manually feel the tension of the abdominal wall, in between the rolls, prior to the sterile draping. With the use of rolls, the table is not flexed and the patient is lying in a neutral prone position, without the need for further adjustments when the grafts or instrumentation are applied later (Fig. 31–4). Other forms of support, such as modified knee-chest positioning, are also useful in decreasing epidural bleeding. A Foley catheter is inserted prior to surgery to en-

sure that bladder distention does not increase intra-abdominal pressure during surgery.

Exposure

The 6- to 7-in incision is made horizontally. For an L4 to L5 PLIF, it is made at the level of the iliac crest, and for the L5 to S1 PLIF the incision is made 1 in below that. Grafts can be removed from the posterior iliac crest through a slight lateral extension of the same incision.

Whenever possible, the integrity of the supraspinous ligaments and the spinous processes is preserved. The presence of spinous processes serves as a lever for the paraspinal muscles to exert their stabilizing influence on the motion segments. Therefore, they should not be removed indiscriminately simply for the sake of better exposure. The inferior laminotomy is performed first, with a Kerrison rongeur. Next, the mesial portion of the inferior facet is removed by sharp dissection with a thin, $\frac{1}{4}$-in osteotome. A horizontal cut is made first, followed by a vertical cut. The mesial half of the inferior facet is removed, and the underlying superior facet, which often appears as a tropism, is exposed (Figs. 31–5 and 31–6).

The mesial half of the superior facet is then removed, either with an osteotome or with a bone punch. With the osteotome, a horizontal cut is made just above the pedicle, followed by a vertical cut up to the lateral limit of the exposure. This is followed by a forceful swiveling rotational action of the osteotome to avulse the remaining tip of the superior

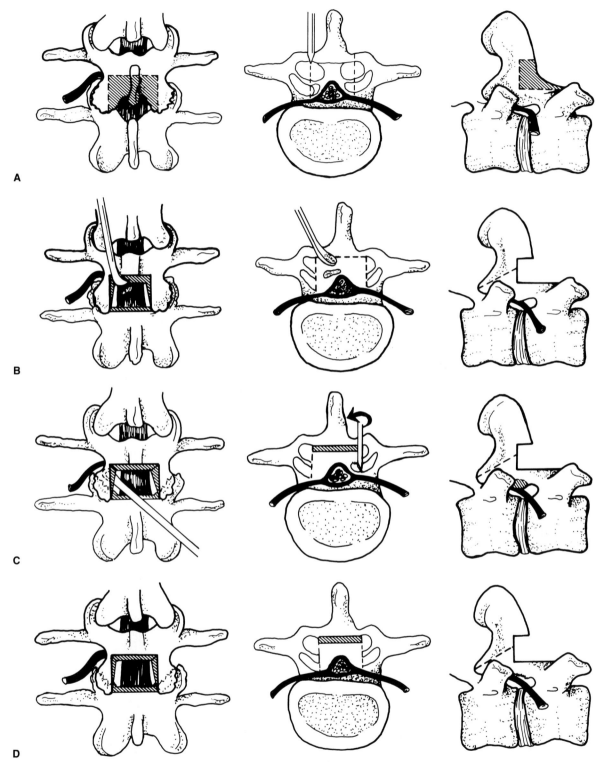

Figure 31–5.   Posterior, axial, and lateral views, showing the steps in the internal decompression of a stenotic spinal canal and the bony exposure for the posterior lumbar interbody fusion. (**A**). Decompressive laminotomy and mesial inferior facetectomy by thin and sharp osteotome. (**B**). Thinning of the lamina by splitting with an osteotome or sonic curette. (**C**). Foraminotomy by mesial superior facetectomy, with avulsion of the tip of the superior facet. (**D**). Spinal canal and foraminal stenosis after decompression.

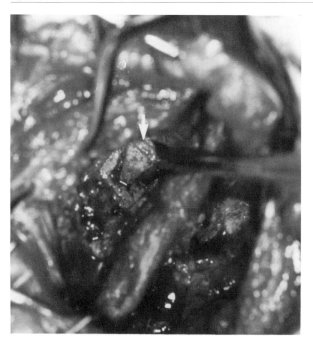

Figure 31–6. Operative photograph. Two Weitlander cerebellar retractors are used for the bony exposure. Note the intact midline structures. Arrow points to the resected mesial inferior facet by thin osteotome; it is being grasped and removed with a straight disk rongeur.

facet, which helps to decompress the intervertebral foramen. The rostral ligamentum flavum, which forms the capsule of the facet, will also come out with the avulsed piece of superior facet. If there is significant spinal stenosis associated with hypertrophy of the lamina and facets, internal decompression for spinal stenosis can be achieved by splitting the lamina with an osteotome, in conjunction with the foraminotomy. The intervertebral foramen and its contents should be exposed and, if necessary, decompressed, preferably from the opposite side of the table. This can be accomplished by an angled bone punch, angled curet, or a sonic angled curet (Figs. 31–7 and 31–8).

The sonic surgery system consists of a hand tool and cutting tip (eg, a curette). Together, they form a resonant structure that is driven by a pair of piezoelectric crystals at approximately 25 000 Hz–sec. The excursions of the tip, typically 0.001 to 0.002 mm, are maintained under a range of loads by the amount of energy (typically 10 W) supplied to the hand tool. The frequency feedback control circuit ensures that efficient resonance is maintained under all tip and load combinations. The sonic curet decreases the resistance between the curette and the bone structures (Fig. 31–9). As in any curetting action on the bone, the tool should be anchored on the bone before any forceful rotatory action is applied. Because the sonic curette generates energy mainly at the tip, the surgeon should avoid touching neural structures with the tip of the instrument, although no demonstrable neural injury was demonstrated in the experimental model. Contact with a metal nerve retractor may reduce the curette's vibration to a lower sonic frequency range, result-

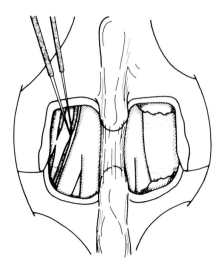

Figure 31–7. Mesial facetectomy with preservation of the spinous processes, supraspinous ligaments, and the lateral facets. Epidural hemorrhage is controlled by means of bipolar coagulation forceps on the left side. On the right side, the epidural hemorrhage is further controlled by Surgicel tampons. Impacted Surgicel tampons also push the nerve root medially and expose the disk space without the use of a nerve root retractor.

ing in increased energy per vibration and a harmless mechanical stimulation of the nerve root.

In patients with dense epidural scarring, the sonic curette is extremely useful for exposing the disk space. The different degrees of resistance to the sonic instrument by different tissues make it easy to curette or chisel off the scar away from its bony attachments. The surgeon first identifies the

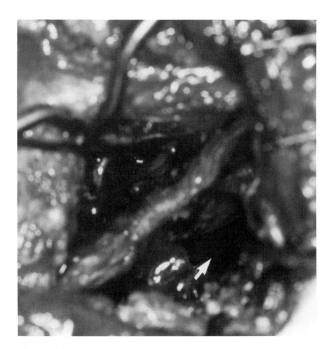

Figure 31–8. Intraoperative photograph showing the exposure into the disk space (arrow). The dural sac is retracted toward the midline by Surgicel tampons, placed epidurally, above and below the entrance to the disk space. Note that no nerve root retractor is needed.

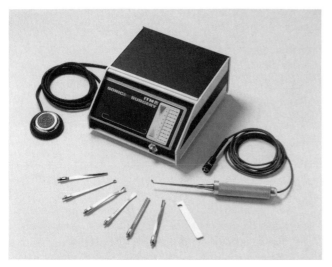

Figure 31–9. Sonic instrument manufactured by I.T.M. of Washington, DC. Control module, handpieces, and assorted curettes, gouges, and osteotomes are shown.

bony pedicle, then strips away all the scar mesially, and finally dissects upward or cephalad to expose the disk space. With this method, it is not necessary to identify the dural sac or the nerve root on a patient who has had multiple previous lumbar surgeries. PLIF is, after all, an intradiskal operation. Once you enter the disk space, you can complete the fusion without tedious and often hazardous dural and neural dissection.

Epidural Hemostasis

The epidural veins should be coagulated by means of bipolar coagulation and then severed. Prior soaking of the Surgicel (Johnson & Johnson, New Brunswick, N.J.) in a double-strength thrombin solution can enhance hemotasis in problematic epidural bleeding. Occasionally, small arterial bleeding in the epidural space may require careful and delicate hemostasis by bipolar coagulation (Fig. 31–7). This is where the advantages of an operative microscope come into play. The use of Surgicel as a temporary tampon, above and below the disk space, displaces the dura and nerve root medially and makes it unnecessary to use a metal nerve root retractor. Surgicel tampons are effective only if a clean cleavage plane is dissected free between the nerve root and lateral wall of the spinal canal. Clean exposure of the mesial surface of the pedicle facilitates the insertion of the inferior Surgicel tampon between the pedicle and the nerve root that exits from the intervertebral foramen one space below. The epidural fat can be debulked by dessication through the gentle application of bipolar coagulation over the adipose tissue; this further increases the exposure of the disk space (Fig. 31–8).

Preparation of the Disk Space

The depth of a lumbar disk space varies from 25 mm under the facet to 35 mm in the center. It is recommended that all intradiskal instruments have a 30-mm marker calibrated to avoid anterior vascular injury. The graft site preparation involved only the central 80% of the disk space. We avoid radical diskectomy too far beyond the medial border of the pedicle.

The disk space is entered by cutting a large square plug from the posterior annulus, which reveals the bony edges of the adjoining vertebral bodies. The adjoining intervertebral rims should be removed with a thin, sharp, $\frac{1}{4}$-in osteotome. The lower cut is generally made with a slight angulation caudally, in accordance with the alignment of the disk space. The normal concavity of the disk space allows removal of approximately 1 cm of the intervertebral rim and the underlying subchondral bone before the osteotome enters the disk space. The thickness of the rim to be removed varies from 2 to 5 mm for the inferior rim and from 0 to 2 mm for the superior rim. Removal of the rims allows wider and straighter access to the disk space.

It is not necessary to remove the disk material in a piecemeal fashion as in a conventional diskectomy. With the exception of a dense annular attachment to the intervertebral rim, there is a distinct cleavage between the cartilage and the endplate that is defined easily after the intervertebral rim has been removed. With a downbite horizontal cutting edge curette, the disk material is scraped from the subchondral endplate along the cleavage plane. With an upbiting-angle curette placed as low as possible (30 mm), the partially detached disk material is then scraped upward and detached totally. The detached disk can then be removed easily with a serrated disk rongeur. An upbite peapod rongeur or Cloward's English bone punch is useful for removal of the disk material from the lateral recess. Total diskectomy should harvest about 30 cc (fill up a 1-oz medicinal glass) (Fig. 31–10).

The midline bar, or the disk under the dural space, requires special attention. With a sharp, pointed cervical osteophyte periosteal elevator, the disk material near the midline is dissected carefully from the posterior longitudinal ligament. After this, downward pressure can be used to remove the remaining intervertebral rim. The midline bar can be removed with a downbite curette and an upbite peapod rongeur. At times the remnants of the midline bar can be removed only after a peg graft has been inserted from the opposite side; the graft pushes and anchors the disk material laterally so that it can be removed with a disk rongeur (Fig. 31–11). When the midline portion of the disk has been excavated, an irrigation solution introduced on one side of the disk space should flow freely to the other side. By the same token, suctioning should be effective if the suction tip is placed in the opposite disk space.

Subchondral bone is not a cortical bone. It has numerous arterial pores whereby the arterial supply to the disk space, through end arterioles, terminates in the subchondral endplates. In a younger person the subchondral endplates are filled with punctated bleeding points, as in the cervical area (Fig. 31–12). However, with advancing age and spondylosis

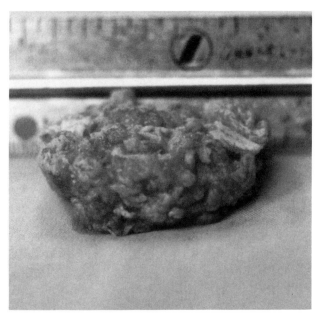

Figure 31–10. The amount of disk material removed from a single level of PLIF is approximately 30 cc. Disk material is detached first, before being removed.

the subchondral endplate becomes sclerotic and acquires the appearance of cortical bone. Thus, the process of thinning of the sclerotic bone is often mistakenly called decortication because anatomically there is no cortical bone, as such, residing within the disk space. Preparation of the grafting bed requires thinning of the endplate to a depth of partially oozing bone. Because the osteogenetic factor is within the grafting material, the autogenous cancellous bone, it is not necessary nor desirable to enter the softer, albeit more vascular, marrow.

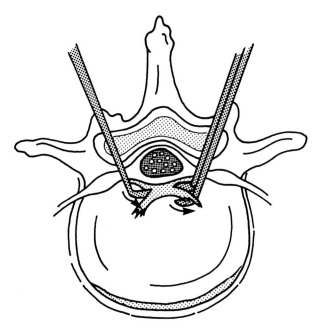

Figure 31–11. Removal of the midline bar of the annulus with either an angled downbite curette or a peapod disk rongeur.

The graft bed within the disk space should have the following characteristics:

1. The bedding construct should be rectangular. For allografts the surfaces prepared must be planed to be geometrically perfect, for there must not be an empty space between the graft-host interface. For high-density autogeneic cortical-cancellous grafting, slight irregularity of the grafting surface is not a significant problem.
2. There should be a keystone undercut that prevents retropulsion; the entrance to the disk space graft bed must therefore be smaller than the centrum of the graft bed (Fig. 31–13).
3. The depth of the bed should be at least 30 mm (average depth of the disk space is 38 mm), and it should occupy the central 80% of the disk space (Fig. 31–14).
4. The prepared bed should not be sclerotic and avascular; nor should it be in the depth of the cancellous bleeding marrow. Soft graft bed thus produced in the marrow enhances settlement within the vertebral body (the Schmorlling effect).

Preparation of the graft bed does not require complete diskectomy. In fact, the various methods described next would remove nearly all the remnant disk material.

FENESTRATION

Penetration of the sclerotic subchondral endplate can be facilitated by tapping a 45-degree-angle sharpened cervical

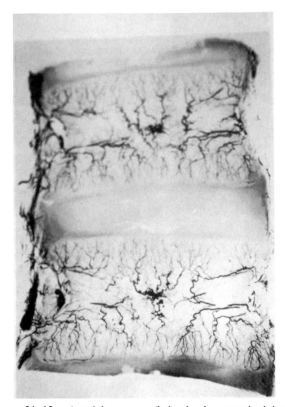

Figure 31–12. Arterial system of the lumbar vertebral body (Crock). Note that the arterial supplies to the subchondral endplates are all end arterioles.

osteophyte periosteal perforator into the cancellous portion of the vertebral body (Fig. 31–15). Either tapping with a hammer or simply a levering action could accomplish the multiple fenestrations. A small curved osteotome, or a Cloward spinous process perforator, could accomplish this in a similar manner.

OSTEOTOME

Cloward advocates the use of sharp and thin osteotomes for preparation of the graft bed. But this method should be reserved for surgeons who are extremely dexterous in the use of this tool. The danger of anterior vascular injury can be a deterrent.

CURETTING

It is possible to prepare the bed with different-shaped curettes. However, unless the instrument is extremely sharp and well maintained, it is advisable that the following two pieces of equipment be made available.

SONIC CURETTE

The energized sonic curette facilitates the curetting action and must be sharpened and well maintained. This instrument is also helpful in sculpturing or undercutting below the intervertebral rim to produce the keystone locking mechanism. The motion of the sonic curette is from side to side, working from the depth of the disk space and gradually working toward the spinal canal (Fig. 31–16).

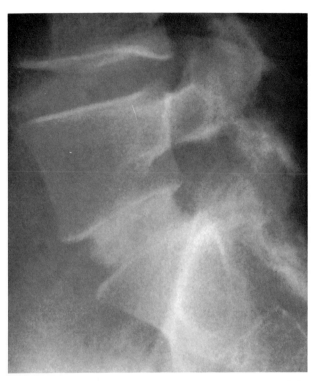

Figure 31–14. A postoperative lateral radiograph shows satisfactory undercutting posteriorly, and the impacted graft occupies the central 80% of the disk space.

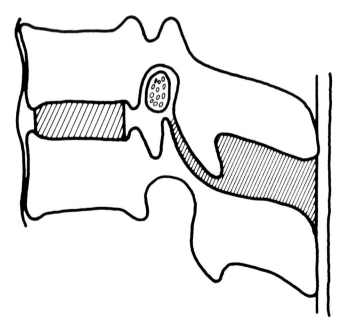

Figure 31–13. Ideal seating of the graft in PLIF. The grafts occupy the central 80% of the disk space. Note the rectangular shape of the bed and the impacted graft as well as the anterior and posterior locking mechanism.

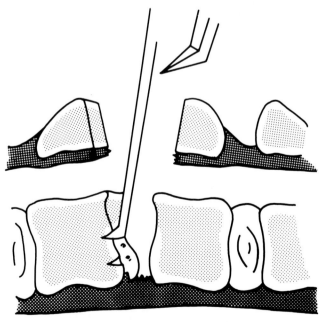

Figure 31–15. Penetration of the subchondral endplate to enhance revascularization. The perforator (top) has a 45-degree angle and a sharpened end. A downward tap on the perforator drives the sharp tip into the cancellous bone of the vertebral body, producing sufficient fenestrations for revascularization.

COLLIS'S DISK SPACE SHAPER (MUELLER)

Collis's disk space shaper is designed to safeguard against anterior penetration through the disk space. The set of instruments is calibrated from 8 to 16 mm as to the width of the cutting edges. The end of the shaper is blunt, and it cannot penetrate through the annulus and anterior longitudinal ligament. The cutting surfaces, however, are located at the distal 5 mm of the disk space shaper, with four cutting edges. By forceful rotation, the cartilage and subchondral endplates can be shaped by a slow peeling process. By gradually increasing of the width of the shaper, a rectangular graft bed can be sculptured effectively. After removal of a fair amount of disk material, the smaller shaper is introduced to a depth of 30 mm. Shearing of the endplates proceeds with 90-degree clockwise and then counterclockwise rotational movements from anterior to posterior. Care should be taken not to cut off the intervertebral rim, thus assuring that the entrance to the disk space is smaller than the center of the prepared bed (the keystone locking effect) (Fig. 31–17).

Graft Preparation

The autogeneic bone graft for the PLIF is removed from the posterior iliac crest through the lateral extension of the horizontal incision. With sharp subperiosteal dissection and electrocoagulation, the lateral portion of the crest and only the posterior surface of the iliac bone is exposed. The posterior half of the lateral muscle attachments to the iliac bone is detached. Total muscle and ligamentous denudation of the iliac crest is to be avoided because it is impossible to reattach them, and this can produce significant postoperative discomfort. A split-thickness unicortical graft is removed with an osteotome. The sheet of graft is usually 5 to 7 cm long, approximately 3 cm wide, and 8 to 10 mm thick (Fig. 31–18). For a two-level PLIF, the amount of graft material harvested can be increased by obtaining a graft block that is 5 cm wide rather than the usual 3 cm wide. After the block of unicortical graft material has been removed, 10 to 12 long strips of cancellous bone are removed with a gouge. A sonic gouge facilitates removal of the cancellous graft material. The graft block is then cut into four to six peg grafts, with the width determined by the measurement of the height of the prepared disk space when distracted maximally and the length determined by the depth of the disk space; usually these peg grafts are 10 by 25 mm. The bleeding of the donor site can be controlled easily by using a sheet of absorbable gelatin sponge Gelfoam (Up-John Laboratories, Kalamazoo, MI) soaked in thrombin.

Graft Insertion

The disk space is distracted by a laminal or vertebral body spreader. The laminal spreader tends to open the disk space posteriorly but may actually close the space anteriorly; a vertebral body spreader distracts the disk space more evenly. The newer model of Cloward's vertebral spreader has three

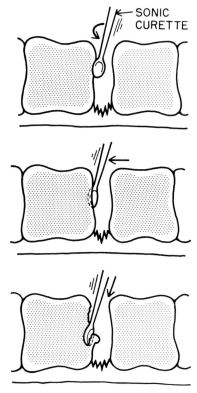

Figure 31–16. Thinning of the subchondral endplate with a sonic curette. This instrument is also helpful in sculpturing or undercutting the intervertebral rim to enhance the mechanism.

long, sharp pins on each side, the combined tip measuring 10 mm. Without modifying and shortening the pins, it would be difficult to insert the spreader within the disk space. The prying action of a blunt-end impactor (Sears or Cloward's Puka stick) within the disk space can distract the disk space sufficiently to allow placement of one of the two large central peg grafts from the opposite side. However, the prying maneuver should be done on both sides before the smaller lateral grafts are inserted.

When the disk space is very narrow, as in spondylosis, it can be entered by hammering a small, straight curette into the disk space. After partial diskectomy on both sides by this curette, the disk space can be opened by placing a 9- or 10-mm Puka stick into each side horizontally. Simultaneous forceful and gradual 90-degree rotations of the two Puka sticks can effect a 9- to 10-mm opening of the disk space.

Ideally, a graft for PLIF is placed in the central 80% of the disk space. Anteriorly, the graft should be adjacent to the annulus, or 2 to 3 mm away; posteriorly, it should be 2 to 3 mm below the adjoining vertebral bodies. If the anterior in-

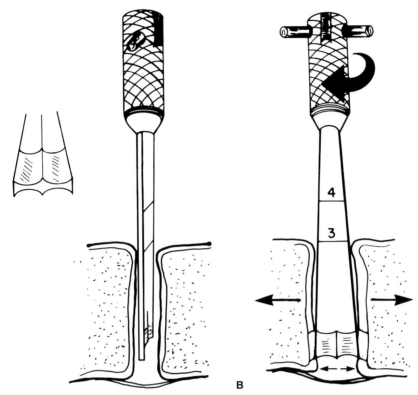

Figure 31–17. Preparation of the graft bed with a Collis's disk space shaper. (**A**). Calibrated disk space shaper is tapped into the disk space to a depth of 3 cm, with the width of the instrument parallel to the width of the disk space. (**B**). Grip the handle, and forcefully shear the remaining disk material and part of the subchondral endplates with 90-degree rotational forces in either direction. Note from the insert that the cutting edges are located on the four sides at the end of the shaper, and the end of the shaper itself is blunt.

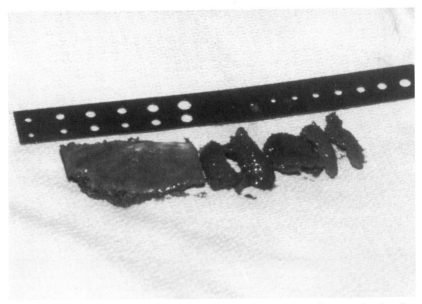

Figure 31–18. A single sheet of a rectangular split-thickness unicortical autograft, measuring 3 × 5 cm and about 8 to 10 mm thick, is removed from the posterior iliac bone, incorporating the posterior half of the iliac crest. Six to twelve cancellous long strips are also removed by gouge (sonic), preferably 12 or more strips for a high-density impaction.

tervertebral rims have been left intact, they form a built-in anterior graft locking mechanism. The posterior keystone effect is established by a shallow undercutting below the vertebral rim.

The entrance to the disk space is more narrow than the prepared graft bed within the disk space. The larger peg graft can be placed in the disk space, with the cortical side of the graft parallel to the subchondral endplates of the vertebral body. Then the graft is grasped firmly with a straight disk rongeur and rotated 90 degrees within the disk space, forcing the cortical plate of the graft to lie parallel to the longitudinal axis of the body, preferably with the disk space distracted from the other side.

We use only moderate-sized peg grafts that can be packed easily into the disk space. The first piece of graft introduced is usually a large cancellous strip, inserted horizontally into the base of the disk space. The larger piece of the peg graft, which is generally 10 to 12 mm wide and 25 to 30 mm long, is then placed in the central portion of the disk space. The graft may be moved toward the midline either by a swiveling action of the Puka stick or by a pushing action from the tip of an upbite disk rongeur. The surgeon should avoid placing the largest possible peg graft within the disk space, because a hard, pounding action to drive in a large graft can be traumatic. Furthermore, with excessive distraction and without proper keystone undercutting below the intervertebral rim, a larger graft may slowly induce posterior graft migration.

The lateral recess is filled with pieces of cancellous bone before the second lateral graft is inserted. Two or three peg grafts are used on each side, depending on the thickness of the graft or the width of the disk space. Every effort should be made to pack cancellous bone strips between each two peg grafts. An osteotome is first placed between the two peg grafts for the initial separation. This is followed with insertion of a Puka stick. A prying and rotating action of the Puka stick further increases the space between the peg grafts. The newly developed space is kept open by inserting an appropriate-size Frazier suction tip (Fig. 31–19). Then a long impactor (tapered, long Sears impactor, filed and rounded after purchase) is used to push the strips of cancellous graft between the peg grafts. The suction tip is removed after sufficient cancellous bone chips or strips have been inserted to keep the peg grafts apart. The surface of the highly impacted, high-density autogeneic cancellous bone grafts should lie 1 to 2 mm below that of the adjoining peg grafts.

It is important that all crevices between the peg grafts, or between the vertebral bodies, be filled with cancellous bone. Before insertion of the central graft, look for residual midline disk material. Then two or three strips of cancellous bone are inserted and pushed toward the midline to fill in all possible space between the two central grafts. A laminal spreader may be used on the side that has already been packed to facilitate graft insertion on the opposite side. High-density autogeneic cancellous grafting is the most osteogenetic portion of the PLIF. It is responsible for achiev-

ing early osteosynthesis or fusion. The success of a PLIF depends to a large measure on insertion and packing of as much autogeneic cancellous or coticocancellous chips into the disk space as possible (Fig. 31–20). If the grafting has been performed properly, the postoperative computed tomography (CT) scan should show the high-density cancellous bone grafts to be as dense (as white) as the cortical plate of the peg graft (Fig. 31–21).

When graft insertion is completed, the exposed portion of the graft should be at least 1 to 2 mm below the undercut surface of the adjoining vertebral bodies (Fig. 31–22). Karlin's offset central canal and the lateral gutter impactors are both useful for countersinking the grafts. To conform to the oval shape of the disk space, the lateral graft should be shorter, smaller, and lie lower than the central graft (Fig. 31–20). Compression force applied in a normal, upright lumbar lordotic curvature and the intact posterior motion segment locks the graft securely within the disk space.

The only tissue in the disk space should be bone graft. Loose or empty spaces will be invaded by fibrous tissue, which will delay fusion (Fig. 31–23). The three most common reasons for failure of fusion at this stage are (1) an inadequate amount of graft material, (2) inadequate size of a graft bed, and (3) spaces between the grafts. In addition, fusion may fail because the autogeneic bone grafts from a patient with osteoporosis are too soft to sustain the disk space

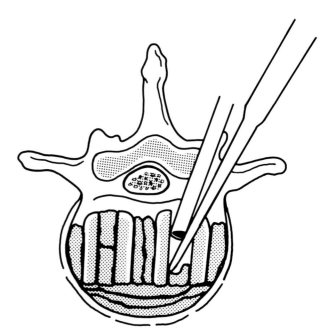

Figure 31–19. Technique for maximal cancellous bone impaction between the unicortical peg grafts. Place an osteotome between the peg grafts and then twist it to create a space. The space can be widened by replacing the osteotome with a Puka stick (blunt-end, osteotomelike impactor, 9 or 10 mm wide, designed by Dr Cloward, for moving the graft in the disk space or using as a distractor). Then use a Frazier suction tip to keep the space open in between the peg grafts. When enough cancellous bone chips have been inserted to keep the peg grafts apart, the suction tip is removed, and more cancellous bone is impacted.

distraction. The addition of two or three stronger allogeneic unicortical peg grafts to the osteopenic autogeneic grafts is recommended for these patients.

Closure

Before the wound closure, a careful search must be conducted to look in the intervertebral foramen for evidence of a loose bone fragment, retropulsed from the lateral most graft.

At the end of the grafting procedure, Surgicel is removed from the epidural space, which is then filled with free fat graft or a thrombin-soaked gelatin sponge (Gelfoam). Duromorph (Elkins-Sinn Inc., Cherry Hill, NJ) (morphine sulfate), 0.75 mg, is injected intrathecally through a number 27 needle. This generally provides excellent postoperative pain relief for 24 to 48 hours.

When the midline structures are intact, there is no dead space and a drain is not necessary. In a repeat surgical procedure, however, especially when the posterior components of the motion segment have been removed, there is a large dead space that should be drained by continuous Jackson-Pratt suction.

A strong wound closure can be obtained by suturing the preserved supraspinous ligaments to the adjoining aponeurosis. If the supraspinous ligaments have been violated, then a number 20 to number 24 wire wrapped around the adjoining spinous processes may help to stabilize the compromised posterior motion segment. For a severely compromised posterior motion segment, an internal fixation device should be considered in conjunction with PLIF.

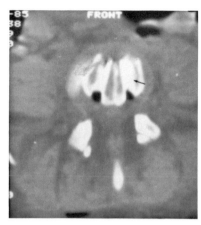

Figure 31–21. Immediate postoperative CT scan shows the high-density cancellous grafts, impacted between the cortical grafts, to be denser than the neighboring cortical peg grafts.

POSTOPERATIVE CARE

Antibiotic Treatment

Every 2 hours during the operation and every 6 hours after the surgery, antibiotics are administered intravenously.

Immobilization

For 4 months after the surgery, the patient should wear Knight's lumbar spinal brace with velcro straps, day and night, except when showering. A Boston Overlap Polyethylene TSL Orthosis may also be used, especially for the hard-to-fit obese person. The patient must be cautioned

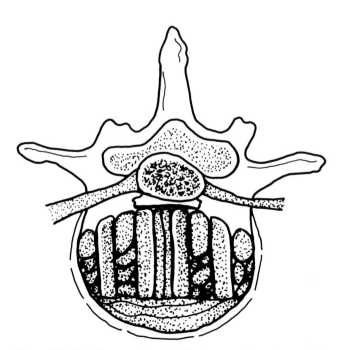

Figure 31–20. Concept of sandwiched autogeneic corticocancellous PLIF, alternating layers of cancellous and unicortical peg grafts. Note the tightness of the impacted grafts and the relatively lower position of the lateral grafts.

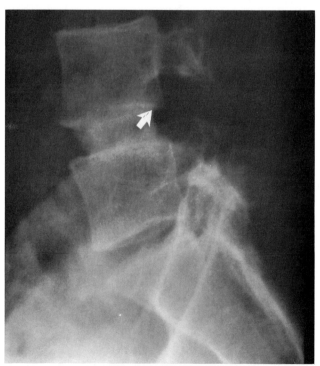

Figure 31–22. A lateral radiograph showing a satisfactory PLIF construct, with the posterior graft lying 2 mm below the undercut surface of the adjoining vertebral bodies.

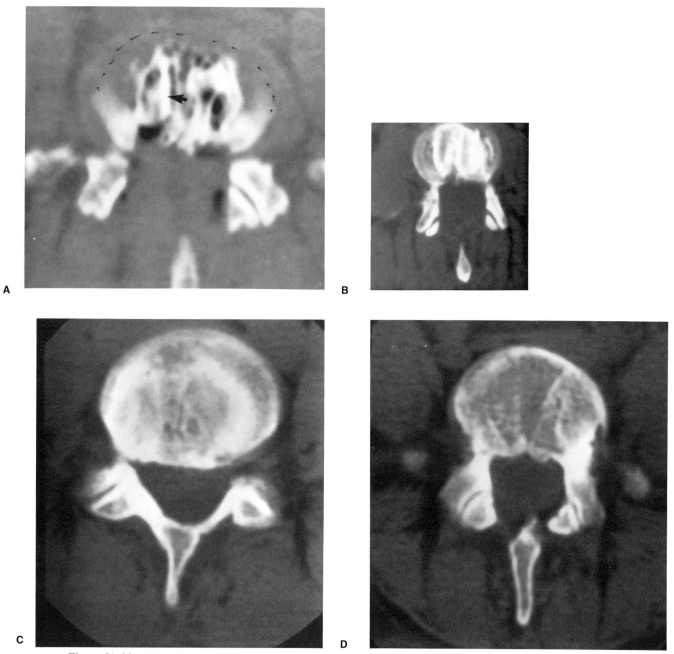

Figure 31–23. Maturing and remodeling processes of PLIF as seen in samples CT scan. (**A**). Immediate postoperative period. (**B**). Four months after surgery. (**C**). One year after surgery. (**D**). Three years after surgery, when the graft assumes the osseous appearance of a vertebral body.

not to flex the lumbar spine during physical activities, especially in getting in and out of bed. When an internal fixation device was used in PLIF, bracing is needed for only a 3-month period. It is recommended that the surgeon be present when the brace is put on for the first time in the hospital after the surgery; this is to ensure that the patient understands the proper application of the brace and the correct way to get up from the bed (from the side).

POSTOPERATIVE TOMOGRAM

Generally, fusion for the autogeneic high-density cancellous PLIF occurs approximately 4 months after surgery. The degree of osteosynthesis is determined on a lateral polytome tomogram done 4 months after surgery. The tomographic demonstration of a homogeneous mix of the graft with the adjoining vertebral bodies is usually sufficient evidence of

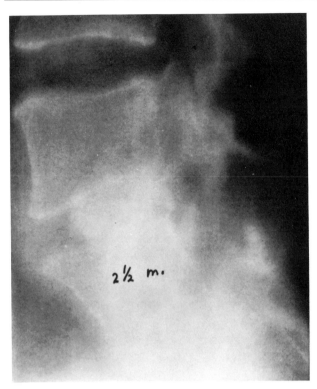

Figure 31–24. Lateral tomogram obtained $2\frac{1}{2}$ months after PLIF. Note evidence of an early, active osteosynthesis of the autogeneic graft. The height of the disk space is maintained.

osteosynthesis (Fig. 31–24). In the CT scan, an early remodeling of the osseous architecture of the vertebra by the graft is the only conclusive radiologic evidence of completed osteosynthesis in PLIF. Complete remodeling (Ring's phenomenon) may be seen as early as 9 months after surgery (Fig. 31–1). Similarly, trabeculation on the lateral radiograph may be seen 1 year after the surgery. Magnetic resonance imaging (MRI) is not helpful in determining the degree of osteosynthesis in PLIF.

ANTI-INFLAMMATORY TREATMENT

The administration of methylprednisolone, 40 mg every 12 hours for 2 or 3 days, decreases the postoperative discomfort by diminishing the tissue edema. Nonsteroidal prostaglandin inhibitors are often used to control the postoperative incisional and graft side discomfort during the period of convalescence.

COMPLICATIONS AND RESULTS

The complications and results of 500 cases of PLIF are presented.[12] The complications were as follows:

1. Infection: There was one superficial case.
2. Thrombophlebitis: There were 24 cases. Twenty-one were diagnosed clinically in the hospital (four verified by venogram) and three were diagnosed clinically after discharge from the hospital (one was fatal due to pulmonary embolism).
3. Myocardial infarction: There were two cases. One was diagnosed 1 week after surgery, and the patient recovered; the other patient died suddenly at home 30 days after surgery.
4. Neurological deficits:
   (a) Foot drop occurred in 25 patients, 12 of whom needed temporary braces. All except three improved, or recovered in 6 months.
   (b) Urinary incontinence occurred in two cases (one mild and one moderate). Both cases improved.
   (c) Anterolateral femoral cutaneous neuritis: This was usually mild and transient and occurred in 6% of patients.
5. Retropulsion: There were four cases of acute retropulsion during the immediate postoperative period. Late retropulsion or pseudoarthrosis occurred in 14 cases; a second PLIF was needed in five and a lateral fusion in nine (seven of whom were in the worker's compensation group).
6. Wrong level: This occurred in two cases.

The results were as follows. In the first 500 cases, fusion was obtained in 88% of cases. In the second 500 cases, the result of fusion was improved to 92%. Forty cases had augmentation with the Variable Serial Placement (VSP) Steffee system, and the fusion rate was 97.5%. Eighty-two percent had a satisfactory clinical result (excellent or good) without the need for pain medication. Functionally, in the noncompensation group, 71% returned to full duty, whereas (as expected) only 39% of the compensation group returned to full duty. In the latter group, fusion success apparently had little correlation with the ability to return to functional recovery.

CONCLUSION

For the complete spinal surgeon, PLIF or any other type of interbody fusion should be a standard procedure in his or her armamentarium. It can be performed safely without injury to the related neural structures. Evidence of arthrodesis, especially for a "floating fusion," with or without the help of internal fixation should be higher than with other comparable lumbar spinal fusion techniques.

REFERENCES

1. Cloward RB. New treatment of ruptured intervertebral disc. Presented at the annual meeting of the Hawaii Territorial Medical Association; 1945.
2. Cautilli RA. Theoretical superiority of PLIF. In: Lin PM, ed. *Posterior Lumbar Interbody Fusion.* Springfield, Ill: Charles C Thomas; 1982:82–93.
3. Lin PM. PLIF complications and pitfalls. *Clin Orthop.* 1985;193:90–102.
4. Urist MR. Bone transplants and implants. In: Urist MR, ed. *Fundamental and Clinical Bone Physiology.* Philadelphia, Pa: JB Lippincott; 1980:331–368.

5. Crenshaw AH, ed. *Campbell's Operative Orthopedic.* 7th ed. Vol 1. St. Louis, Mo: CV Mosby; 1987:15, 17, 60.

6. Goldner JS, Wood KE, Urbaniak JR. Anterior lumbar discectomy and interbody fusion. In: Schmidek HH, Sweet WH, eds. *Operative Neurosurgical Techniques 2nd ed.* Vol 2. New York: Grune & Stratton; 1988:1421–1436.

7. Evans JH. Biomechanics of lumbar fusion. *Clin Orthop.* 1985;193:38–46.

8. Lin PM. Techniques and complications of PLIF. In: Lin PM, Gill K, eds. *Lumbar Interbody Fusion.* Rockville, Md: Aspen Publications; 1989:171–209.

9. Lin PM. Clinical indications for lumbar interbody fusion. In: Lin PM, Gill K, eds. *Lumbar Interbody Fusion.* Rockville, Md: Aspen Publications; 1989:36–53.

10. Lin PM. A technical modification of Cloward's posterior lumbar interbody fusion. *Neurosurg.* 1977;1:118–124.

11. Lin PM. Technique of posterior lumbar interbody fusion. In: Lin PM, ed. *Posterior Lumbar Interbody Fusion.* Springfield, Ill: Charles C Thomas; 1982:94–139.

12. Lin PM, Cautilli RA, Joyce MF. Posterior lumbar interbody fusion. *Clin Orthop.* 1983;180:154–168.

32 Simmons Plating System for Segmental Stabilization

James W. Simmons, M.D., F.A.C.S.

INTRODUCTION

The Simmons plating system (Smith and Nephew Spine, Memphis, Tenn) was designed to enhance decompression and stabilization of the spine. It is one of several instrumentation systems developed in the 1980s. Over the course of the decade, improvements in posterior spinal fixation instrumentation, especially those incorporating the pedicle, brought reconsideration of arthrodesis techniques. Although all fusion techniques are enhanced by the plating system, the author's preference is the posterior lumbar interbody fusion (PLIF) procedure accompanied by the bolt/plate construct.

Before instrumentation, the strongest early proponent of PLIF in the United States was Ralph Cloward,[1] who in 1947 reported on 100 cases wherein the procedure was incorporated in the treatment of ruptured lumbar disks. Enthusiasm for the procedure, however, was stronger outside the United States, with Crock[2] in Australia, James and Nisbet[3] in New Zealand, LeVay[4] in England, and Junghanns and Schmorl[5] in Germay reporting refinements to the procedure in the 1950s and 1960s. Their attempts incorporated the use of a variety of graft methods (tibial grafts for body-to-body fusion, osseous packs with distraction) and expanded the range of indications for the procedure to include spondylolisthesis. In the 1960s in the United States, Wiltberger[6] used iliac and tibial dowel grafts for PLIF with good results in 70% of cases. Later, Christoferson and Selland[7] placed lamina in the intervertebral disk space after diskectomy. Lin[8] refined Cloward's technique and renewed interest in its applications. Ma[9] and Collis[10] introduced new instruments and reported on the use of allograft bone. Simmons[11] reported on the use of autograft chips obtained at the time of laminectomy.

The advantages of instrumentation include formation of three-column stability, with allowance for wider decompression, prevention of graft dislodgement, and improved fusion rate. Instrumented PLIF affords biomechanical advantages, including load sharing and graft protection while disk height and interpedicular distance are maintained by the instrumentation. This, in turn, allows earlier patient mobilization, shorter hospital stays, and freedom from brace requirements.

THE SIMMONS PLATING SYSTEM

Design Considerations

The Simmons plating system is applicable for spinal stabilization with placement of bone graft material in any of a number of fusion techniques: posterolateral (intertransverse), anterior lumbar interbody (ALIF), and PLIF. In the author's center, it has been incorporated most often into PLIF procedures.

Description of Components

The system was designed to maximize the attributes of versatility, stability, and simplicity. To that end, components are available in a wide range of sizes, for application in various degrees of constraint of any given construct, and with component adaptations that make the system easy to apply (Fig. 32–1).

Components include bolts, screws, standard washers, contoured washers, oblique washers, offset bolts, and plates. Sizes of components are as follows: bolts come in a 5.5-mm diameter (lengths 30 to 35 mm), a 6.4-mm diameter (lengths 30 to 50 mm in 5-mm increments), and a 7.0-mm diameter (lengths 30 to 55 mm in 5-mm increments). Screws include a 5.5-mm diameter (30-, 35-, and 40-mm lengths) and a 6.4-mm diameter (lengths 30 to 50 mm in 5-mm increments). Offset bolts are supplied as a 6.5-mm diameter (lengths 30 to 50 mm in 5-mm increments) and a 7.0-mm diameter (30- to 50-mm lengths). Plate lengths range from 40 to 200 mm in 10-mm increments with the addition of a 65-mm length. Tools for assembling and affixing the Simmons plating system are available in autoclave-safe trays.

Components can be assembled for a variety of constructs, ranging from a relatively unconstrained all-screw construct to the highly constrained all-bolt and crossplate construct (Fig. 32–2).

Special consideration has been given to the design of individual components to increase ease of placement and reduce mechanical causes of failure. Bolts are precut. Screws and bolts are cannulated for use by surgeons preferring a cannulated technique; biomechanical testing reveals that cannulation reduces the strength of bolts by only 3.8%. The tapered shank of the bolt increases the overall bolt strength

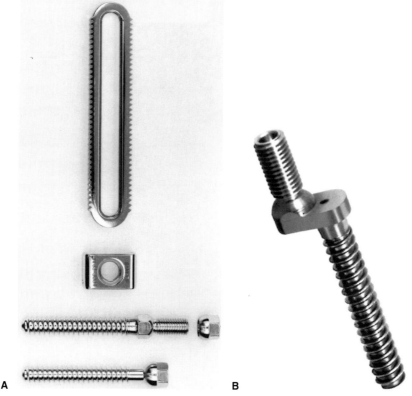

Figure 32–1. Simmons plating system components. (**A**). Top to bottom: Plate, washer, bolt with Spiralock locking nut, screw. (**B**). Offset bolt.

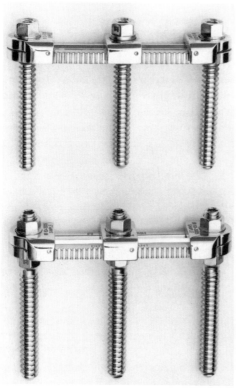

Figure 32–2. Assembled components of the Simmons plating system. Top: Assembled screw construct. Bottom: Assembled bolt construct.

and eliminates the stress-riser effect at the most common point of breakage in older systems. Bolts and screws have a large minor diameter with a relatively decreased pitch of threads, effectively increasing the strength of the bolt and screws without diminishing pullout strength. Stress shielding and bolt fatigue are reduced by the large radius at the bolt-plate interface, which allows micromotion. Finally, the self-locking Spiralock nut can be tightened and loosened as needed without diminishing the self-locking function.

It was noted through biomechanical testing that the Simmons plating system demonstrated a lower bending strength than three other plating systems.[12] The static strength of a construct is dependent on the material properties and geometry of the individual system components. The Simmons plating system was designed to provide as low a profile as possible. The Simmons plate, with a thickness of 4 mm, can be bent intraoperatively to accommodate changes in spinal geometry, yet there is no report of plate breakage or additional bending in vivo. A clinical investigational device exemption (IDE) study involving 413 patients revealed five screw/bolt breakages. These breakages resulted from fatigue fracture or external trauma; therefore, static bending strength of spinal system constructs has not been shown to be clinically relevant.

Construct flexibility and stiffness also were determined in the study. It was noted that the Simmons plating system was less stiff, and therefore more flexible, than the other plating systems. The optimal stiffness necessary for a spinal construct is not known. Although it is necessary for a system to provide adequate spinal stability, excessive stiffness may result in stress shielding. This was taken into consideration in the design of the Simmons plating system. Micromotion was intentionally built into the system at the bolt-plate interface, not only to decrease stress-shielding effects but also to increase bolt fatigue strength.

Construct Selection

An all-bolt construct is the most rigid of the systems, particularly when crossplates are employed. A screw construct used alone or in conjunction with bolts is considered an unconstrained system. At the author's center, the all-bolt system is used in the lumbar spine when instrumentation accompanies a PLIF procedure. The all-bolt system without the crossplate and employing large-diameter bolts best provides the micromotion required to mimic the elasticity of bone, thereby stimulating osteogenesis. With use of the all-bolt system and its micromotion capability, the stress-shielding effect is less likely to occur and diminish the chances for adequate fusion.

Use of a Simmons construct employing screws alone or in combination with bolts is best limited to lateral fusion in the lumbar spine and posterior thoracic fusion. The screw construct is easy to use in the thoracic spine, with the mechanics of the screw and plate serving as a reduction device for thoracolumbar fractures.

The advantage of using the pedicle for fixation is its allowance for segmental spinal stabilization. In conjunction with PLIF, utilizing the plate with the bolt and/or a screw construct or a combination of bolt and screw, it is sufficient to include only the involved segments of the spine in the fusion procedure. For fracture dislocation and other spine and spinal cord injuries requiring stabilization, two or three levels above and below the involved segment may be incorporated in the fusion to allow the paralytic patient to advance into a rehabilitation program.

INDICATIONS FOR PLIF

Many investigators have identified low back pain with or without sciatica secondary to abnormalities of the motion segment or functional spinal unit as the clinical hallmark of spinal instability. Any of a number of spinal abnormalities, or a combination of them, can cause the clinical constellation that may warrant fusion: degenerated disk, disk protrusion, disk herniation, spinal stenosis, postlumbar laminectomy-diskectomy syndrome, spondyloylysis or spondylolisthesis, failed back surgery syndrome, and pseudarthrosis.

Our indications for PLIF[13] are a combination of pathophysiological, functional, and lifestyle requirements: (1) spinal stenosis unresponsive to nonoperative measures, particularly subarticular or foraminal stenosis requiring partial or complete facetectomy; (2) segmental instability unre-

sponsive to nonoperative measures, if radiographically definable (primary sagittal or rotational instability may be difficult to quantify or define); and (3) diskogenic disease unresponsive to job or activity modifications, including chemically induced disk pain.

Several investigators have cited PLIF as the most biomechanically satisfying stabilizing process. Lin,[14] for example, found that PLIF reconstitutes the normal anatomic relationship between the motion segment and the neural structures, restoring anatomic alignment of disk space and motion segment. Further, Lin found that degenerative changes of the fused segment are halted with PLIF, although this had been found to increase the range of motion of adjoining segments, possibly stimulating their degenerative changes. Total diskectomy performed in the course of PLIF prevents recurrent lumbar disk herniation at the fused level.

Lin[14] and Cautilli[15] cited the advantage of exposure of a wide area of bone surface and adequacy of blood supply through the cancellous portion of the vertebral body once the cortical plate has been removed. The procedure allows for complete visualization of the area of nerve root compression and provides complete access for removal of compression areas centrally and laterally, at the foraminal trough.

Evans[16] uses the "flagpole" model to describe the biomechanical advantages of PLIF. In this model, the central graft placement represents the flagpole, with the facets, remaining annulus anteriorly, and posterior ligamentous restraints representing surrounding guy wires. This construct, according to Evans, balances both compressive and torsional forces.

Additional advantages are obtained when instrumentation with interpedicular fixation is an adjunct to PLIF. Specifically, after significant facetectomy or sacrifice of posterior ligaments, instrumentation reestablishes the natural construct. In addition, the combination of interbody corticocancellous grafts with interpedicular fixation forms a load-sharing construct, protecting both graft and screw from failure. Instrumentation enhances all of the attributes of the PLIF.

PATIENT SELECTION AND DIAGNOSIS

A history of persistent low back pain with or without sciatica is characteristic. In response to this clinical presentation, definitive diagnosis should be made relating to the anatomic structure involved, the lesion, the morphological changes, instability, and extent of neurological involvement. Also to be considered is the need to distinguish between instability and physiological mobility. Even normative values of intervertebral mobility in asymptomatic patients may present ranges of translation that exceed the criteria for pathologic instability.[17,18] Therefore, the need to correlate clinical with radiographic findings is emphasized.

Clinically, instability has been defined as "the patient with back problems who with the least provocation steps from the mildly symptomatic to the severe episode."[19] The patient may complain of a feeling of "giving way" or "slipping out." A series of torsion-type injury mechanisms may be described. Some investigators have reported hypertrophied muscle, palpable catches on flexion, and uncoordinated muscle contractions as physical signs. Abnormal lumbar motion may be either translational or rotational. Instability may be apparent in quality or coupling of movements rather than quantity.

For those patients who do not present with a clear, single-root, unilateral syndrome as a source of their pain, magnetic resonance imaging (MRI) is a valuable initial screen. Torsion and compression testing as described by Farfan[20] may be useful adjuncts to the standard neurological examination. Provocative diskography is useful for localization of pain (especially the awake diskogram).

Primary radiographic signs often are elusive. Abnormal translation has been used to identify lumbar instability most frequently, with Knutsson[17] finding more than 3 mm of translation in the sagittal plane to be abnormal. Posner and colleagues[18] defined the limits of translation in flexion of 8% at L1 to L5, 6% at L5 to S1, and 9% in extension at all levels. They found absolute values somewhat less than Knutsson's 3 mm. An abnormal translational lateral shear may also be seen. Rotational abnormalities may be demonstrated in side-bending x-ray films showing the spinous process at the abnormal segment rotating toward the convexity.[21] Rotational abnormalities may also appear as double density of the uncinate processes on the lateral projection.[21] However, the pairing of translation and rotation may obscure segmental instability so that quantifying the abnormality becomes impossible.

Secondary radiographic signs of segmental instability should be considered when primary signs are absent or obscure. Secondary signs include the vacuum disk sign, Macnab traction spur,[22] spondylolisthesis,[23] retrolisthesis,[24] or previous total laminectomy.[25]

OPERATIVE TECHNIQUE

Variations in the Performance of PLIF

With the patient placed prone on the Andrews spinal table, posterior elements are exposed to initiate the process of instrumentation placement. Lateral imaging with C-arm fluoroscopy is used to confirm position and provide reference for placement of pedicle bolts. Pedicles are broached with care at an angle corresponding to that shown on fluoroscopy. Upon completion of preparation of the bed and probing of all pedicles to be included in the fixation, the pedicles are tapped. Placement of the bolts is then done. The bolts at S1 engage the promontory. Thereafter, the appropriate plates are selected and bent to maintain the lumbar lordosis. The plate is fixed on the bolts with the system's washer and locking nut mechanism. The PLIF technique, as used in the author's center, follows placement of instrumentation.

Many variations exist in performance of PLIF, especially in the use of bone graft material. Cloward[1] originally used autogenous iliac plugs and later adopted the use of allograft iliac plugs. James and Nisbet[3] used autogenous fibula. Jaslow[26] used a peg of bone in the intervertebral disk space and chips from the posterior elements place posteriorly. Wiltberger[6] used iliac dowels and had used split fibular plugs. Christoferson and Selland[7] fashioned a graft from a portion of the lamina and medial facet. Proponents of chips as alternatives for struts, dowels, or plugs include Briggs and Milligan[27] and Ma.[9] The latter devised an injection instrument for firm impaction of corticocancellous chips approximately 5 mm below the posterior border of the vertebral body. Hutter[28] employed a keystone modeling of the intervertebral disk space to encompass a graft of autogenous chips. Blume and Rojas[29] fashioned corticocancellous bone from the iliac crest fitted to the carefully sculpted endplates placed over corticocancellous chips. Lin and associates[30] used a combination of autograft and allograft bone blocks to fill the disk space.

RESULTS

No universally accepted standards exist to measure results after spinal fusion. Investigators report results based on presence or absence of radiographic evidence of solid union, although such a parameter does not necessarily reflect long-term postoperative spinal stability. Stability may indeed be afforded by fibrous union rather than by radiographic evidence of bony union. Figures 32–3, 32–4, and 32–5 show pre- and postoperative radiographic findings in three patients undergoing PLIF and Simmons plating system instrumentation.

A prospective clinical study of the Simmons implant in conjunction with PLIF is in progress. Results of PLIF alone, without instrumentation, have been reported previously by the author,[13,31] with solid fusion in 91% of cases. Cloward has reported 92% successful fusion with PLIF alone.[32] Lin et al reported 88%[33] and Ma[9] reported an 85% rate of solid union.

Reports of PLIF in conjunction with instrumentation have come from Steffee and Sitkowski[34] (PLIF with plates instrumentation), who, in 1988, reported 100% solid union in their series.

COMPLICATIONS

All spine surgery techniques carry the risks of blood loss, epidural bleeding, nerve root injury, intra-abdominal vascular injury, pseudoarthrosis, instability, graft resorption, infection, epidural scar, arachnoiditis, dural tears, graft retropulsion, and adjacent-level degeneration.

Complications implicated particularly after PLIF include nerve root injury, epidural scar, dural tears, graft retropulsion, and adjacent-level degeneration.[10,35–37] However, plates give immediate stabilization, enhance

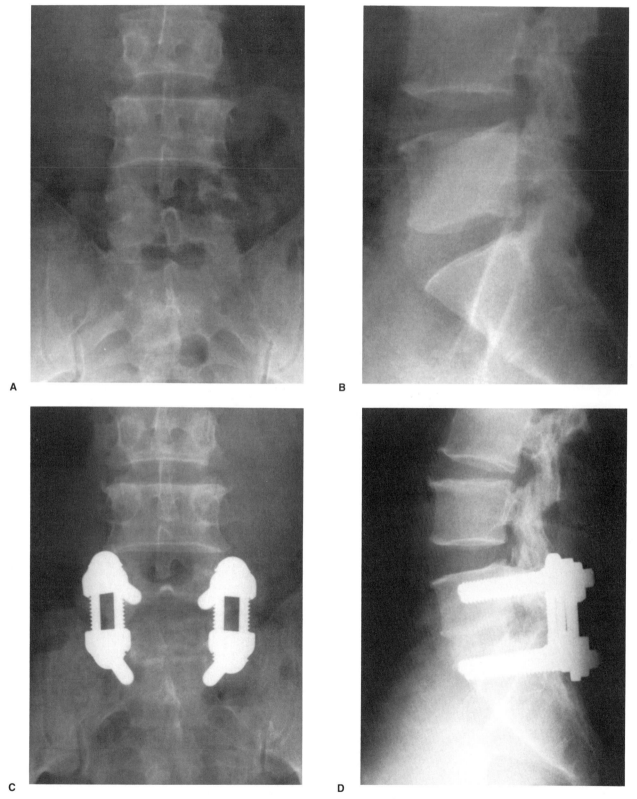

Figure 32–3. (**A**) and (**B**). Preoperative films from a 50-year-old male with incapacitating low back pain with sciatica secondary to a painful herniated nucleus pulposus at L5, confirmed with diskography. (**C**) and (**D**). A decompressive laminectomy and foraminotomy were done with stabilization by a Simmons bolt and plate construct and a body-to-body composite graft. Note that the S1 bolts purchase on the promontory.

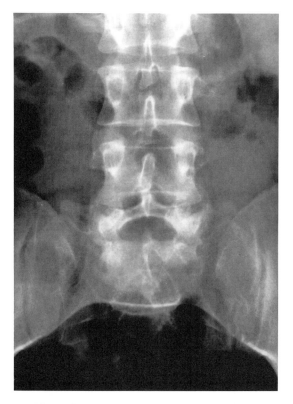

A

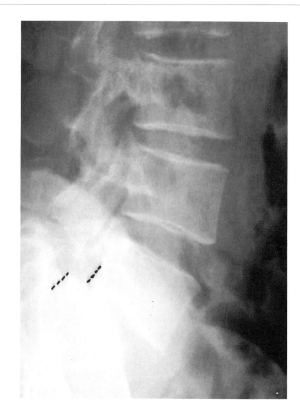

B

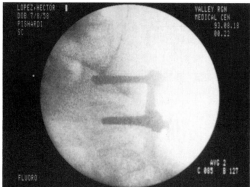

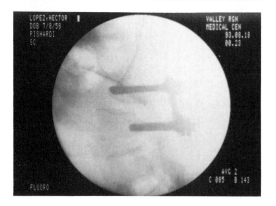

C

Figure 32–4. (**A**) and (**B**). A 33-year-old male with a painful grade II spondylolisthesis demonstrated on the plain films. (**C**). The C-arm fluoroscopic films show the reduction of the spondylolisthesis. The top image shows the bolts in place with the S1 bolt fixed firmly and tightened with the torque wrench. The bolts are purchasing on the promontory for a more stable purchase. The L5 bolt is attached loosely with the washer on the plate. The bottom image shows the reduction and the S1 washer fixed firmly on the plate prior to diskectomy and insertion of the graft material into the L5 intervertebral disk space. (**D**) and (**E**). The plain films with the Simmons system in place show good reduction with composite graft (chipped autograft from the posterior element and allograft plugs).

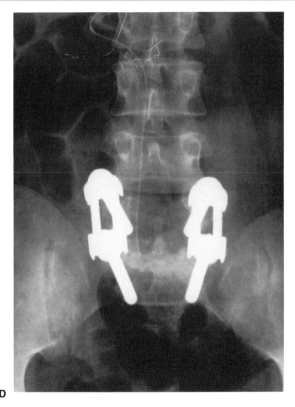

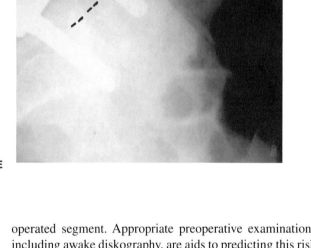

D   E

Figure 32–4 Continued.

fusion rates, and contribute to a reduction in eventual nerve root injury.

Nerve root injury can be avoided by careful decompression and retraction. Having sufficient lateral disk exposure with ample facetectomy, made possible by the plating system, protects the existing and traversing nerve roots at the time of graft impaction. Nerve roots should be inspected for impingement after graft impaction; and certainly if lower-extremity movement occurs during graft impaction, roots should be inspected carefully for entrapment.

Epidural scarring has been particularly troublesome with PLIF. The addition of segmental plate fixation prevents excessive neural traction from epidural scar mass. Fat grafting, gentle retraction, and consistent hemostasis are procedures designed to reduce occurrence of epidural scarring.

Graft retropulsion has been reported subsequent to PLIF. Careful endplate shaping, graft sizing, and countersinking of graft material should prevent this complication. The addition of pedicle fixation to the PLIF procedure reduces occurrence of this complication.

Degeneration of adjacent levels has been observed as a consequence of the high degree of stability afforded to the

operated segment. Appropriate preoperative examinations, including awake diskography, are aids to predicting this risk. It is important to spare the facets adjacent to the fused segment to avoid subsequent degeneration of adjacent levels. Pseudoarthrosis can occur after PLIF, as it does with other surgical attempts at spinal fusion. It can be minimized by use of the instrumentation.

CONCLUSIONS

A posterior lumbar interbody fusion, with or without instrumentation, is a technically difficult operation. Most potential postoperative problems can be eliminated using spinal instrumentation. With the addition of instrumentation to the basic PLIF procedure, a number of disadvantages of the PLIF procedure are alleviated. Patient response after surgery is enhanced, given the reduced hospitalization time, more rapid rehabilitation, earlier return to work, and decreased morbidity by early ambulation afforded by PLIF with instrumentation.

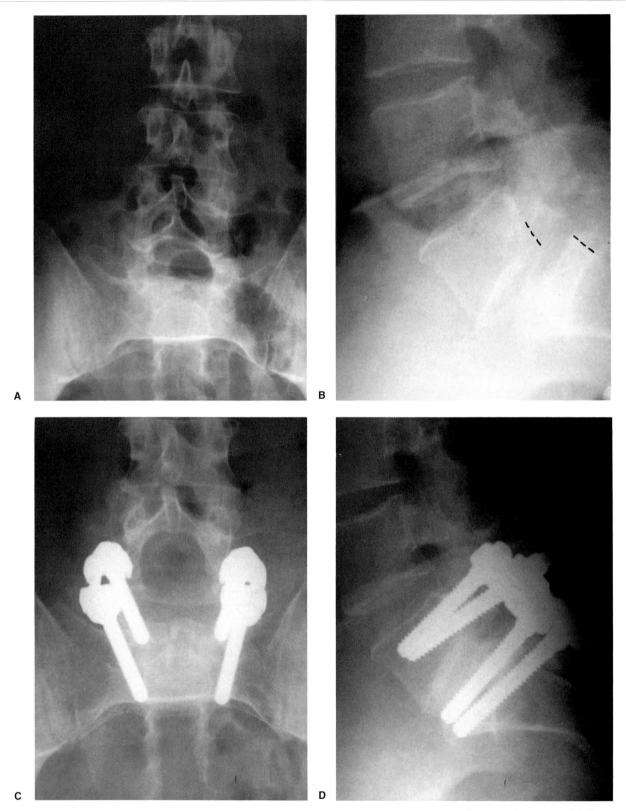

Figure 32–5. (**A**) and (**B**). Preoperative radiological appearance of a 35-year-old male with a painful L5 spondylolisthesis. (**C**) and (**D**). The plain films show the grade I spondylolisthesis with the Simmons implants in place. The plating system is affixed well in the body of L5 with the bolts at S1 purchasing on the promontory. Extensive decompression was performed, and autogenous chips were placed anteriorly with allograft plugs placed posteriorly.

REFERENCES

1. Cloward RB. The treatment of ruptured lumbar intervertebral discs by vertebral body fusion: indications, operative technique, after care. *J Neurosurg.* 1953;10:154–168.

2. Crock HV. *Practice of Spinal Surgery.* New York: Springer-Verlag; 1983.

3. James A, Nisbet NW. Posterior intervertebral fusion of lumbar spine. Preliminary report of a new operation. *J Bone Joint Surg.* 1953;35B:181–187.

4. LeVay D. A surgery of surgical management of lumbar disc prolapse in the United Kingdom and Eire. *Lancet.* 1967;1:1211–1213.

5. Junghanns H, Schmorl GL. *The Human Spine in Health and Disease.* 2nd ed. New York: Grune & Stratton; 1971:35.

6. Wiltberger BR. The dowel intervertebral-body fusion as used in lumbar-disc surgery. *J Bone Joint Surg.* 1957;39A:284–292.

7. Christoferson LA, Selland B. Intervertebral bone implants following excision of protruded lumbar discs. *J Neurosurg.* 1975;42:401–405.

8. Lin PM. A technical modification of Cloward's posterior lumbar interbody fusion. *J Neurosurg.* 1977;9:118–124.

9. Ma GW. Posterior lumbar interbody fusion with specialized instruments. *Clin Orthop.* 1985;193:57–63.

10. Collis JS. Total disc replacement: a modified posterior lumbar interbody fusion. *Clin Orthop.* 1985;193:64–67.

11. Simmons JW. Posterior lumbar interbody fusion with posterior elements as chip grafts. *Clin Orthop.* 1985;193:85–89.

12. Cunningham BW, Sefter JC, Shono Y, et al. Static and cyclical biomechanical analysis of pedicle screw spinal constructs. *Spine.* 1993;18:1677–1688.

13. Simmons JW. Posterior lumbar interbody fusion. In: Frymoyer JW, ed. *The Adult Spine: Principles and Practice.* New York: Raven Press; 1991:1961–1987.

14. Lin PM. *Introduction of PLIF: Biomechanical Principles and Indications.* Springfield, Ill: Charles C Thomas; 1982:3.

15. Cautilli RA. Theoretical superiority of posterior lumbar interbody fusion. In: Lin PM, ed. *Posterior Lumbar Interbody Fusion.* Springfield, Ill: Charles C Thomas; 1982:82–93.

16. Evans JH. Biomechanics of lumbar fusion. *Clin Orthop.* 1985;193:38–46.

17. Knutsson F. The instability associated with disc degeneration in the lumbar spine. *Acta Radiologica.* 1944;25:593–609.

18. Posner I, White AA III, et al. A biomechanical anslysis of the clinical stability of the lumbar and lumbosacral spine. *Spine.* 1982;7:374–389.

19. Paris SV. Physical signs of instability. *Spine.* 1985;10:277–279.

20. Farfan HF. *Mechanical Disorders of the Low Back.* Philadelphia, Pa: Lea and Febiger; 1973.

21. Dupuis PR, Yang-Hing K, Cassidy JD, et al. Radiologic diagnosis of degenerative lumbar spinal instability. *Spine.* 1985;10:262–276.

22. Macnab I. The traction spur: an indicator of segmental instability. *J Bone Joint Surg.* 1971;53A:663–670.

23. Penning L, Blickman JR. Instability in lumbar spondylolisthesis: a radiologic study of several concepts. *Am J Radiol.* 1980;134:293–301.

24. Frymoyer JW, Selby DK. Segmental instability. Rationale for treatment. *Spine.* 1985;10:280–286.

25. Bradford DS. Spinal instability: orthopedic perspective and prevention. *Clin Neurosurg.* 1980;27:591–610.

26. Jaslow IA. Intercorporal bone graft in spinal fusion after disc removal. *Surg Gynecol Obstet.* 1946;82:215–218.

27. Briggs H, Milligan PR. Chip fusion of the low back following exploration of the spinal canal. *J Bone Joint Surg.* 1944;26A:125–130.

28. Hutter CG. Spinal stenosis and posterior lumbar interbody fusion. *Clin Orthop.* 1985;193:103–114.

29. Blume HG, Rojas CH. Unilateral lumbar interbody fusion (posterior approach) utilizing dowel grafts. *J Neurol Orthop Surg.* 1981;2:419–430.

30. Lin PM, Cautilli RA, Joyce MF. Posterior lumbar interbody fusion. *Clin Orthop.* 1983;180:154–168.

31. Simmons JW. Posterior interbody fusions. Paper presented at the Seventh Annual Meeting of the International Society for the Study of the Lumbar Spine; 1980; New Orleans, La.

32. Cloward RB. Posterior lumbar interbody fusion updated. *Clin Orthop.* 1985;193:16–19.

33. Lin PM. Posterior lumbar interbody fusion technique: complications and pitfalls. *Clin Orthop.* 1985;193:90–102.

34. Steffee AD, Sitkowski DJ. Posterior lumbar interbody fusion with plates. *Clin Orthop.* 1988;227:99–102.

35. Macnab I, Dall D. The blood supply of the lumbar spine and its application to the technique of intertransverse lumbar fusion. *J Bone Joint Surg.* 1971;53B:628–635.

36. Cotler JM, Star AM. Complications of spinal fusion. In: Cotler JM, Cotler HB, eds. *Spinal Fusion: Science and Technique.* New York: Springer-Verlag; 1990:361–387.

37. Smith GJ. Complications of lumbar spine surgery. Presented at the 8th Annual Meeting, North American Spine Society; Oct. 14–16, 1993; San Diego, Calif.

33 The Rogozinski Spinal Rod System for Fixation of the Lumbosacral Spine

Chaim Rogozinski, M.D., Abraham Rogozinski, M.D.

SYSTEM EVOLUTION

The Rogozinski spinal rod system (Smith and Nephew Spine, Memphis, Tenn) was designed to remedy instrumentation problems compounding the inherent difficulties in performing spinal surgery. Design proceeded from a desire to achieve an implant with a high level of safety and efficacy in conjunction with a high degree of user friendliness. Ideally, such a system would be sufficiently strong to enhance arthrodesis; it would allow early mobilization of patients without the need for external bracing, and it would eliminate the occurrence of complications commonly associated with spinal instrumentation.

Since it was first implanted in a patient in 1988, the authors' application of the system has undergone an evolution over the course of 200 cases. Initially, the system was utilized in 54 cases incorporating nonsegmental fixations using laminar hook attachments. Subsequently, laminar hook attachment capturing the cephalad segment was utilized with pedicle screws in combination with hooks at S1 for segmental fixation. This so-called hybrid construct was employed in 19 cases. In 1990, pedicle screws were first employed in segmental fixation of vertebrae above S1. In this application, the system has evolved to its present level to be used as posterior instrumentation of the lumbar spine in the course of posterolateral or simultaneous combined anteroposterior procedures. Results were tabulated as part of an FDA investigational device study for the first 150 patients and are reported herein. (The system has a 510K approval for hybrid or all-hook constructs; use of pedicle screws at levels other than the sacrum is investigational.)

Because of the modularity of the system, various levels of rigidity can be achieved. The results have revealed significantly higher rates of fusion with the more rigid fixation procedures—posterolateral fusion with pedicle screws and combined anteroposterior procedures with pedicle screws posteriorly and dowel grafts anteriorly. As a consequence, implants using only nonsegmental laminar hooks have been abandoned by the authors and all-screws constructs are used predominantly with occasional use of hybrid constructs.

Various spinal surgery centers throughout the United States have employed the system for lumbosacral and thoracolumbar spine stabilization procedures since 1990, during which time the system has been used to accompany posterolateral spinal fusion as well as interbody fusion (posterior and anterior). Newer applications such as an anterior instrumentation have been investigated recently.

SYSTEM COMPONENTS

The system inventory (Fig. 33–1) includes rods, pedicle screws, hooks, couplers, set screws, and cross bars. Various configurations are possible and are comprised of screws or hooks attached to bilateral rods linked by cross bars at each level, forming a quadrilateral or ladder-shaped configuration.

Pedicle Screws

In the case of pedicle screw fixation, screws are placed bilaterally in the central axis of the pedicles. Pedicle screws are connected independently to the rods via various-sized cross bars, thus eliminating the need to align screws in the frontal and sagittal plane. Pedicle screws are supplied in lengths from 35 mm to 60 mm in 5-mm increments. Three sizes are available: 6.4-mm major with a 4.8-mm minor diameter; 5.5-mm major with a 4.8-mm minor diameter; and 7.0-mm major with a 5.4-mm minor diameter.

Hooks

Hooks may be used alone or in pairs to sandwich laminae above and below. In addition, they may be used as a double anchor in the sacrum along with sacral pedicle screws. The hooks, which are open backed, are closed with modified cross bars called hook bars.

Hooks are supplied in 7-mm and 11-mm aperture sizes with three designs—upangle, downangle, and neutral—to achieve tricortical laminar capture. The volume occupied by the hook within the canal, when appropriately seated on the lamina, is 2 mm, representing the thickness of the hook pad. This minimizes the likelihood of iatrogenic stenosis encountered with previous hook designs.

Rods and Cross Bars

Rods are smooth, measure 6.4 mm in diameter, and are flared at one end. They are supplied in lengths of 50 to

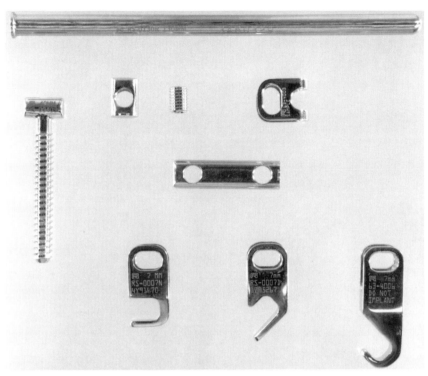

Figure 33–1. Rogozinski spinal rod system components. Rod (top); hooks (bottom) with three hook designs—neutral, downangle, upangle; bone screw (left); cross bar (center); hook bar (below rod, left); coupler (below rod, right); and set screw (below rod, center) used to secure cross bars.

300 mm in 10- or 20-mm increments. The rods are intended to be contoured intraoperatively to fit a lordotic curve or kyphoscoliotic deformity.

The contralateral rods are connected by cross bars to enhance rigidity of the construct when faced with torsional stresses on the implant and to increase significantly the pullout strength of individual screws (Fig. 33–2). Cross bars are supplied in 10-mm to 55-mm lengths in 3-mm increments. The smallest cross bars, called hook bars, are used to close laminar hooks. Cross bars and hook bars incorporate a self-locking mechanism (Spiralock) that prevents vibratory loosening.

Couplers and Set Screws

The system is designed to provide a top-loading construct. Screws are seated within an open-backed coupler and hooks are themselves open backed to facilitate ease of insertion and construction of the implant. Only when the surgeon is satisfied with placement of hooks and screws is rod attachment performed and the implant completely assembled and tightened down with torquing of set screws (Fig. 33–3). However, set screws may be loosened for readjustment of components even after torquing, making the implant forgiving of last-minute modifications or allowing for implant removal, if the need arises.

INDICATIONS AND SURGICAL CRITERIA

The system is indicated whenever internal fixation is desired for spinal arthrodesis to correct chronic hypermobility, in-

stability, or deformity of the spine. A number of diagnoses fall within this category: degenerative disk disease, facet arthropathy, pseudoarthrosis of previous fusions, spondylolisthesis, and scoliosis. Typically, patients are referred because of mechanical instability of the spine in combination with persistent pain despite treatment trials of at least 6 months and because of the failure of other methods of fixation or postlaminectomy syndrome.

In the series of 150 procedures outlined herein, diagnostic categories were as follows: degenerative disk disease alone or associated with herniated nucleus pulposus and–or spinal stenosis, 56%; failed back surgery syndrome accompanied by degenerative disk disease or iatrogenic defects, 29%; failed back surgery syndrome with pseudarthrosis, 8%; and spondylolisthesis, 7%.

In all cases, patients have undergone rigorous attempts at conservative treatment before they are considered surgical candidates. Conservative treatment measures include physical therapy and reconditioning, judicious use of selected analgesics, use of nonsteroidal anti-inflammatory drugs, and attempts at epidural steroid and trigger-point injections. Trials of thoracolumbosacral orthoses are attempted in some, when indicated.

Patients whose pain and physical limitations remain unacceptable to them and who request consideration for surgery are referred for baseline isokinetic testing and extensive psychological evaluation. Those who smoke are required to discontinue the practice before surgery because smoking has long been identified as affecting fusion nega-

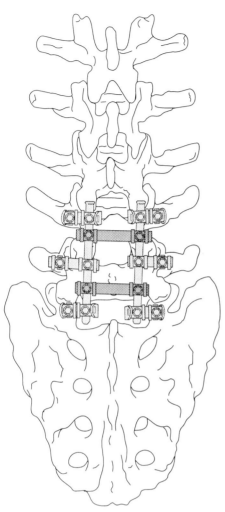

Figure 33–2. Illustration of a two-level instrumented spine. Cross bars connect the bilateral rods to provide a ladder-shaped configuration that increases pullout strength and enhances rigidity of the construct to withstand torsional stresses.

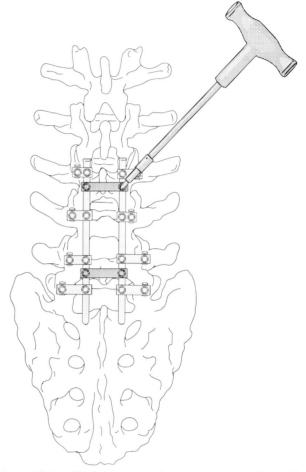

Figure 33–3. Final tightening of the construct is performed by torquing set screws with a torque wrench preset at 50 in-lb of torque. Note the advantage of top-loading set screw placement.

tively.[1] Cessation of smoking is confirmed by preoperative carboxyhemoglobin levels titrated for both urban and rural dwellers, as dictated by local demographics.

Preoperative Radiologic Evaluation

All patients are evaluated by plain radiographs and magnetic resonance imaging (MRI) of the lumbar spine. Gadolinium-enhanced studies are obtained in patients who have undergone previous operation. Provocative diskography and computed tomography (CT) scans are performed in most patients; those whose pathology warrants further investigation have at least one additional study performed from among the following: myelography, bone scans, stress films, selected nerve root blocks, or electromyogram/nerve conduction studies.

OPERATIVE TECHNIQUE

General Exposure for Posterior Lumbosacral Fusion

Our technique for a three-level instrumentation (L3 to S1) using pedicle screws is described. Participants in an American Academy of Orthopedic Surgeons Summer Institute[2] have recommended direct visualization of the pedicle by limited decompression. This is our preference, and this technique is presented. Use of the Rogozinski spinal rod system in a hybrid configuration of screws and hooks has been described elsewhere.[3] Instrumentation should not be considered a substitute for meticulous surgical technique in performing a spinal arthrodesis.

Patients are positioned on an Andrews frame. Thermal blankets are placed over the head, upper thoracic region, and arms. Draping includes a self-adhesive plastic hip drape that acts as a greenhouse to contain body heat and moisture. A midline incision is made and extends one and one half levels proximal and distal to the anticipated fusion level. (This

PEDICLE

Medial   Lateral

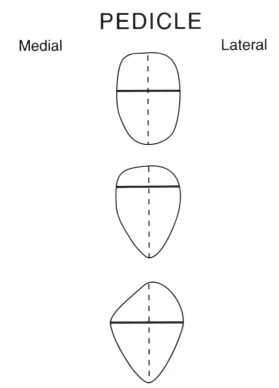

Figure 33–4. Various pedicle shapes in cross section. The solid line represents the pedicle equator, which is the widest portion of the pedicle. Note that this is not necessarily the point midway between the superior and inferior extent of the pedicle.

length allows lateral retraction of the wound so that an adequate convergent angle can be applied on the pedicle screw trajectory.)

A lateral radiograph is taken to establish the degree of lordosis on the frame and to confirm operative levels. The resultant radiograph is used to establish the cephalad-caudad tilt of the pedicles in the sagittal plane. The superior endplates' inclination closely parallels this axis in the sagittal plane to assist pedicle preparation.

Dissection proceeds laterally and subperiosteally to the tip of the transverse processes and is carried initially extracapsular to the facet joints. Complete capsulectomies are then performed at the intervertebral levels to be incorporated in the fusion. This allows better control of capsular bleeders and minimizes blood loss. Prior to capsulectomy, the paraspinal muscles have been mobilized laterally off the intertransverse fascial ligament. Once adequate exposure has been obtained, retraction of the soft tissue is achieved using very large Gelpi-type retractors to avoid foreshortening the wound or compromising paraspinal muscular blood flow. Any work within the canal, such as bony decompression or disk exploration, is undertaken as needed.

Technique for Pedicle Screw Instrumentation
After completing the exposure, attention is directed at visu-

alization of the pedicles in preparation for instrumentation. Small bilateral laminotomies are performed at each instrumented level. This is achieved by first elevating the ligamentum flavum in a subperiosteal manner off the margins of the laminae. Positioning the lamina spreader may facilitate this. Thereafter, the dura is visualized, and a Kerrison rongeur is used over cottonoid pledgets to form the laminotomy, which is lateralized to the medial wall of the pedicle by unroofing the subarticular recess.

With the medial wall of the pedicle exposed, the exiting nerve root and dural sac are retracted medially to allow better visualization of the pedicle. The entry point into the pedicle is determined by palpating the superior, medial, and inferior wall of the pedicle from within the canal by the use of a right-angle nerve hook. Once done, the superior and inferior margins of the pedicle are marked on the facet and pars regions, respectively, with an electrocautery mark. The nerve hook is used as a stylus within the canal to determine the widest pedicle diameter, typically at the point where the medial wall is most convex. This should correspond to the equator of the pedicle and thus is the optimal location for initiating entry (Fig. 33–4). At this point, with three sides of the pedicle visualized, the entry point is established. (The relationship of the transverse process to its adjoining facet provides additional visual cues and guidance.)

A high-speed burr is used to decorticate the bone overlying the anticipated entry point in the central axis of the pedicle. The pedicle probe is then advanced into this opening. The intraoperative lateral roentgenogram is used to guide the cephalad-caudad trajectory in the sagittal plane. Pedicle convergence angle and depth are ascertained from preoperative MRI scan or CT scan films. Typically, the probe is driven 20 to 25 mm to completely cannulate the pedicles.

One of the advantages of the open pedicle technique is the ability to perform the following confirmatory tests to evaluate the possibility of cutout into the canal through the pedicle: (1) The medial pedicle wall is visualized directly as described earlier, and (2) a suck test is performed wherein a small neurosucker is placed into the cannulated pedicle and the blood fluid level is observed within the laminotomy. Normal saline may be placed within the canal if the field is dry. If suction fails to evacuate the fluid (blood or saline), the test is deemed negative (ie, the pedicle walls are deemed intact adjacent to the canal). A reamer is then placed into the pedicle and driven to approximately 50% depth of the vertebral body, as guided by the intraoperative lateral roentgenogram. The reamer trajectory and integrity of the lateral wall of the pedicle and vertebra are palpated with a flexible pedicle feeler probe to perform a four-quadrant test. If the trajectory is acceptable, a calibrated x-ray guide pin is placed into the pedicle to the depth of the reamer, usually 30 to 40 mm. The bore is plugged with a small pledget to tamponade back bleeding.

Once each pedicle is prepared and marked, a repeat lateral radiograph is taken to reconfirm trajectory and depth of the pedicle markers. If the guide wire position and trajectory within the pedicle are radiographically acceptable, each pedicle marker is removed and a screw is chosen for later application. To determine the appropriate screw length, once the appropriate depth of penetration is determined, the surgeon should add an extra 5 mm to the calculation so that the screw head sits proud. At this adjusted length, the screw head is not impinging on the most cephalad facet joint. But in the more caudad screws, maintaining the screw head proud by 5 mm ensures that the screw head and rod are level. This adjustment maintains a top-loading application of set screws and facilitates construction of the implant.

An instrument nurse records the depth of guide wire penetration and then the size and length of each screw at each vertebral level. Each pedicle is then tapped to an appropriate depth. The bore is again plugged with a cottonoid pledget to maintain hemostasis (and assist in easier identification of the prepared pedicles after decortication).

With pedicle preparation completed, decortication is undertaken prior to insertion of any implants. This allows more aggressive decortication and easier access to bone surfaces for decortication. Decortication is performed aggressively to include the transverse processes, the facet, and the pars region of each level. We prefer to use Capener gouges and a large cup curette that works well to "banana peel" the processes to expose the cancellous portion. The facets at the fusion-level interspaces are osteotomized obliquely in the frontal plane to allow incorporation of facets into the arthrodesis. Bony remnants are discarded. The ala of the sacrum is osteotomized axially with the anterior bony and soft-tissue attachment intact. It is flipped 90° into the L5 to S1 interspace. Following decortication, cancellous graft (previously removed from the iliac crest) is packed into the prepared fusion bed. Only one half of the total graft material is used initially. The spinous processes at the fusion levels can be removed and the bone used to increase graft volume.

Pedicle screws are readied for insertion. The prepared pedicles are found by following the cottonoid strings and removing them sequentially followed by placement of the screws. Not all screw threads will be engaged. This allows the T head of the most cephalad pedicle screws to sit above the nonfused facet, thereby sparing injury to that joint. Upon placement of all pedicle screws and alignment of the T head with the long axis (Fig. 33–5A), the appropriate-length rods are selected and contoured symmetrically for lordosis. Only one rod is inserted at a time. The fixation is begun with the smallest transverse cross bar loosely premounted in a lateral direction on the rod. This cross bar is then inserted into the coupler of the most medially based pedicle screw, regardless of its corresponding vertebral level. (All other screws are more lateral, and there is an infinite variety of cross-bar sizes to span the rest of the construct.) The contoured rod is maintained parallel to the long axis. The set screw is placed over the lateral hole of the cross bar within the pedicle screw

coupler; the set screw is advanced only halfway. The remainder of the ipsilateral pedicle screws are attached to the rod in any sequence via couplers and variable-length transverse cross bars (Fig. 33–5B). (All cross bars should be oriented with the dimple or notch in the dorsal position to engage the self-locking mechanism of the set screws.) The process is repeated on the contralateral side, again beginning with the most medial pedicle screw as the initial rod attachment site. We keep the system very loose or "sloppy" at this point, engaging only half of the threads of the set screws. This is critical to ensure adequate tolerance for easier component connection. A caliper is utilized to measure the distance between rods and assist in choice of an appropriate-length cross bar to connect the bilateral rods. A minimum of two transverse cross bars is used, forming a ladder configuration. The cross bars are placed as far apart as possible. We use and recommend a 3- to 5-mm overhang of the rod distal to the last coupler to ensure proper containment within the coupler. Set screws are tightened provisionally with a hex screwdriver with simultaneous counterclockwise stabilization of the construct via a rod holder.

As the construct is assembled, at no time has the surgeon had to alter pedicle screw placement to accommodate design constraints of the device. Final tightening of set screws is performed with a torque wrench preset to apply 50 in-lb of torque. The remainder of the graft material is impacted into both gutters.

Any structural correction required should be effected after provisional tightening and final torquing. For example, a disk space collapse often occurs because of degeneration with secondary foraminal stenosis. We apply distraction at these collapsed levels to reconstitute foraminal height and physiologically effect a foraminotomy. By employing this method, an indirect decompression can be effected rather than a more radical decompression.

At this juncture, 0.5 mg of preservative-free morphine is injected into the subarachnoid space for postoperative pain control. A 27-gauge needle is used and is placed at a more proximal level than that laminotomized to reduce the possibility of subsequent dural leak. A deep drain is inserted and the wound is closed in layers. Patients are mobilized out of bed on the first postoperative day. They do not receive postoperative corsets, braces, or orthoses. Figures 33–6 and 33–7 show all-screw constructs of the Rogozinski spinal rod system in place.

Combined Simultaneous Anteroposterior Approach
Typically, the posterior portion of the procedure is performed first. The anterior procedure is performed under the same anesthesia. In the authors' center, a vascular surgeon performs the exposure via an anterior retroperitoneal approach. Freeze-dried femoral rings are presently used as interbody dowels. Figure 33–8 shows radiographs of a patient having received combined simultaneous anteroposterior arthrodesis with a Rogozinski all-screw construct in place posteriorly.

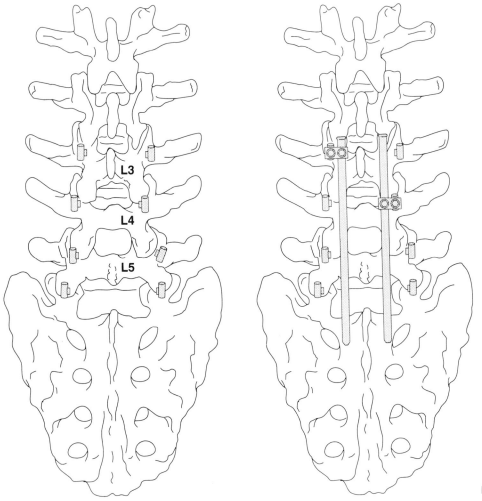

Figure 33–5. (**A**). T heads in position prior to placement of rods and cross bars. (T heads would normally be positioned in a coupler at this point but are deleted here to better highlight positioning of pedicle screw heads.) The screw in L3 on the left is the most medial and will thus be the first point of attachment to the left rod. On the right, L4 is the most medial and should be the first rod attachment site. Always use the 10-mm cross bar (shortest available) to begin rod attachment to this most medial screw. Note also that the right L5 pedicle screw is malrotated and should be adjusted. (**B**). The rod on the left is first attached to L3 followed by attachment of the rod on the right to L4. (As described in A, the screws in L3 on the left and L4 on the right are the most medial and thus are the first attached to the rods on their respective sides.)

POSTOPERATIVE MANAGEMENT

At present, most patients are discharged to home after 3 to 4 postoperative days unless complications intervene. This postoperative stay has declined since the first patient in the series received nonsegmental instrumentation with an arthrodesis. At that time, hospital stay after surgery averaged 14 days. Currently, patients are discharged to home earlier, with the hospital stay averaging 5 days. Typically, patients return to the outpatient clinic for suture removal and reexamination on the 10th postoperative day. Most patients are advised at that time to begin a walking program (1 mile a day by week 6, up to 2 miles per day by week 12) and are advised that they may resume driving.

Pain control is afforded through a tapering regimen of oral analgesics (oxycodone for 2 to 3 weeks, hydrocodone for 6 to 8 weeks, and propoxyphene at around 12 weeks). Prescribed oral analgesics are discontinued by 4 months.

Progress is assessed initially at 6-week intervals if the patient's course is uncomplicated. Radiographs are taken and evaluated at 6 and 12 weeks (anteroposterior, lateral views). If the fusion appears solid radiographically, a reconditioning program is begun. This occurs in most cases on the 12th to 16th postoperative week. Reconditioning continues for 8 to 12 weeks. Anteroposterior and lateral films are repeated at the conclusion of the reconditioning program. Patients return at 52 weeks, and thereafter at yearly intervals, if their course has been uncomplicated.

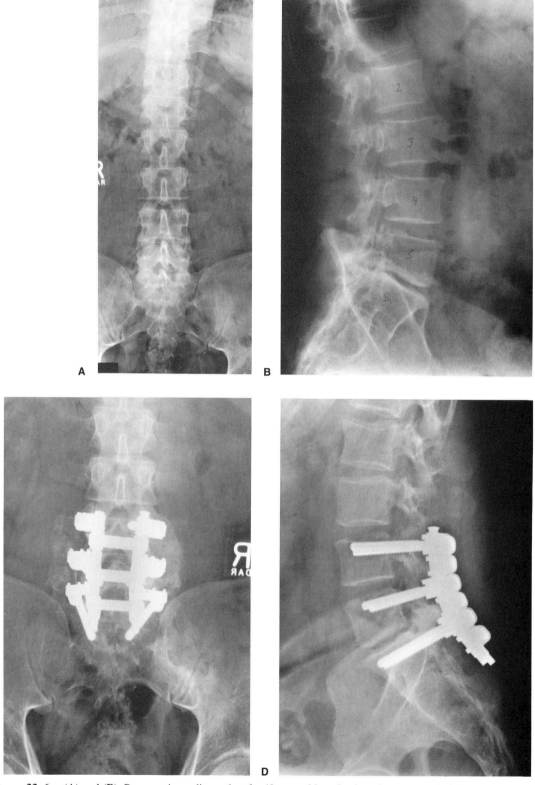

Figure 33–6.   (**A**) and (**B**). Preoperative radiographs of a 49-year-old car hauler who presented with two prior diskectomies of L5 to S1 and L4 to L5. He had chronic low back pain, left sciatica, and bowel control problems subsequent to surgeries. (**C**) and (**D**). He underwent posterolateral fusion and instrumentation with the Rogozinski system from L4 to S1 with excellent relief of pain; he requires no analgesics. He has returned to full-time work with modified activity.

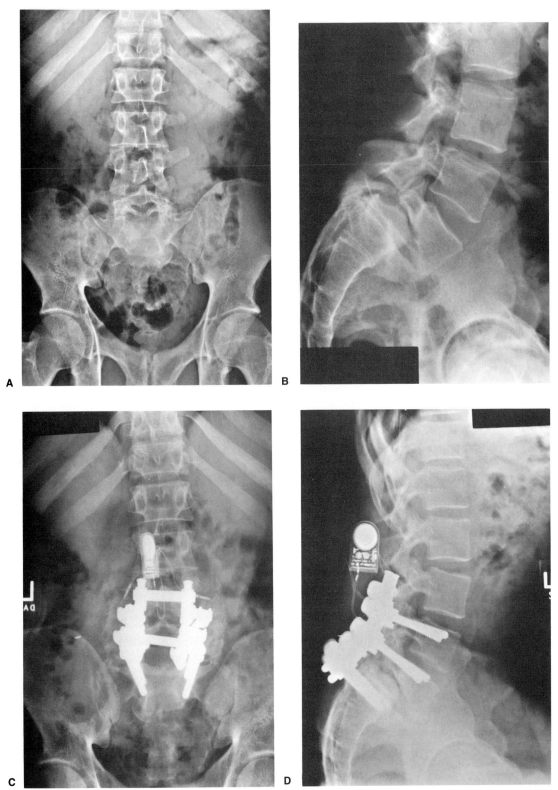

Figure 33–7. (**A**) and (**B**). Preoperative radiographs of a 30-year-old male laborer. He denied any prior back problems and presented with predominantly bilateral leg pain following a work injury. A grade IV spondylitic spondylolisthesis was observed radiographically. He remained symptomatic despite participation in an aggressive pelvic stabilization program. Diskograms confirmed a symptomatic degenerative disk at L4 and L5. (**C**) and (**D**). Posterolateral fusion was performed at L4 to S1 with Rogozinski instrumentation. Reduction of the slip angle was achieved with instrumentation under SSEP monitoring. Postoperatively, he has had complete relief of leg pain and has returned to unrestricted activities.

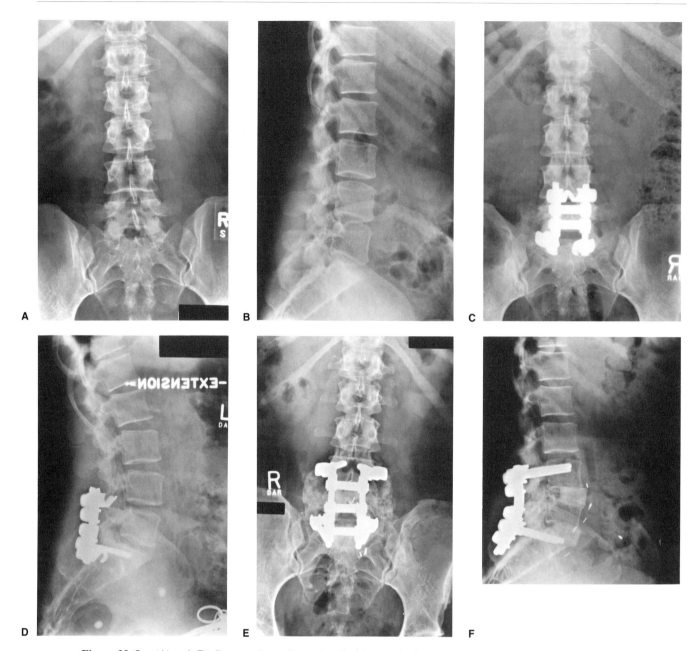

Figure 33–8. (A) and (B). Preoperative radiographs of a 38-year-old female who developed left sciatica following an injury. She had previously undergone diskectomies of L4 to L5 and L5 to S1. Her left leg pain returned several months after diskectomy and was associated with progressive low back pain. Diskograms demonstrated symptomatic degenerative disks and residual herniated nucleus pulposus. (C) and (D). One year later, she underwent a posterior spinal fusion from L4 to S1 with instrumentation. Subsequently, she developed nonunion. (E) and (F). One and one half years subsequent to the initial instrumentation, a simultaneous anteroposterior spinal fusion was performed at L4 to S1. One-year follow-up films demonstrate good incorporation of the anterior femoral rings and posterolateral fusion.

Table 33–1.   Results of Fusion in 150 Procedures, by Construct Type.

TYPE (*n*)	FUSION (*n*/%)	NONUNION (*n*/%)
All screws (60)	54/90%	6/10%
Hybrids (hooks and screws) (19)	16/84%	3/16%
Nonsegmental (hooks) (54)	30/56%	24/44%
Combined anteroposterior (17)	16/94%	1/6%

RESULTS

Overall Results in 150 Cases, Various Procedures

In a recent review of clinical results with the system, in 150 cases with an average follow-up period of 98 weeks, use of the Rogozinski system accompanied by bone graft has produced solid union as follows: 90% in constructs using pedicle screws; 84% using screw/hook combinations (so-called hybrid constructs); 94% of combined simultaneous anterior-posterior fusion; 56% using all-hook constructs in nonsegmental fixations (Table 33–1). Because of the superior results observed in all-screw fixations, the authors prefer pedicle screw fixation of constructs, and, when indicated, pedicle screw attachment posteriorly in combination with freeze-dried dowel grafts anteriorly.

Consistent with the reports of other investigators,[4–7] nonunions were found to correlate with a number of factors: smoking, previous failed back surgery, banked bone graft, and less rigid (ie, nonsegmental) implants (Table 33–2).

Table 33–2.   Nonunions in 150 Cases, Various Procedures.

PROCEDURES RESULTING IN NONUNION: 34	
Variables	
Fixation method	
Nonsegmental (hooks)	71% (24/34)
All screws or hybrids	26% (9/34)
Combined anteroposterior	3% (1/34)
Smoking	
Smoker pre- and postop	71% (24/34)
Nonsmoker	29% (10/34)
Graft type	
Banked bone	47% (16/34)
Previous back surgery	41% (14/34)

Observations surrounding smoking were consistent with previous reports that postoperative smoking contributed to nonunion. However, because patients in this series were required to have ceased smoking at least 2 months preoperatively (as confirmed by carboxyhemoglobin levels), it was possible to compare three groups: those who never smoked, those who smoked preoperatively and quit permanently before surgery, and those who resumed smoking after surgery. In the series of 150 patients, no difference was found in fusion rates of nonsmokers and preoperative-only smokers, whereas those who resumed smoking postoperatively constituted 71% of nonunions.

Results in All-Screw Constructs

Table 33–3 shows clinical results in 60 cases of posterolateral fusion using pedicle screws with a minimum of 52 weeks' follow-up (with one exception: a 22-week follow-up, discussed later). Solid union, as evidenced by trabeculation of bone graft across the operative levels and absence of motion on stress films, occurred in 54 of 60 cases (90%) overall.

Table 33–3.   Clinical Results in 60 Cases of Lumbosacral Fusion Using Pedicle Screws.

PATIENT PROFILE
Average age: 38.6 years (range 21–59 years)
Gender: 38 male, 22 female
Average blood loss: 461 mL (range 175–1500 mL)
Insurance status: 52 worker's compensation; 8 private insureds
OVERALL FUSION RATE
54 cases solid union (90%); 6 cases nonunion (10%)
FUSION RATE BY LEVEL
One level: 29 solid union (97%); 1 nonunion
Two levels: 23 solid union (85%); 4 nonunion
Three levels: 1 solid union (50%); 1 nonunion
Four levels: 1 solid union (100%)
PATIENT-REPORTED PAIN RELIEF AT 1 YEAR: 10-POINT SCALE*
(Average % improvement or decline, pre- and postop)
Patients with solid union: +20.4% improvement
    (range –2% to +100%)
Patients with nonunion: +16% improvement
    (range 0 to +50%)
*4 patients incomplete data either pre- or postop scores, not counted
RATE OF RETURN TO WORK
Patients with solid union
    45% at full or modified activity
    38% cleared to return; looking for work
    18% disabled or not seeking work
Patients with nonunion
    66% at full or modified activity
    0% cleared to return
    33% disabled or not seeking work

COMPLICATIONS

No deep infections have occurred in the series of 150 procedures (Table 33–4). Fixation failure occurred in one early case when the rod was cut too short and slipped free of its attachment. It is recommended that rods be cut to extend 3 to 5 mm distal to the last coupler to prevent such disengagement. No other fixation failures occurred; there were no occurrences of fatigue failure, component fracture, pedicle fracture, or screw pullout. In one case, a patient suffered a neurological sequela when a preexisting grade 4 foot drop was found to have dropped a grade in the course of postoperative follow-up.

Table 33–4. Complications.

COMPLICATION	NUMBER (PERCENT)
Major complications (Fixation Related)	**2 (1.3%)**
Fixation failure	1 (0.7%)
Neurological sequela	1 (0.7%)
Deep infection	0
Medical complications	**11 (7%)**
Pneumonia	2 (1.3%)
Embolism	2 (1.3%)
Bronchitis	3 (2%)
Deep-vein thrombosis	2 (1.3%)
Polyneuropathy	1 (0.7%)
Atelectasis	1 (0.7%)
Urinary retention	1 (0.7%)
Orthopedic complications	**6 (4%)**
Trochanteric bursitis	3 (2%)
Knee effusion	1 (0.7%)
Acromial bursitis	1 (0.7%)
Patellar tendinitis	1 (0.7%)
Wound complications	**18 (12%)**
Superficial wound dehiscence	4 (3%)
Seroma	14 (9%)
Positional complications	**5 (3%)**
Dental	1 (0.7%)
Skin	2 (1.3%)
Neuropraxia	1 (0.7%)
Compartment syndrome	2 (1.3%)
Repeat surgery	**16 (11%)**
Anterior-posterior procedure for augmentation of fusion or exploration of pseudarthrosis	5 (3%)
Posterior augmentation or exploration of pseudarthrosis	6 (4%)
I&D of seroma	3 (2%)
Fasciotomy (for compartment syndrome)	1 (0.7%)
Embolectomy	1 (0.7%)

In the first year of the series, a number of complications occurred that were attributed to intraoperative positioning. Neuropraxia of the brachial plexus occurring in two patients resolved completely after observation and required no subsequent treatment. An anterior tibial compartment syndrome occurred in one patient, necessitating fasciotomy. Fasciotomy was also performed in a second patient following plaque embolism; treatment was undertaken because of impending compartment syndrome. One patient displayed an acute exacerbation of neglected periodontal disease and required subsequent periodontal attention. Another suffered a superficial decubitis of the chin. Increased attention to padding and positioning by surgeons and anesthesia personnel has been successful in preventing recurrences of positioning complications.

Two patients in the series died subsequent to surgery. One, a 43-year-old female, succumbed to melanoma discovered subsequent to spinal surgery. Her clinical and radiographic course as a result of her spinal fusion were positive, with complete relief of leg and back pain and radiographically solid union. Follow-up was 22 weeks—the only patient in the series followed less than 52 weeks. A second patient, a 36-year-old male, had graft resorption subsequent to surgery. His postoperative course was complicated by ongoing narcotic dependency, and he died after exploration of his fusion by another surgeon.

Repeat spinal surgery was conducted in 16 cases, necessitated by continued clinical presentation of instability, with pain accompanied in some cases by radiographic appearance of pseudarthrosis. Reoperation consisted of augmentation of instrumentation and–or exploration of pseudarthrosis. Failure to fuse occurred subsequent to reoperation in four of these cases.

DISCUSSION

Any discussion of outcome after spinal surgery must account for the many variables all too familiar to surgeons specializing in the spine. Whether positive outcome of surgery can be attributed to an instrumentation system, growing expertise of the surgeon, or more precise patient selection may be impossible to determine absolutely.

Conclusions to be drawn from the use of the Rogozinski spinal rod system are that in patients with a surgically correctable pathology, the system used for segmental fixation provides sufficient stiffness and strength to promote fusion. In vivo, use of the system in 150 procedures, as presented herein, has resulted in no system failures, component breakage, or screw pullout that would suggest inherent inadequacy in strength or stiffness. It was noted, however, that nonsegmental constructs provide inadequate fixation to enhance fusion.

A number of factors were observed to contribute to nonunion. Among them are insufficient rigidity of fixation (ie, nonsegmental fixations), postoperative smoking, and multiple previous failed back surgeries. A number of factors likewise were observed to contribute to union: The best results are obtained in patients with segmental one- or two-level fusions or anteroposterior procedures. Patients who smoked preoperatively but did not resume the practice postoperatively achieved a fusion rate nearly as high as that for nonsmokers.

The literature shows a growing consensus that fixation with pedicle screws is achieved safely when performed by experienced surgeons using impeccable technique in screw placement. The authors believe the Rogozinski system is so designed that it conforms to the patient's anatomy rather than having anatomy subjugated to instrumentation, and this, in turn, frees the surgeon to position screws in the most accurate and safe trajectory within the pedicle. In addition, the cross connecting of rods by cross bars in a quadrilateral configuration renders the implant a load-sharing device that avoids preloading and enhances fixation capability, especially torsionally.

As a result of experience with the system, the authors feel confident that surgeons will find that it enhances performance of fusions and, ultimately, contributes to improved clinical outcome.

REFERENCES

1. Brown CW, Orme TJ, Richardson HD. The rate of pseudarthrosis (surgical nonunion) in patients who are smokers and patients who are nonsmokers: A comparison study. *Spine.* 1986;11:942.

2. American Academy of Orthopaedic Surgeons Summer Institute, San Diego, Calif; 1988.

3. Rogozinski C, Rogozinski A. The Rogozinski spinal rod system: a new internal fixation of the spine. In: Arnold DM, Lonstein JE, eds. *Spine: State of the Art Reviews.* Philadelphia, Pa: Hanley & Belfus; 1992:107–120.

4. Horowitch A, Peek RD, Thomas JC Jr, et al. The Wiltse pedicle screw fixation system: early clinical results. *Spine.* 1989;14: 461–467.

5. Lorenz M, Zindrick M, Schwaegler P, et al. A comparison of single-level fusions with and without hardware. *Spine.* 1991; 16(suppl 8):5455–5458.

6. Esses SI. The AO spinal internal fixator. *Spine.* 1989;14: 373–378.

7. Dickman CA, Fessler RG, MacMillan M, et al. Transpedicular screw-rod fixation of the lumbar spine: operative technique and outcome in 104 cases. *J Neurosurg.* 1992;77:860–870.

34 Thoracic and Lumbar Fractures: Management Analysis

Patrick W. Hitchon, M.D., James C. Torner, Ph.D., Souheil S. Haddad, M.D., Kenneth A. Follett, M.D., Ph.D.

INTRODUCTION

There are no universally accepted guidelines for the treatment of thoracic and lumbar fractures. Whereas operative management has been favored by some,[1–5] others have advocated nonoperative recumbency.[6–9] Although operative and nonoperative approaches in the treatment of these fractures have often been analyzed and compared,[10–16] the advantages of one approach over the other have not always been self-evident or consistent in terms of benefits in recovery or deformity. It does, however, appear that surgical management has been associated with shorter periods of bed rest.[13,14,16] Because thoracic and lumbar fractures are complex in terms of the elements of the spine involved, the neurological deficit, and the subsequent stresses, it is not entirely surprising that opinions vary regarding any one particular case. Decisions are further influenced by the experiences and judgment of the managing team.

In an attempt to arrive at a set of functional guidelines for the management of these fractures, we elected to conduct a retrospective study of our patient population with thoracic and lumbar fractures. The surgery for decompression and stabilization was performed by one neurosurgeon (P. W. H.). When recumbency was the treatment, that was the decision of any one of the six members of our neurosurgical team. The recumbency patients go back to 1984. The surgical patients, on the other hand, go back to February 1987. In the study, we elected to collect and analyze clinical and radiological data regarding all patients.

CLINICAL MATERIALS AND METHODS

Admission

Since 1984 a total of 120 patients with thoracic and lumbar fractures were admitted to The University of Iowa Hospitals and Clinics, the majority on the neurosurgical service. In all, there were 86 males and 34 females. The mean age was 30 years ± 15, with a range of 13 to 80 years. Forty-eight percent of these injuries were automobile related. Motorcycles constituted only 13% of the causes, and falls made up 23%. Although information was not available in 8%, it appears that only 17% involved in car or truck accidents were wearing seatbelts. Upon admission, 29% of patients had been consuming alcoholic beverages, but in 18% this information was unavailable. Associated injuries at the time of admission consisted of head injuries in 19%, chest injuries (pulmonary contusions, hemo-, or pneumothorax) in 19%, rib fractures in 8%, extremity fractures in 8%, abdominal injuries in 6%, and other spinal injuries in 4%.

Radiological studies of the spine consisted of plain films, computerized axial tomography (CT), and magnetic resonance imaging (MRI). Angulation of the spine was assessed on lateral films using the first intact endplate rostral to the fracture and the first intact endplate caudal to the fracture. Using axial CT scans, the residual canal was measured in the anteroposterior (AP) diameter and expressed as a percentage of the canal rostral to the fracture site. Fractures were classified based on criteria adopted from Denis et al[17] into burst (57) with anterior- and middle-column disruption, flexion/compression with anterior-column compression (32), fracture dislocation with three-column disruption and dislocation (30), and one distraction injury secondary to a slice fracture.

Clinical performance scoring was assessed upon admission and follow-up using the Frankel Grading System[7]:

- Grade 1/A: Complete motor and sensory paralysis below the lesion
- Grade 2/B: Some sensory preservation, but complete motor paralysis below the lesion
- Grade 3/C: "Motor useless," some motor preservation below lesion, but not functional
- Grade 4/D: "Motor useful," incomplete but useful motor function below lesion. Can walk with or without aids.
- Grade 5/E: Normal motor and sensory function.

Statistical analysis of this retrospective observational study was done utilizing chi-square tests for comparison of frequency counts of categorical variables, Kruskal-Wallis tests for comparison of ordinal categorical data (ie, Frankel scores), and analysis of variance for continuous variables. Multivariate analysis of variance was used for comparison of surgery and recumbency when differences were observed at admission (ie, angulation at admission). Significance was determined at a probability level of 0.05.

RESULTS

Admission

The most common spinal segment involved with fracture was that of T12 to L1 (46), followed by the lower thoracic (35) between T7 and T11, the lumbar spine between L2 and L5 (21), and finally the upper thoracic (18) between T1 and T6. As expected, and as shown by others, the level of fracture correlated strongly with the extent of neurological deficit ($P < .001$) (Fig. 34–1). Sixty-one percent of T1 to T6 and 69% of T7 to T11 fractures had a Frankel score of 1. On the other hand, 100% of L2 to L5 and 83% of T12 to L1 fractures had a Frankel score of 4 or 5. In addition, the spinal segment appears to have correlated strongly with the type of fracture ($P < .001$). Thus burst fractures constituted 76% of L2 to L5 and 72% of T12 to L1 fractures. On the other hand, flexion-compression fractures and fracture dislocations constituted 94% of T1 to T6 and 71% of T7 to T11 fractures. A positive correlation was also noted between the Frankel score upon admission and the fracture type ($P < .001$) (Fig. 34–2). Seventy-nine percent of burst fractures had a Frankel score of 4 or better, whereas 67% of fracture dislocations had a score of 1. Flexion-compression fractures were associated with Frankel scores of 4 or 6 in 66% of cases yet in 31% were associated with a Frankel score of 1. In addition, a significant correlation was noted between spinal angulation ($P = .0012$) and the residual spinal canal ($P = .0001$) when compared to performance (Figs. 34–3 and 34–4). The greater the degree of angulation or the more severe the canal compromise, the worse the neurological deficit upon admission.

Based on the general medical and neurological condition and the radiological findings of each patient, the decision was made to operate in 61 cases and recommend nonoperative recumbency in 59. The mean Frankel score of patients treated with surgical stabilization and decompression was 2.6 ± 1.6, whereas that for patients treated with recumbency was 3.9 ± 1.7 ($P < .001$) (Fig. 34–5). Whereas 47% of patients treated surgically had a Frankel score of 2, 3, or 4, 24% of patients treated with recumbency had a Frankel score of 1, and 59% had a score of 5.

Concerning the spinal level, there appeared to be no significant difference in the frequency of surgery or recumbency at the various levels ($P = .219$). Fracture types in patients treated with recumbency were divided equally between burst and flexion-compression fractures. On the other hand, patients treated with surgery were divided equally between burst fractures and fracture dislocations. This difference in management based on fracture type was significant ($P < .001$). Spinal angulation at the fracture site in the surgical group (13.0 ± 13.1) was twice that encountered in the recumbency group (6.5 ± 10.0) ($P = .003$) (Fig. 34–6). In terms of the residual canal, the difference between the surgical and the recumbency groups was also significant ($P = .0001$) with a mean of 41% in the surgical group versus 73% in the recumbency group.

In those who underwent surgery, it was performed at 16 ± 24 days, or at the earliest opportunity when deemed appropriate. Intraoperative blood loss was estimated at 1100 ± 800 cc; hence transfusions in the perioperative phase within 1 to 3 days following surgery were necessary in only 45% of patients. Harrington distraction rods with sublaminar wires were used in 30, Luque rods or rectangles in 18, transpedicular screws and plates in six, ISOLA rods and hooks in three, Weiss springs in one, and no instrumentation was utilized in three. At the time of surgery 74% of patients underwent spinal canal decompression in addition to reduction, stabilization, and fusion. This decompression was accomplished through the costotransversectomy or extracavitary

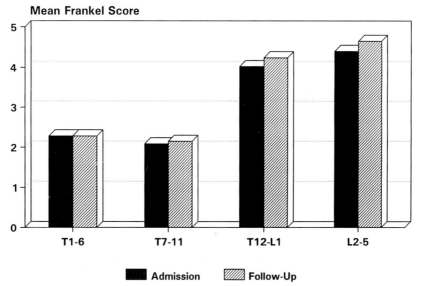

Figure 34–1. A significant correlation is noted between the level of the fracture and the Frankel score ($P < .001$). The slight improvement in Frankel score was significant in those patients treated with surgery.

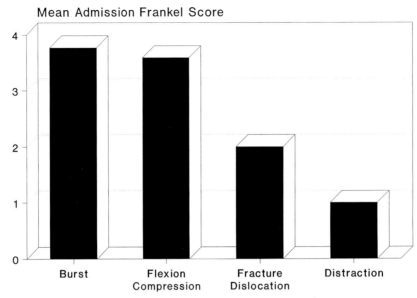

Figure 34–2. A significant correlation is noted between the type of fracture and the Frankel score upon admission ($P < .001$). Burst and flexion-compression fractures do significantly better than fracture dislocations or those associated with distraction.

approach in 16, and through the transpedicular approach in 29. In the former, the patients underwent an anterior interbody fusion with rib or iliac autologous bone. All the rest had a posterolateral transverse process fusion.

OUTCOME

In spite of surgical intervention, one of the intentions of which was to expedite mobility and discharge, the hospital stay for the surgical group (37 ± 21) was not statistically different from that of patients treated with re-

cumbency (40 ± 18). On the other hand, the days of bed rest to which surgical patients were confined (26 ± 12) was significantly shorter than that of patients treated with recumbency (33 ± 12) ($P = .002$). Two patients contracted pneumonia in the surgical group compared to four in the recumbency group. Urinary tract infections were twice as common in the surgery group as they were in the recumbency group (19 versus 10). Seven patients developed deep-vein thrombosis in the operative group and only one in the nonoperative. There was one case each of pulmonary embolism in either group; it resulted

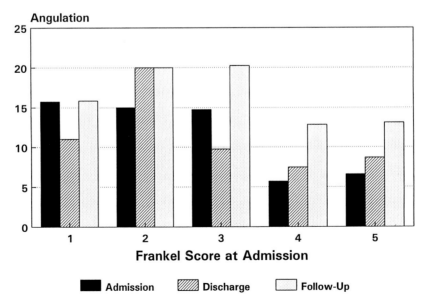

Figure 34–3. A significant correlation is noted between the extent of angulation upon admission and the Frankel score ($P = .0012$). These results further suggest that the angulation on follow-up increased in those patients with a higher Frankel score; this, however, did not attain significance.

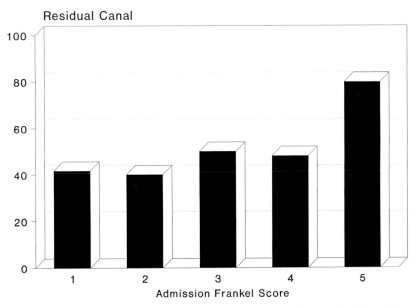

Figure 34–4. A significant correlation is encountered between the residual spinal canal and Frankel performance score ($P = .0001$).

in death in the surgical group in spite of an inferior vena cava filter.

In the surgical group, however, six patients necessitated a second operation: one for inadequate decompression, two for progressive angulation, one for twisting of Harrington rods in the lumbar spine, one for rostral hook slippage following a second trauma 18 months later, and a sixth for cauda equina traction that recovered following decompression. There was one wound infection in the surgical group that necessitated eventual rod removal for failure to control the infection. An elderly woman with ankylosing spondylitis developed a wound dehiscence that was treated successfully with eventual healing. There was one death in the surgical group secondary to a pulmonary embolism postoperatively.

Upon discharge, angulation in the recumbency group had progressed from 6.5 ± 10.0 to 10.0 ± 10.0 (Fig. 34–6). The surgical group, on the other hand, had shown a decrease in kyphotic angulation from 13.0 ± 13.1 to 8.7 ± 10.2. At follow-up, both groups progressed in their angulation, with the recumbency increasing to 12.5 ± 10.8 and the surgical to 15.6 ± 10.6, values that are not significantly different ($P = .14$). The final increase in angulation over admission was $2.6°$ in the surgical group, significantly smaller than the $6°$ increase of the recumbency group ($P = .0195$). The angulation at follow-up did not seem to be affected by whether or not a decompression had been performed ($P = .15$). The difference in angulation between admission and discharge measured $-5.2°$, $2.6°$, and $6.3°$ in those patients without decompression (16), those with a transpedicular decompres-

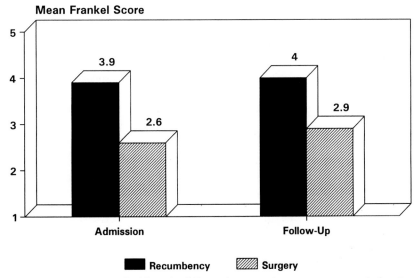

Figure 34–5. The Frankel score was significantly different between the two groups, surgical and recumbency, both upon admission and discharge. The improvement in performance of the surgical group alone was significant ($P = .0005$).

sion (29), and those with a costotransversectomy (16), respectively. This trend of progressive angulation with more aggressive decompression was statistically significant (P = .024).

The mean and median interval to follow-up was approximately 1 year in both surgical and recumbency groups. At latest follow-up, the Frankel score of the surgical group had improved by 0.3 from 2.6 ± 1.6 upon admission to 2.9 ± 1.7 (P = .0005) (Fig. 34–5). The recumbency group, however, had started out 1.3 Frankel points above the surgical group and improved by only 0.1 points from 3.9 ± 1.7 upon admission to 4.0 ± 1.7 (P = .07). As on admission, the Frankel scores of the surgical and recumbency groups at follow-up remained different (P = .001).

A questionnaire was forwarded to patients in both groups and inquired about the presence of spasms, pain, or employment (Fig. 34–7). The response rate was 77%. Whereas 36% of the recumbency group suffered spasms, the rate was 70% in those patients treated with surgery (P = .001). In regard to pain, 50% of the recumbency group and 58% of the surgical group respondents complained of pain requiring occasional medications (P = .443). In regard to employment, approximately one quarter of both groups was unemployed. The remainder were able to return to either the same job or to a different one (60%). Forty-six patients of the surgical group responded to a questionnaire regarding the benefits of surgery. Whereas 42 believed the operation was worthwhile, four denied or were unsure of the advantages of the operation. Thirteen (22%) of those patients who underwent instrumentation had it removed 1 or more years later for discomfort, hook slippage, or prominence.

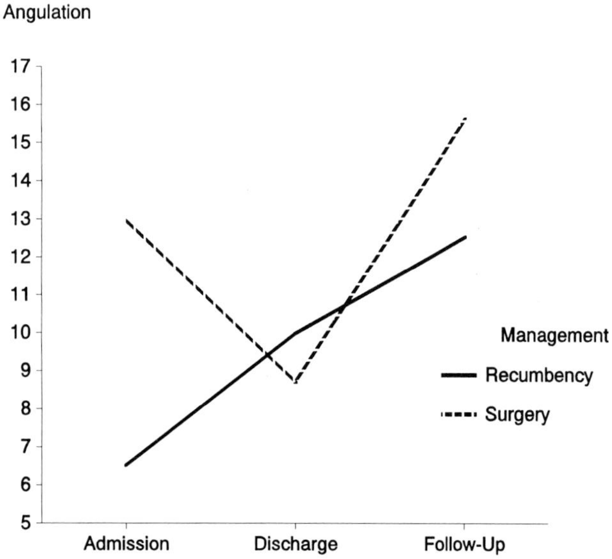

Figure 34–6.   The difference in angulation on admission between the surgical and recumbency groups was significant (P = .003). At discharge, at a mean of 6 weeks from admission, the two groups were similar. Likewise at latest follow-up, although the angulation of the surgical group was approximately 3° greater than the recumbency, the two were not dissimilar.

DISCUSSION

Based on the preceding analysis, it appears that a major determinant of posttraumatic neurological deficit is the level of injury. The more rostral, the more likely it is to be associated with a neurological deficit. This observation is similar to the retrospective studies conducted by Frankel,[7] Willen,[18] Benzel,[1] Gertzbein,[4] and Hadley.[11] Fractures with dislocation were also far more likely to be encountered with severe neurological deficit and paraplegia than burst fractures and flexion-compression fractures. This is also not unanticipated considering the forces necessary for fracture dislocations as opposed to the less forceful injuries in flexion-compression and burst fractures.[4,12,13,17] The more severe injuries, and in particular those resulting in fracture dislocations, are also accompanied by a greater degree of spinal angulation and compromise of the spinal canal. A positive correlation was encountered in our study between angulation, canal compromise, and the Frankel score. These correlations were both significant and similar to those encountered by others.[4,18,19]

Our analysis of 61 operative cases reveals one death, one wound dehiscence, one case of increased neurological deficit secondary to cauda equina traction, one infection, and five reoperations. The patient with increased deficit did require a second decompression with full recovery. Furthermore, the incidence of urinary tract infections and deep-vein thrombosis was higher in the operative (19 and 7) than in the nonoperative group (10 and 1). This is probably related to the lower Frankel score of the former (2.6 ± 1.6 versus 3.9 ± 1.7). The operative series was also associated with a greater degree of angulation (15.7 ± 10.6) compared to the recumbency group of 12.5 ± 10.8. It is to be recalled, however, that upon admission the angulation of the operative group (12.9 ± 13) was twice that of the recumbency group (6.5 ± 10.0) (Fig. 34–6). Thus, our philosophy has been to reserve surgical intervention primarily for patients with partial neurological deficit who may benefit from decompression[1,2,4,5,10,13,20] (Fig. 34–8).

Surgical intervention resulted in only a 1.7° overall increse in angulation over admission, whereas the recumbency group increased by 6°; this difference between the two groups was significant (P = .019) (Fig. 34–6). It is due to this observation that surgery has also been undertaken in patients with severe angulation or dislocation whether intact or paraplegic (Fig. 34–8). We continue to believe that the benefits of surgical intervention are more likely to be encountered in patients with partial neurological deficit . In our series, a significant (P = .0005) improvement in Frankel score of 0.3 was encountered in the surgical group compared to 0.1 in the recumbency (P = .07) (Fig. 34–5). In addition to reduction and stabilization, decompression of neural elements is paramount if neurological improvement is to be achieved. Decompression through a costotransversectomy, although associated with a greater increase in angulation at follow-up (6.3°) than through a transpedicular approach (2.6°), may have to be adopted particularly in the thoracic

FOLLOW-UP QUESTIONNAIRE

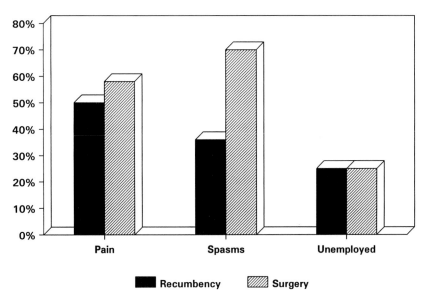

Figure 34–7. Whereas the frequency of pain was similar in the two groups, spasms were twice as frequent in patients treated with surgery as compared to those treated nonoperatively. One quarter of both groups is unemployed.

spine. This increase in angulation may be secondary to the amount of bone removal and destabilization that takes place with costotransversectomy vis-à-vis the transpedicular route. These changes, however, should not deter the surgeon from pursuing the approach best suited for the particular patient.

It is not surprising that the frequency of spasms (Fig. 34–7) encountered with surgery exceeds that of patients treated with recumbency (35 versus 15) because the former group is also associated with a greater degree of angulation

upon admission (12.9 ± 13° versus 6.5 ± 10) and a smaller residual canal (40.7 ± 24.6 versus 73.1 ± 26.3 mm). The algorithm illustrated in Figure 34–7 is to be adopted with flexibility and is not intended to be rigid and unwavering. Spinal instrumentation, even when indicated, can be associated with grave complications.

Acknowledgment. The authors acknowledge the help of Gatana Stoner, Susan Piper, and Karen VanDenBosch, coordinators of the Upjohn Head Injury Tirilazad Trials and the

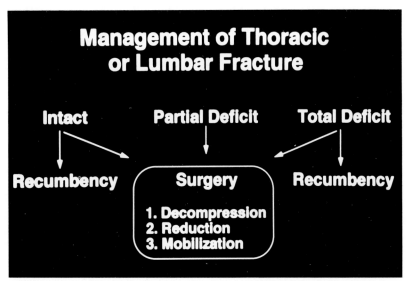

Figure 34–8. Whereas the majority of patients who are intact or complete following thoracic or lumbar fracture are treated with recumbency, the majority of those with partial deficit are treated operatively. Operative intervention contributes to decompression of neural elements, reduction of dislocation, and early mobilization.

National Acute Spinal Cord Injury Study—Part III, in the collection of the data. The authors also thank Judy Huston for the preparation of this manuscript.

REFERENCES

1. Benzel EC, Larson SJ. Functional recovery after decompressive operation for thoracic and lumbar spine fractures. *Neurosurgery.* 1986;19:772–778.

2. Bohlman HH, Freehafer A, Dejak J. The results of treatment of acute injuries of the upper thoracic spine with paralysis. *J Bone Joint Surg.* 1985;67A:360–369.

3. Dickson JH, Harrington PR, Erwin WD. Results of reduction and stabilization of the severely fractured thoracic and lumbar spine. *J Bone Joint Surg.* 1978;60A:799–805.

4. Gertzbein SD, Court-Brown CM, Marks P, Martin C, Fazl M, Schwartz M, Jacobs RR. The neurological outcome following surgery for spinal fractures. *Spine.* 1988;13:641–644.

5. Transfeldt EE, White D, Bradford DS, Roche B. Delayed anterior decompression in patients with spinal cord and cauda equina injuries of the thoracolumbar spine. *Spine.* 1990;15:953–957.

6. Bedbrook GM. Spinal injuries with tetraplegia and paraplegia. *J Bone Joint Surg.* 1979;61B:167–284.

7. Frankel HL, Hancock DO, Hyslop G, et al. Value of postural reduction in the initial management of closed injuries of the spine with paraplegia and tetraplegia. *Paraplegia.* 1969;7:179–192.

8. Davies WE, Morris JH, Hill V. An analysis of conservative (non-surgical) management of thoracolumbar fractures and fracture-dislocations with neural damage. *J Bone Joint Surg.* 1980;62A:1324–1328.

9. Guttmann L. Surgical aspects of the treatment of traumatic paraplegia. *J Bone Joint Surg.* 1949;31B:399–403.

10. An HS, Vaccaro A, Cotler JM, Lin S. Low lumbar burst fractures: comparison among body cast, Harrington rod, Luque rod, and Steffee plate. *Spine.* 1991;16(suppl):S440–S444.

11. Hadley MN, Browner CM, Dickman CA, Sonntag VKH. Compression fractures of the thoracolumbar junction: a treatment algorithm based on 110 cases. *BNI Quarterly.* 1989;5:10–19.

12. Holdsworth F, Chir M. Fractures, dislocations, and fracture-dislocations of the spine. *J Bone Joint Surg.* 1970;52A:1534–1551.

13. Jacobs RR, Asher MA, Snider RK. Thoracolumbar spinal injuries: a comparative study of recumbent and operative treatment in 100 patients. *Spine.* 1980;5:463–477.

14. Osebold WR, Weinstein SL, Sprague BL. Thoracolumbar spine fractures: results of treatment. *Spine.* 1981;6:13–34.

15. Weinstein JN, Collalto P, Lehmann TR. Thoracolumbar "burst" fractures treated conservatively: a long-term follow-up. *Spine.* 1988;13:33–38.

16. Willen J, Lindahl S, Nordwall A. Unstable thoracolumbar fractures: a comparative clinical study of conservative treatment and Harrington instrumentation. *Spine.* 1985;10:111–122.

17. Denis F. The three column spine and its significance in the classification of acute thoracolumbar spinal injuries. *Spine.* 1983;8:817–831.

18. Willen J, Anderson J, Toomoka K, Singer K. The natural history of burst fractures at the thoracolumbar junction. *J Spinal Disorders.* 1990;3:39–46.

19. Hashimoto T, Kaneda K, Abumi K. Relationship between traumatic spinal canal stenosis and neurological deficits in thoracolumbar burst fractures. *Spine.* 1988;13:1268–1272.

20. Maiman DJ, Larson SJ, Benzel EC. Neurological improvement associated with late decompression of the thoracolumbar spinal cord. *Neurosurgery.* 1984;14:302–307.

Index

DATE DUE

DEMCO, INC. 38-3012